AF902674

Cancer and Work in Asia Volume 2

Motoki Endo • Mitsue Saito • Go Muto
Editors

Cancer and Work in Asia Volume 2

Perspective from Basic and Clinical Medicine

Springer

Editors
Motoki Endo
Department of Public Health
School of Medicine, Dokkyo Medical University
Mibu, Tochigi, Japan

Mitsue Saito
Department of Breast Oncology
Graduate School of Medicine, Juntendo University
Tokyo, Japan

Go Muto
Department of Hygiene and Public Health
Tokyo Women's Medical University School of Medicine
Shinjuku, Tokyo, Japan

Department of Hygiene
Kitasato University School of Medicine
Sagamihara, Kanagawa, Japan

ISBN 978-981-95-6536-8 ISBN 978-981-95-6537-5 (eBook)
https://doi.org/10.1007/978-981-95-6537-5

© The Editor(s) (if applicable) and The Author(s), under exclusive license to Springer Nature Singapore Pte Ltd. 2026

This work is subject to copyright. All rights are solely and exclusively licensed by the Publisher, whether the whole or part of the material is concerned, specifically the rights of translation, reprinting, reuse of illustrations, recitation, broadcasting, reproduction on microfilms or in any other physical way, and transmission or information storage and retrieval, electronic adaptation, computer software, or by similar or dissimilar methodology now known or hereafter developed.
The use of general descriptive names, registered names, trademarks, service marks, etc. in this publication does not imply, even in the absence of a specific statement, that such names are exempt from the relevant protective laws and regulations and therefore free for general use.
The publisher, the authors and the editors are safe to assume that the advice and information in this book are believed to be true and accurate at the date of publication. Neither the publisher nor the authors or the editors give a warranty, expressed or implied, with respect to the material contained herein or for any errors or omissions that may have been made. The publisher remains neutral with regard to jurisdictional claims in published maps and institutional affiliations.

This Springer imprint is published by the registered company Springer Nature Singapore Pte Ltd.
The registered company address is: 152 Beach Road, #21-01/04 Gateway East, Singapore 189721, Singapore

If disposing of this product, please recycle the paper.

Foreword

Cancer and Work in Asia is a unique two-volume book which provides comprehensive information about cancer and the challenges that cancer provides in the workplace from a specifically Asian perspective. This is important because just under 50% of the world's cancer and 60% of the mortality from cancer comes from this region. Yet, less research has been done into return-to-work challenges in this region than in Western countries and so a text which brings the latest knowledge all together is indispensable.

Learnings from Western cultures don't always fit well into the culture and perspective of Asia. Also, this region encompasses the whole range of socio-economic groupings. A great strength of this book is that it features specific chapters from 22 countries in the region. This enables comparisons of the outcomes of strategies related to cancer and the workplace and returning to work after cancer to be made and allows countries of similar socioeconomic groups to be compared, be that high- or low-income countries.

One volume focuses on public health and return to work. Workers need to know about the modifiable lifestyle factors that will impact on their risk of cancer. This book highlights lifestyle factors including smoking and avoiding passive smoking, alcohol consumption, diet and exercise. It also documents which countries have screening programs for breast, bowel and cervical cancer and shows differences, for example, parts of India screen for oral cancers and Korea for stomach cancer. HPV and hepatitis B vaccines are available in some countries and not others.

Occupational exposures to cancer-causing chemicals in the workplace are also modifiable risk factors. Workplaces can manage the environment to lower occupational exposure to carcinogens, encourage the wearing of personal protective equipment and ensure that their workers are educated about the health consequences of their workplace.

There are insightful chapters on return-to-work. Work is related to having a purpose in life and contribution to make, raising self-esteem. However, the experience of having a life-threatening illness can change people's values and priorities, so they may not want to continue the same job as before their diagnosis, although most do return to their previous workplaces. There can be physical and cognitive barriers to returning to a previous job caused by the cancer and its treatment and the level of support from their employer and fellow employees can be key to successfully returning to their workplace. A flexible approach and good communication ideally includes individualised counselling in the workplace which is reported as very helpful. A chapter on the specific challenges of adolescents and young adults returning to work and how to provide for their special needs provides important insights into how to help them reach their potential.

In documenting strategies for employers to facilitate returning to work for employees, it is recommended that educating themselves and the workforce about cancer is useful. In a second volume, this book provides all of the information that would be required. Starting with explanations on the nature of cancer, its genetics, immunology and how it spreads around the body, the incidence of various cancers is explored. How cancer is diagnosed, and the scans required to detect it and follow the progress of the treatment, shows the ongoing requirements for monitoring the cancer. The spectrum of treatments including surgery, radiotherapy and pharmacotherapies, chemotherapy, hormone therapy, targeted therapy and immunotherapy are covered in the text. A chapter on evidence-based clinical guidelines shows how to standardise the management of cancers across the world. These general chapters are followed by chapters on the management of common cancers.

Most important for caring for people returning to work after cancer are the chapters on supportive care including psycho-oncology, the financial challenges that patients face with cancer treatment and not working, ongoing rehabilitation and the longer-term issues faced by survivors of cancer.

The editors of these volumes are internationally recognised practitioners and researchers whose expertise covers the fields of basic research, clinical oncology and public health. They have achieved a comprehensive range of topics written by authors expert in clinical and basic oncology from all over Asia.

This book will provide employers with essential education about cancer and how to best support employees with cancer in facilitating their return to work. Examples of strategies to achieve this from many Asian countries provide a spectrum of ideas on what to put in place. Since the advice includes providing information about cancer to other employees, these volumes will also be a source of the information that employers can use, or which can be directly accessed by other employees and their colleagues with cancer. These volumes bring into one place updated information on cancer and work which will be invaluable to help professionals ranging from oncologists, oncology nurses and occupational professionals to the multiple disciplines involved in the provision of supportive cancer care including social workers, psychologists, dieticians, exercise practitioners, physiotherapists, occupational therapists and those involved with rehabilitation and survivorship care.

Adjunct Professor, Faculty of Health and Medical Sciences
University of Adelaide
South Australia

Ian A. M. Olver, MD PhD

Preface

The advancements in cancer research have been remarkable, transforming cancer from an incurable disease to one that can be treated if detected early. Even when discovered at a more advanced stage, treatments can extend life, and methods to alleviate the pain caused by cancer and its treatments are continually being explored. Guidelines have been developed and regularly updated to reflect these advancements.

However, a significant challenge remains: how to live after being diagnosed with cancer. In modern society, regardless of the country, people work to live and often find purpose and means of living through their jobs. Now that it is possible to live with cancer, people work to continue their treatment and seek treatment to be able to work more. Even if they are undergoing medical treatment and taking a long-term sick leave, people who find some meaning in working may want to return to their workplace in the future.

To fulfill these desires, social security systems in some countries, support from local communities and families, and understanding from workplaces are essential.

Rather than learning about it for the first time after being diagnosed and panicking, we aim to spread understanding of cancer throughout society. Specifically, we want colleagues, superiors, subordinates, or oneself to have the correct basic knowledge and know what actions to take when someone in the workplace is affected. This project was planned together with Dr. Endo and Dr. Muto. With the cooperation of public health and epidemiology researchers from various Asian countries, domestic clinicians and medical researchers in Japan, and cancer survivors, this book was created. Although there may be many shortcomings in the first edition, we hope to refine it into a more sophisticated educational book for the general public with the cooperation of our readers. Finally, we would like to express our heartfelt gratitude to the editors at Springer who patiently accompanied us until the completion of this work.

Tokyo, Japan Mitsue Saito, MD PhD MBA

Contents

Part I

Basic Medicine in Cancer

What Is Cancer? 1 Cancer Incidence

1

Tatsuro Irimura and Mitsue Saito

Abstract

There are two types of so-called cancer: one is a malignant solid tumor, which includes carcinoma and sarcoma, and the other is blood cancer, such as leukemia or malignant lymphoma. The primary distinction lies in their origin: carcinomas emerge from epithelial cells, while sarcomas arise from connective tissues. In this introductory chapter, the biology of cancer cells is outlined, focusing on carcinoma. What is the difference between the growth of cancer cells and normal cells? How does our body suppress the growth of emerging cancer cells? What are the reasons for the failure to eliminate cancer cells? How do cancer cells damage our bodies? Although no complete answers to these fundamental biological questions can be provided, it is important to keep these questions in mind to understand and to effectively treat cancer.

Keywords

Carcinogenesis · Oncogene · Immune escape · Tumor microenvironment · Dormancy · Cancer stem cell

1.1 Cell Divisions and Cancer

A multicellular organism, such as a human, is developed from a fertilized egg, which is a single cell. The human body is known to consist of 40 trillion cells, which are the results of cell divisions. During development and ontogeny, cells of our body divide and change their properties during and after cell divisions and eventually form functional organs. Our body at the adult stage, *i.e.*, after completion of development and growth, essentially consists of three types of cells regarding their characteristics of cell division. Cells of the first group never divide once the body has completed its development, such as neurons. Cells of the second group do not usually divide but maintain the capacity to divide when it is necessary, such as hepatocytes and breast epithelial cells. Cells of the third group keep dividing throughout our lives, such as bone marrow cells and intestinal epithelial cells. Importantly, cell divisions are strictly regulated throughout life so that the growth of any of these cells does not lethally damage other cells or impair body functions.

It is commonly said that cancer is a result of the uncontrolled growth of cells. Uncontrolled growth of cancer cells is not simply due to continuous divisions. Physiological proliferations of cells, as mentioned above, are stopped by many mechanisms. One of the predominant mechanisms of senescence is apoptosis due to the shortening of telomeres, the capping structure of chromosomal DNA [4]. Cells without telomeres undergo apoptosis, programmed cell death. Cancer cells escape from such a mechanism through the extension of telomeres by activating telomerase and continuously proliferate.

1.2 Genetic Basis of Carcinogenesis

It is widely accepted that cancer cells acquire properties such as uncontrolled proliferation in a process called carcinogenesis. Carcinogenesis is always associated with genetic changes. There are genes that play important roles in carcinogenesis (Fig. 1.1). These are oncogenes, which regulate cell divisions, and suppressor oncogenes, which are engaged with antagonizing the oncogene functions and with the repair of damaged genes [11, 15]. Alterations in these genes, such as mutations and amplifications due to exposure to radiation, chemical carcinogens, or oncogenic viruses, are the primary causes of carcinogenesis. Hereditary genetic differences,

T. Irimura
Division of Glycobiologics, Department of Breast Oncology, School of Medicine, Juntendo University, Bunkyo-ku, Tokyo, Japan
e-mail: t-irimura@juntendo.ac.jp

M. Saito (✉)
Department of Breast Oncology, Graduate School of Medicine, Juntendo University, Bunkyo-ku, Tokyo, Japan
e-mail: mitsue@juntendo.ac.jp

© The Author(s), under exclusive license to Springer Nature Singapore Pte Ltd. 2026
M. Endo et al. (eds.), *Cancer and Work in Asia Volume 2*, https://doi.org/10.1007/978-981-95-6537-5_1

Fig. 1.1 Oncogenes and suppressor oncogenes are often associated with cancer. *SCLC* small cell lung cancer, *NSCLC* nonsmall cell lung cancer

Oncogenes	gene function	mechanism of activation	affected cancer
BCR-ABL	growth factor receptor	translocation	chronic myelocytic leukemia
MYC	regulation of cell cycle	amplification, translocation	SCLC
RAS	signal transduction leading to cell proliferation	point mutation	pancreatic ductal ca NSCLC, colorectal ca
HER2	growth factor receptor	amplification	breast ca, stomach ca

Suppresser oncogenes	gene function	mechanism of inactivation	affected cancer
P53	DNA repair induction of apoptosis	point mutation	breast ca, colorectal ca, stomach ca, soft tissue cancer, and many others
BRCA1/2	DNA repair	mutation, promoter methylation	breast ca, ovarian ca
APC	suppression of Wnt signal	deletion, mutation	colorectal ca

termed predispositions, sometimes facilitate this process. It is widely accepted that accumulations of mutations in multiple genes take place before carcinogenesis [2]. Accumulations of mutations are lifelong events, and the incidence of carcinogenesis increases upon aging in general. Thus, hereditary genetic backgrounds may be associated with cancers that develop at younger ages. The reason why a mutation at the level of our genome, which is carried by all the cells in our body, appears to strongly influence carcinogenesis in only a few specific organs in most cases of hereditary cancer is not fully understood.

1.3 Tissue Microenvironment and Immunological Surveillance

During aging, genetic alterations and resultant abnormal growth of cells may always take place, but not all of them result in cancer. A cancer cell becomes a tumor only when microenvironmental supports, such as nutrition, growth factors, and extracellular scaffolds, are provided, though cancer cells become refractory to some of these conditions upon cancer progression [14]. It is well known that cancer cells get access to and even induce vasculature to maintain nutritional support. This process is termed tumor angiogenesis [3]. Connective tissue and basal lamina are distributed throughout our body, and the cells present in the tissue, such as fibroblasts, other resident cells, and even resident bacteria, indirectly influence the growth of cancer cells through inflammation, which can either lead to the establishment or the elimination of a tumor.

Another important issue is the fact that our immune system always surveys the body for the presence of newly formed abnormal cells. These processes, generally described as immunological surveillance, were first proposed by Burnet [1] and later experimentally confirmed by Smyth and co-workers [13] through the understanding of natural immune systems. Products of mutated genes expressed by proliferating cells are potentially recognized by the immune system as nonself, and specific immune responses could participate in the elimination of cancer cells. However, some cancer cells may be less sensitive to being attacked by the immune system. On such occasions, cancer cells sustain growth, and the elimination phase turns into an equilibrium phase. When tumors are established, cancer cells apparently develop mechanisms to escape from immunological surveillance. Only recently were new medicines such as immune checkpoint inhibitors developed to block these escape mechanisms so that host immunity alone or in combination with other therapeutic modalities can effectively recognize, attack, and eliminate cancer cells in a responsive subset of patients [10].

1.4 Malignant Progression

Tumor cells change their properties and become more malignant while they grow, which is termed malignant progression. Three important acquired properties during malignant progression are resistance to drug therapy, metastasis, and the systemic effects on the metabolism of the body called cachexia. These acquired properties form persistent obstacles that interfere with effective cancer treatments and result in huge inconveniences and harm for patients. The causes of these three properties are not necessarily genetic changes, as is always the case with carcinogenesis, but rather they are induced by the phenotypic versatility of cancer cells, although it is believed that the role of genetic changes in malignant progression differs among cancers of different organs.

A variety of mechanisms are involved with increased resistance to drug therapy, including efficient excretion of anticancer compounds and resistance to apoptosis [9]. Most of these mechanisms are thought to be based on cellular versatility. Cancer cells are a mixture of phenotypically heterogeneous cell populations. During the treatment of cancer with therapeutic compounds, sensitive cancer cells are eliminated. However, a small subset of resistant cancer cells survives and grows even in the presence of therapeutic compounds and later becomes dominant. While these subsets do not usually carry genetic changes, resistance to molecularly targeted therapeutic compounds is sometimes mediated just by mutations of the target molecules.

Metastasis is the growth of cancer cells at locations that can be far away from the organ in which the cancer originally derived. Metastatic growth damages the functions of vital organs, such as the lung, liver, brain, or bone, and is the primary cause of death due to cancer. Metastasis is a result of the heterogeneity of cancer cells due to their phenotypic versatility. Some metastatic cancer cells show the capacity to leave the primary tumor sites, travel within our body through the vasculature, extravasate, and establish a secondary growth in a distant organ microenvironment. Studies revealed the molecular basis engaged with each unit process of metastasis. These characteristics are considered within a spectrum of phenotypic versatility, and genetic changes are not usually involved in how and why a cancer cell metastasizes. Metastatic phenotypes may be temporally acquired in response to microenvironmental factors. This process is often referred to as epithelial-mesenchymal transition (EMT) because many cancer cells having epithelial origins transform themselves into motile and invasive mesenchymal-like cells upon interactions with other cells. Further information and references regarding cancer metastasis can be found in Chap. 2 in this book.

Cachexia is a condition characterized by an elevated metabolism caused by inflammatory cytokines [12]. The body levels of these inflammatory cytokines increase by secretion from cancer cells and from inflammatory cells activated as a consequence of the immune recognition of cancer cells. The process may be considered as a part of the natural immune response to cancer cells; however, it becomes evident in the late stages of cancer. During cachexia, degradation of fat and skeletal muscle proteins occurs, and the body becomes insulin-resistant. As a result, so-called wasting syndrome with significant weight loss, fatigue, and impairment of other body functions is observed in some patients with advanced cancer.

1.5 Dormancy and Cancer Stem Cells

Cancer cells may survive within our body for many years without forming a detectable tumor. This is sometimes termed dormancy and probably corresponds to the equilibrium conditions mentioned in Sect. 1.3. Such conditions pose a significant clinical problem because they are the cause of the recurrence of cancer after an initially successful treatment. The mechanisms of dormancy and tumor recurrence from dormant cancer cells remain mysteries happening beneath the surface, though it is likely that at least a certain number of cancer cells disseminate before the primary tumor is clinically diagnosed, and not all of them are sensitive to adjuvant drug therapy, which is recommended by guidelines to prevent recurrence of tumors based on scientific evidence. Evidence is established through reliable clinical studies and approved by a consensus of expert panels. It is strongly hoped that detailed genetic and other approaches will unveil the microscopic and molecular world beneath and improve cancer therapy in the near future.

The hypothesis that there is a cancer stem cell population hiding somewhere in the body may explain the dormancy and recurrence after successful surgery with adjuvant drug therapy [8]. A cancer stem cell population could be defined as a slow-growing subset of cancer cells. Cell divisions by cancer stem cells give rise to slow-growing cells, which maintain the cancer stem cell population, and to faster-growing, proliferative cells, which then may form growing tumors. Cancer stem cells are known to be resistant to chemotherapeutic drugs or radiotherapy because of their low proliferation rates. In other words, highly proliferating cells are sensitive to chemotherapy and radiotherapy in general. It is also likely that cancer stem cells remain unscathed by host immunological surveillance. Thus, cancer stem cells may stay alive and dormant even when all the proliferative cancer cells have been eliminated. These cancer stem cells have the potential to form metastases, and therefore, recurrence and distant metastasis formation after considerable periods may be explained by the growth of tumor-forming cancer cells out of hiding cancer stem cells initiated by many mechanisms, including, for instance, age-associated weakening of the immune system (Fig. 1.2).

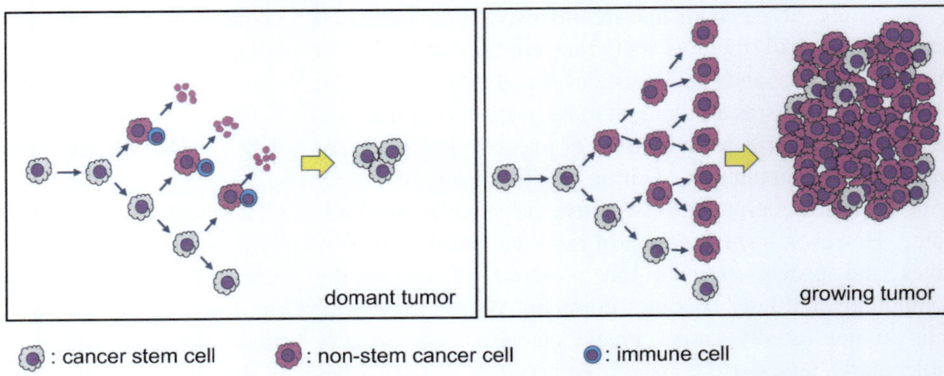

Fig. 1.2 Hypothetical scheme of cancer stem cells and the mechanistic basis of dormancy

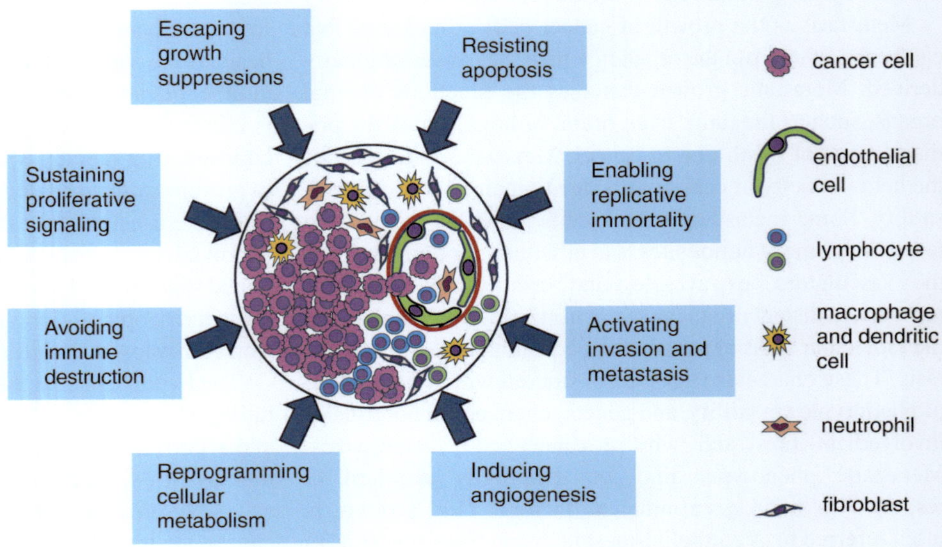

Fig. 1.3 The hallmarks of cancer. Shown are the acquired capabilities that allow cancer cells to grow, spread, and avoid destruction. Hanahan and Weinberg first proposed cancer hallmarks in 2000 [6]. Revised versions were subsequently proposed later [5, 7]

1.6 Conclusions

Cancer is caused by accumulations of genetic alterations in our cells, particularly in genes for molecules that control cellular proliferation. There are mechanisms supporting and antagonizing cancer cell growth within the cells. Also, the tissue microenvironment supports or suppresses the growth of cancer cells. The host immune system always attempts to eliminate cancer cells. However, cancer cells develop ways to escape from host immunological surveillance. Cancer cells are phenotypically versatile, always undergo malignant progression, and attack the host by developing resistance to therapy, metastasizing to different organs, and eventually inducing cachexia. These natures are summarized and illustrated in a scheme termed the hallmarks of cancer, shown in Fig. 1.3.

References

1. Burnet FM. Immunological aspects of malignant disease. Lancet. 1967;1:1171–4.
2. Fearon ER, Vogelstein B. A genetic model for colorectal tumorigenesis. Cell. 1990;61:759–67.
3. Folkman J. Tumor angiogenesis. Adv Cancer Res. 1985;43:175–203.
4. Greider CW. Mammalian telomere dynamics: healing, fragmentation shortening and stabilization. Curr Opin Genet Dev. 1994;4:203–11.
5. Hanahan D. Hallmarks of cancer: new dimensions. Cancer Discov. 2022;12:31–46.
6. Hanahan D, Weinberg RA. The hallmarks of cancer. Cell. 2000;100:57–70.
7. Hanahan D, Weinberg RA. Hallmarks of cancer: the next generation. Cell. 2011;144:646–74.
8. Maccalli C, Rasul KI, Elawad M, Ferrone S. The role of cancer stem cells in the modulation of anti-tumor immune responses. Semin Cancer Biol. 2018;53:189–200.

9. Mimeault M, Hauke R, Batra SK. Recent advances on the molecular mechanisms involved in the drug resistance of cancer cells and novel targeting therapies. Clin Pharmacol Ther. 2008;83:673–91.
10. Peggs KS, Quezada SA, Korman AJ, Allison JP. Principles and use of anti-CTLA4 antibody in human cancer immunotherapy. Curr Opin Immunol. 2006;18:206–13.
11. Pierotti MA, Dragani TA. Genetics and cancer. Curr Opin Oncol. 1992;4:127–33.
12. Rubin H. Cancer cachexia: its correlations and causes. Proc Natl Acad Sci U S A. 2003;100:5384–9.
13. Smyth MJ, Godfrey DI, Trapani JA. A fresh look at tumor immunosurveillance and immunotherapy. Nat Immunol. 2001;2:293–9.
14. van Kempen LC, Ruiter DJ, van Muijen GN, Coussens LM. The tumor microenvironment: a critical determinant of neoplastic evolution. Eur J Cell Biol. 2003;82:539–48.
15. Varmus HE. The molecular genetics of cellular oncogenes. Annu Rev Genet. 1984;18:553–612.

What Is Cancer?: 2 Cancer Metastasis

2

Tatsuro Irimura

Abstract

Metastases are tumor foci growing at distant sites from the original tumors. In many cancers, metastases cause inconvenience and pain for the patients and are often responsible for therapeutic failures. Ninety percent of cancer-related deaths are known to be due to metastasis. Therefore, it is often remarked that if metastasis is conquered, then cancer can be conquered. Metastasis, present at the time of the initial diagnosis or discovered during the therapy, significantly changes how the disease is dealt with by clinicians and their patients. Despite advances in the understanding and treatment of primary tumors, the treatment of metastatic cancer remains a big challenge. The purpose of this chapter is to outline the biology of cancer metastasis in a broad context and to discuss why, how, when, and where metastases occur. In this chapter, the readers will understand the biological basis of metastasis as a process having both specific and stochastic elements reminiscent of embryogenesis, morphogenesis, and even evolution, and as an inefficient result of many consecutive processes taking place throughout all the stages of cancer. Based on these clinical and biological features, it is true that cancer is potentially intractable because it acquires metastatic capability. Thus, cancer is malignant due to metastasis.

Keywords

Metastasis · Seed and soil hypothesis · Epithelial-mesenchymal transition · Metastatic pre-conditioning Organ-selective metastasis

T. Irimura (✉)
Division of Glycobiologics, Department of Breast Oncology, School of Medicine, Juntendo University, Bunkyo-ku, Tokyo, Japan
e-mail: t-irimura@juntendo.ac.jp

2.1 Metastasis—Why?

2.1.1 Seed and Soil Hypothesis

Biological understanding of cancer metastasis was founded on the "Seed and Soil Hypothesis" proposed by the British surgeon Stephen Paget in 1889. In his report published in The Lancet entitled "Distribution of secondary growths in cancer of the breast," he conducted necropsies in 735 fatal cases and concluded that the causes of metastases are not sporadic but rather that specific mechanisms are involved [20]. He noted that a large number of cases, 241 in his cohort, had cancer in the liver, but only 17 had cancer in the spleen, though liver and spleen are supposed to receive similar numbers of blood-borne tumor cells that have escaped from the primary sites. Such disproportion was not observed for pyemia or bacterial colonization. This observation clearly indicates that the nature of the organ microenvironment, i.e., the soil, plays an equally important role as the nature of the tumor cells, i.e., the seeds, in the formation of metastases. In another comparison based on reported data, he noted that bone was another frequent site of metastasis of breast cancer, whereas not a single case of bone metastasis was seen among 903 autopsies done on cancers of the stomach and pylorus. Thus, the importance of the nature of the tumor cells and the seeds in determining the sites of the metastatic growth is clearly revealed by Paget's clinical observations.

2.1.2 Biological Basis for Why Cancers Metastasize

More than 130 years have passed since Paget's report, and the seed and soil hypothesis has been accepted as fact, yet the essential question of why tumor cells metastasize remains unanswered. Like any other biological creature, unicellular or multicellular, bacteria, plants, or animals, cancer cells migrate and colonize when they can do so. Plant seeds migrate by a variety of means and colonize if they can find

© The Author(s), under exclusive license to Springer Nature Singapore Pte Ltd. 2026

M. Endo et al. (eds.), *Cancer and Work in Asia Volume 2*, https://doi.org/10.1007/978-981-95-6537-5_2

proper soil. Cancer cells do the same and apparently evolve to acquire ways for initiating and sustaining metastatic growth, unfortunately.

2.2 Metastasis—How?

2.2.1 Experimental Investigations of Metastasis

Experimental investigations on the mechanisms of cancer metastasis in model animals, particularly the specific elements in the process, were initiated by Isaiah J. Fidler. He reproduced lung metastasis of melanoma by intravenously injecting syngeneic melanoma cells into mice. Several out of 10^5 melanoma cells colonized the lung, and tumor foci were visually detectable 3 weeks later [4, 5]. Melanoma cells were placed in cultures, and the cells were intravenously injected again. By repeating this cycle 10 times, he was able to obtain variant cells that were highly metastatic to the lung. Fidler proposed in 1978 that metastasis results from a cascade of events (depicted in Fig. 2.1), and that highly metastatic cells are capable of efficiently performing all these steps, like decathlon champions [4, 5]. His experiments also clearly indicated that metastasis is an inefficient process and stochastic elements are also involved. Cellular and molecular phenotypes associated with highly metastatic subpopulations of tumor cells opened up new directions of research on metastasis. Another important notion was that malignant tumors consist of heterogeneous populations of tumor cells in their metastatic capacity, as they are also heterogeneous regarding other biological phenotypes. How this heterogeneity arises is discussed later.

By characterizing these highly metastatic cells representing a subpopulation of tumor cells, the cellular and molecular basis for the specific aspects of lung metastasis formation were extensively explored. The selected highly lung metastatic melanoma cells are shown to express high levels of extracellular matrix degradation enzymes such as metalloprotease and heparanase, apparently responsible for the

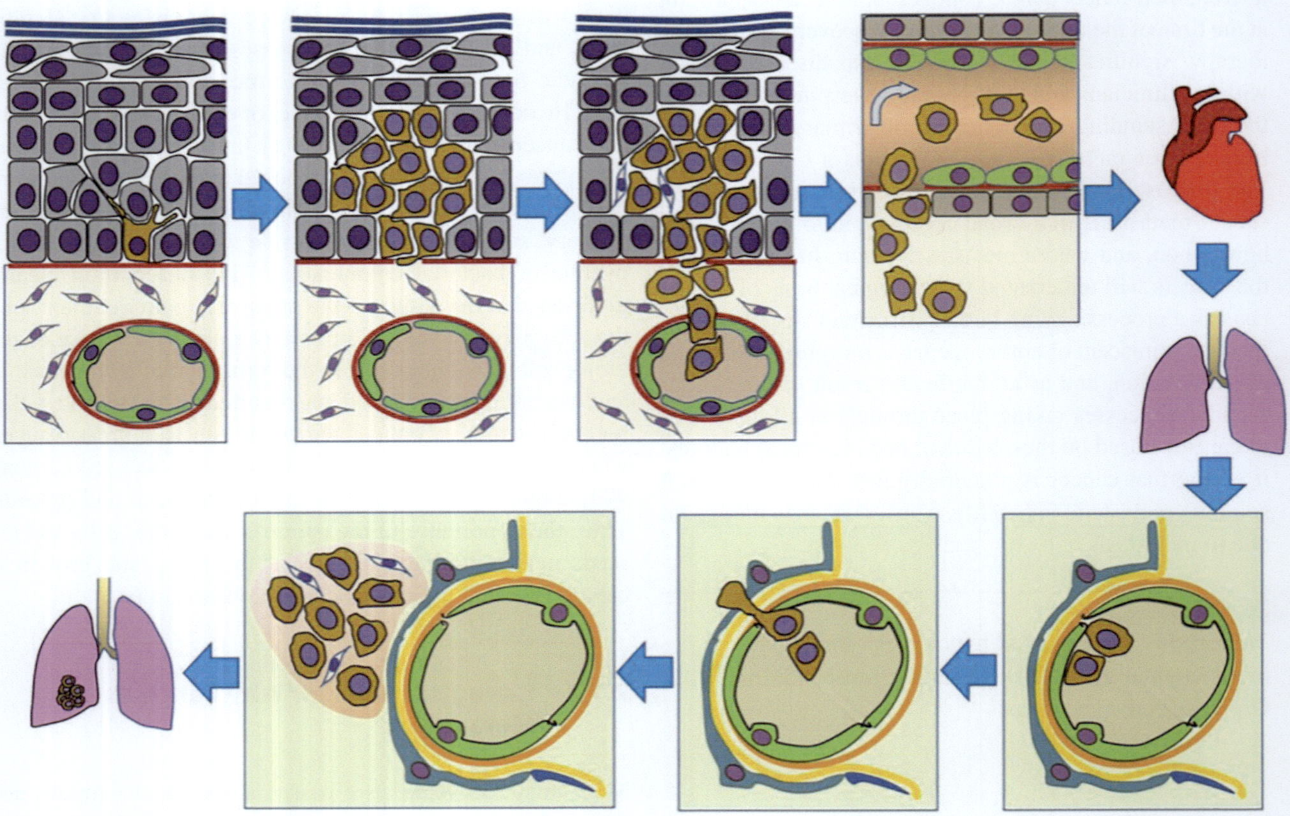

Fig. 2.1 Cascade of events leading to the metastasis of tumor cells as originally proposed by Fidler [5]. This scheme is drawn to show the events in lung metastasis of skin melanoma. A melanocyte (shown as a brown cell in the upper left panel) undergoes malignant transformation and grows into a tumor, melanoma. Some tumor cells invade the basement membranes and migrate into blood vessels. These cells travel through the bloodstream to the heart and then to the lungs. The cells attach to the endothelium of a microcapillary and invade the alveolar space. If the tumor cells are able to establish a focus with host cells, such as fibroblasts, a metastatic tumor, which can be detected by imaging tools, forms

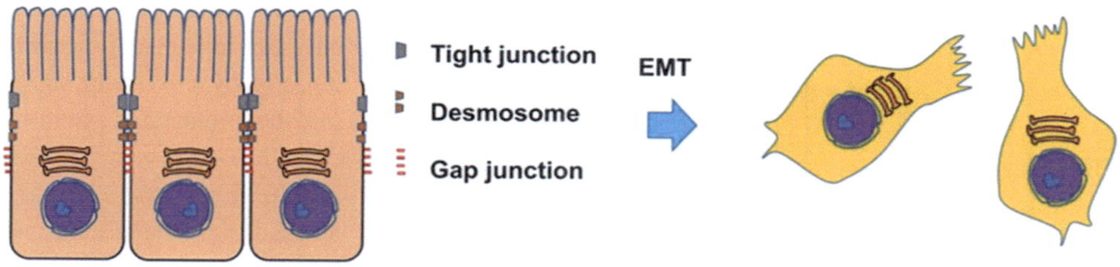

Fig. 2.2 Epithelial-mesenchymal transition (EMT) commonly takes place during embryonic development. Apical-basal polarity and tight associations with adjacent cells are lost during EMT [3]

highly efficient basement membrane breakdown important for tumor cell invasion [16]. As a strong confirmation, melanoma cells selected in vitro for their invasive capacity through basement membranes turned out to be metastatic to the lung in vivo, as reported by Hart [7]. Other studies by Nicolson and coworkers revealed that organ-selective metastatic variants of the same melanoma can be obtained [19]. Organ-selective elements in the process of metastasis formation are further discussed in Sect. 2.4.

2.2.2 Regulation of Metastatic Phenotypes

Studies on metastases in experimental animals revealed a variety of important biological hallmarks of metastatic tumor cells in addition to extracellular matrix degradation. These features are useful to interpret clinicopathological observations from mechanistic contexts and to elucidate the regulatory mechanisms of metastatic traits. These traits, i.e., hallmarks of metastatic tumor cells, include (1) high levels of degradative capacity of basement membranes and cellular motility, both of which are necessary to metastasize across tissue barriers, (2) capacity to adhere to vascular walls or to form emboli in microcapillaries for tumor cells to stay at distant organs after travelling through vasculatures, (3) unique properties to communicate with cells in distant organ sites through signaling substances such as chemokines, cytokines, growth factors, and exosomes, all facilitating cellular trafficking from the primary sites to distant sites, and (4) properties of tumor cells to communicate with the host organ microenvironment to establish tumor tissue regardless of the organ. It is widely accepted that cancer cells arise as a result of multiple genetic changes leading to the dysregulation of cell growth. Such changes in the regulation of cell growth are important for tumor cells to be metastatic, but additional properties, as listed above, are also essential.

It is important to keep in mind that each of these hallmarks and substances involved in the metastatic cascade is not unique to malignant cells but is expressed and used in the maintenance of homeostasis by a variety of somatic cells, particularly cells in the immune system. It is not surprising to find that metastatic tumor cells simultaneously acquire many of these metastatic traits through altered networks of gene expression and/or epigenetic changes, which are not direct consequences of the malignant transformation of cells caused by the genetic changes. Metastatic capacity can be regarded as the intrinsic personality of a malignant tumor cell, or such a property can be triggered in the course of tumor growth. Many malignant tumors are derived from epithelial cells. Normal somatic epithelial cells adhere to and communicate with adjacent cells. Even malignant cells having epithelial origins often maintain such properties. However, they sometimes lose this property and become non-epithelial-like cells. It is likely that a systematic change in gene expression occurs during this process, which is termed epithelial-mesenchymal transition (EMT) [3], depicted in Fig. 2.2. EMT is an event common in embryogenesis and pathogenesis [12]. How and when EMT takes place during cancer progression and formation of metastases is discussed in Sect. 2.3.2.

2.2.3 Metastatic Phenotypes Involved with Genetic Changes and Host Immunity

In some cases, advanced stages of cancer are associated with multiorgan metastases. Mechanisms leading to multiorgan metastasis are not fully understood. However, two important changes appear to be taking place at such advanced stages of cancer. The first is the accumulation of additional mutations in cancer cells. It is likely that the generation of clonal variations within cancer cell populations becomes highly frequent [23]. Such genetic and phenotypic diversification supports metastases to a variety of organs with different microenvironments. Diversification through genetic changes and selective adaptation are essential elements of evolution. For this reason, metastasis is often referred to as an evolutionary process, although no gene or any particular mutation has been identified to be essential in driving metastases [1]. The second is the deterioration of the immune system, which makes it easier for tumor cells to escape immune surveillance and spread. At the same time, organ microenvironments are remodeled and/or destroyed everywhere in the body, and tumor cells become prone to growing anywhere. Therefore, the question of how metastasis occurs does not have a simple answer. It is true that we have just begun to understand the details of the specific and stochastic aspects of the biology of metastasis.

2.3 Metastasis—When?

2.3.1 The Cascade of Events

Clinically, "When does metastasis occur?" is a burning question to provide the best treatment to patients. However, this is not a simple question to answer clinically as well as biologically. Malignant tumors break through the basement membranes according to the pathological definitions. They are often detected even in blood vessels or lymphatic vessels when the tumor sections are carefully examined at the time of the initial surgical resection. Therefore, it is reasonable to speculate that some tumor cells have initiated the process of the metastatic cascade already when a malignant tumor is discovered. Because metastasis is an inefficient process, the initial process has to be repeated numerous times before the second stage becomes the determining point. Then, the tumor cells form so-called micro-metastases. These micro-metastases may become established metastases by multi-factorial interactions between the tumor cells and the host tissue microenvironment. As the metastatic cascade shown in Fig. 2.1 consists of multiple steps, the mechanistic basis for these seed and soil characters of metastasis is complex. It should be understood that cancer patients are potentially at any stage of the metastatic cascade when the primary tumor is discovered. Changes in gene expression and epigenetic changes in the tumor cells are assumed to be associated with an increased metastatic propensity. However, when exactly they take place is difficult to predict. Changes in the micro-environment also potentially promote metastatic processes directly by providing supportive soil and indirectly by fueling the metastatic phenotypes of tumor cells. All of these cross-talks are sometimes forwarding and sometimes reversing the metastatic cascade. If there is any critical event that drives the metastatic cascade forward, then it should be considered as a therapeutic target to prevent metastasis. It is worth keeping in mind that the metastatic cascade is not like a downstream flow after a dam is broken, although the word "cascade" is used. It is more like an uphill obstacle race, and therefore metastasis is known as an inefficient process.

2.3.2 EMT in Cancer Metastases

EMT is a process to arm tumor cells with a variety of tools useful in the obstacle race. As depicted in Fig. 2.3, EMT may take place on a variety of occasions in the metastatic cascade and plays important roles in pushing the process forward [14]. A more difficult question is what initiates EMT.

Intrinsic changes within the tumor cells, microenvironmental factors, and their combinations are likely to trigger the process. Changes in gene expression and epigenetic changes are important intrinsic elements. EMT is also known as a consequence of physical and biochemical changes in the microenvironment. Hypoxia is a condition known to be induced by a low-oxygen microenvironment and to change

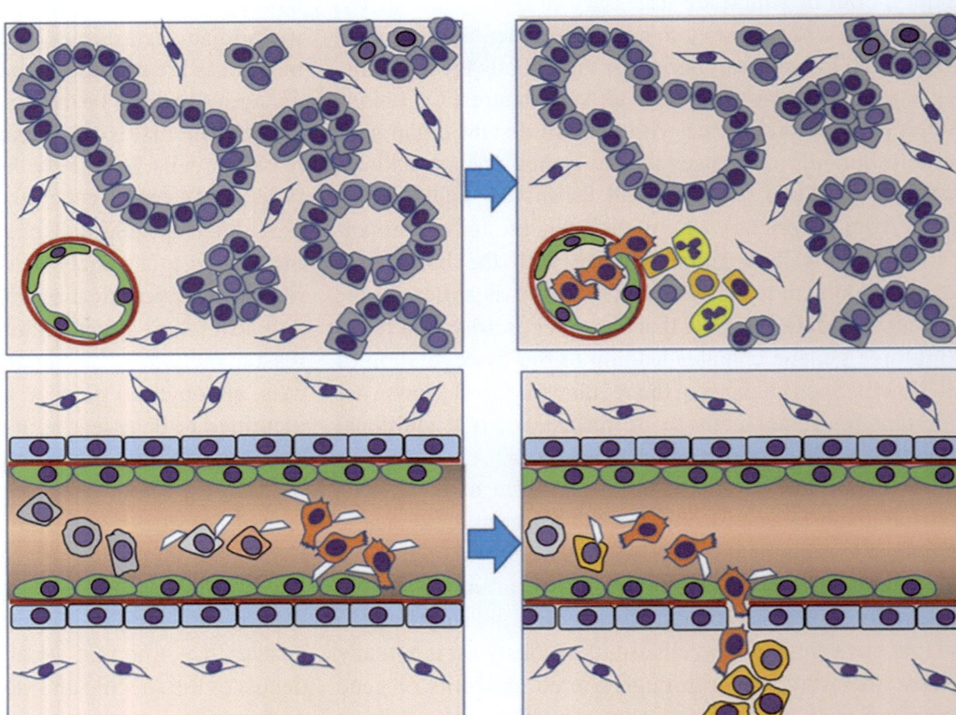

Fig. 2.3 Epithelial-mesenchymal transition (EMT) by tumor cells promotes invasion and metastasis. In the upper panels, EMT (grey to orange change) is shown to be initiated by the effect of inflammatory cells (cells in yellow color), and the cells undergo vascular invasions. In the lower panels, blood-borne circulating tumor cells undergo EMT, sometimes through their interaction with platelets (shown as white pieces). These tumor cells exhibit increased capacity to adhere to endothelial cells and invade through the basement membranes

gene expression properties of tumor cells [22]. When tumors grow large and vascular formation is not sufficient, hypoxic portions of a tumor increase, and tumor cells undergo various changes in gene expression and epigenetic gene regulation. These changes enable tumor cells to migrate into oxygen-rich environments and to adapt and grow in an oxygen-depleted environment.

The other important changes that potentially induce EMT of tumor cells are immune and inflammatory responses. This is a complex issue because external EMT inducers such as TGF-β and other cytokines also modulate immune response and inflammation [13]. Furthermore, stimulation of inflammatory processes and immune responses is initiated by a variety of events, including infection and the onset of metabolic and other disorders. All of them have the potential to promote the metastatic cascade and should be considered as important determinants of when metastasis occurs.

2.3.3 Cancer Cell Evolution

Genomic alterations are always considered as important origins of the phenotypic heterogeneity of tumor cells, which is the basis of metastasis as a result of diversification and selection. Such assumptions proposed in the early days of metastasis research were proven to be true through extensive analysis of cancer genomes in a large number of clinical specimens [1]. Birkbak and McGranahan's review, based on many such investigations, also revealed important genomic changes that appear to be taking place during the formation of metastases in different cancers. The first important notion that there is no single or limited number of genes that drive metastases was already mentioned above. There are many additional mutations during cancer progression toward metastasis formation; almost all of them do not look like the driver but rather passengers. Second, metastases are sometimes monoclonal and sometimes polyclonal, i.e., derived from multiple clones. These analyses also strongly suggest that metastases to the same organ site have taken place many times at early and late stages of the growth of the primary tumors. In some cases, undetectable micrometastasis remain dormant for many years, then get activated to become metastatic foci [2]. Thus, the final answer to the question of when metastasis occurs is "at any moment."

2.4 Metastasis—Where?

2.4.1 Organ-Selective Metastases

We now come back to one of the central issues of the seed and soil hypothesis. Although both blood and lymphatic flows are essential routes through which tumors disseminate, biological aspects that are not fully understood determine the tendency of where metastatic tumors grow. Tumor cells of gastrointestinal origin travel through the portal vein to the liver and tend to form metastases in the liver. The predominant site of uveal (ocular) melanoma metastasis is the liver, whereas skin melanoma metastasizes to the lung and the brain, which is not fully explained by the circulatory connections [24]. It is obvious that both the intrinsic properties of the tumor cells and the microenvironment where metastatic tumors grow play important roles.

2.4.2 Importance of Vascular Endothelium

It was Garth L. Nicolson who emphasized the importance of vascular endothelial cells as the determinant of metastatic organ tropism in an early stage of research on the biology of metastasis [18]. The unique natures of vascular endothelium in the brain (blood–brain barrier), liver (sinusoid), and lymph node (high endothelial venule) are well described. While these and other unique natures of endothelial cells are used to target therapeutic agents to specific organs, the understanding of organ-selective metastases through the nature of the endothelium is not well developed [8]. However, the importance of specific adhesive interactions between tumor cells and endothelial cells is further supported by notions that endothelial cell surface molecules play crucial roles in the homing of circulating cells in the immune system [15]. Metastatic tumor cells use molecular mechanisms similar to leukocyte migration, and the roles of tumor cell surface carbohydrates in cancer cell adhesion and invasion were noted [11, 17] (Fig. 2.4).

In addition, the formation of tumor vasculature was shown to be essential for tumor growth and metastasis, and its prevention became a target of cancer therapy [6, 25].

2.4.3 Metastatic Preconditioning

A mechanism called metastatic preconditioning, which elevates the potential of vasculatures of distant organs to serve as the site of distant metastasis, was proposed by Hiratsuka and coworkers [9, 10] (Fig. 2.5).

They reported that cytokines released by the primary tumor induced the expression of enzymes responsible for extracellular matrix degradation and inflammatory proteins S100A8 and S100A9 specifically in the vasculatures of the lung but not in other organs such as the liver or kidney [10]. These proteins seem to be responsible for changing the endothelia in the lung to promote colonization of myeloid cells and to form a premetastatic niche for the tumor cells to colonize. Whether the organ selectivity of metastases to other

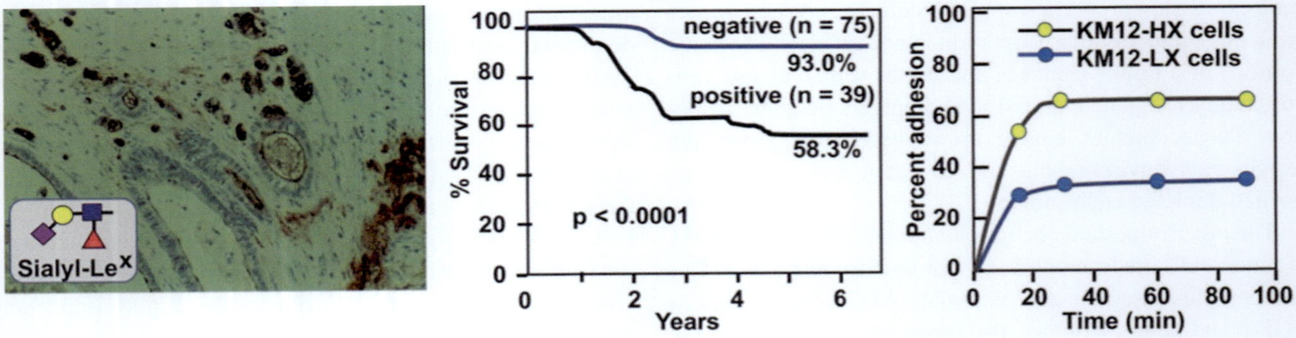

Fig. 2.4 Colon carcinoma cells are heterogeneous in the expression of carbohydrate antigens such as sialyl-Lewis X (Sialyl-Le^X) antigen. As shown in the left panel, brown staining by monoclonal antibody FH6 is associated with invading cells. Patients with high levels of staining had poor survival (middle panel) [17]. Colon carcinoma variant cells selected for high sialyl-Lewis X antigen expression (KM12-HX cells) exhibited a higher adhesion rate to tumor necrosis factor-activated endothelial cells than low-expressing (KM12-LX) cells (right panel) [11]

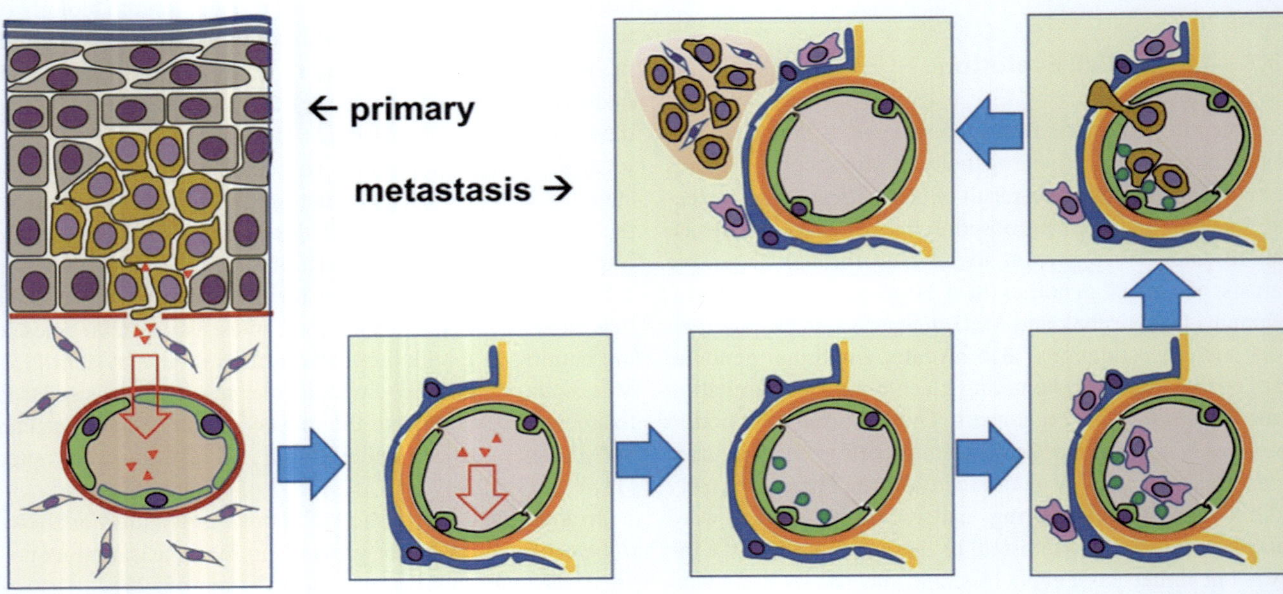

Fig. 2.5 A primary tumor can send signals to the future site of metastasis to form the "soil" suitable for the growth of tumor cells [10, 21]. This so-called metastatic preconditioning is mediated by inflammatory cytokines from tumor cells (shown as small red triangles), which modulate some endothelial cells of microvasculatures (shown by the appearance of green dots, which represent expression of S100A8/A9) to recruit inflammatory macrophages (pink cells) and promote adhesion and invasion of tumor cells. These macrophages seem to further aggravate the vicious cycle

organs is determined through a similar mechanism needs further evaluation. Lyden and coworkers extended the notion of preconditioning by proposing that the tumor cell-derived exosome, which is armed with non-coding RNA, DNA, and other tumor cell-derived substances, travels to endothelia of distant sites and changes the properties of these endothelia [26].

2.5 Concluding Remarks and Future Directions: Prevention, Diagnosis, and Therapy of Metastasis

Malignant tumors are invasive by definition. When they give rise, tumor cells start spreading. These cells may be eliminated, stay dormant, or step forward in the metastatic cascade. Naturally, it would be best to prevent metastasis before the cascade is completed. Therefore, eradication of both the tumor cells at the primary site and all tumor cells, which might be at a variety of stages in the metastatic cascade, disseminating throughout the body, has to be achieved to prevent metastasis. What the biology of metastasis can tell us is that it is difficult to know at which stage(s) of the metastatic cascade a patient is when cancer is diagnosed or at which stage(s) he/she is during and after the therapy of the primary tumor; and there are cases where metastases might be present but are not found. In the future, it is going to be paramount to define such premetastatic stages by utilizing combinations of novel biomarkers and to effectively interfere with the metastatic cascade using compounds and drugs yet to be found, to ultimately achieve the complete cure of cancer.

References

1. Birkbak NJ, McGranahan N. Cancer genome evolutionary trajectories in metastasis. Cancer Cell. 2020;37:8–19.
2. Blasco MT, Espuny I, Gomis RR. Ecology and evolution of dormant metastasis. Trends Cancer. 2022;8:570.
3. Boyer B, Thiery JP. Epithelium-mesenchyme interconversion as example of epithelial plasticity. APMIS. 1993;101:257–68.
4. Fidler IJ. Selection of successive tumour lines for metastasis. Nat New Biol. 1973;242:148–9.
5. Fidler IJ. The pathogenesis of cancer metastasis: the 'seed and soil' hypothesis revisited. Nat Rev Cancer. 2003;3:453–8.
6. Folkman J. Role of angiogenesis in tumor growth and metastasis. Semin Oncol. 2002;29:15–8.
7. Hart I. The selection and characterization of an invasive variant of the bi 6 melanoma. Am J Pathol. 1979;97:587–600.
8. Hennigs JK, Matuszcak C, Trepel M, Korbelin J. Vascular endothelial cells: heterogeneity and targeting approaches. Cells. 2021;10:2712.
9. Hiratsuka S, Nakamura K, Iwai S, Murakami M, Itoh T, Kijima H, Shipley JM, Senior RM, Shibuya M. MMP9 induction by vascular endothelial growth factor receptor-1 is involved in lung-specific metastasis. Cancer Cell. 2002;2:289–300.
10. Hiratsuka S, Watanabe A, Aburatani H, Maru Y. Tumour-mediated upregulation of chemoattractants and recruitment of myeloid cells predetermines lung metastasis. Nat Cell Biol. 2006;8:1369–75.
11. Izumi Y, Taniuchi Y, Tsuji T, Smith CW, Nakamori S, Fidler IJ, Irimura T. Characterization of human colon carcinoma variant cells selected for sialyl Lex carbohydrate antigen: liver colonization and adhesion to vascular endothelial cells. Exp Cell Res. 1995;216:215–21.
12. Kalluri R, Neilson EG. Epithelial-mesenchymal transition and its implications for fibrosis. J Clin Invest. 2003;112:1776–84.
13. Lopez-Novoa JM, Nieto MA. Inflammation and EMT: an alliance towards organ fibrosis and cancer progression. EMBO Mol Med. 2009;1:303–14.
14. Lu W, Kang Y. Epithelial-mesenchymal plasticity in cancer progression and metastasis. Dev Cell. 2019;49:361–74.
15. Nakache M, Berg EL, Streeter PR, Butcher EC. The mucosal vascular addressin is a tissue-specific endothelial cell adhesion molecule for circulating lymphocytes. Nature. 1989;337:179–81.
16. Nakajima M, Irimura T, Di Ferrante D, Di Ferrante N, Nicolson GL. Heparan sulfate degradation: relation to tumor invasive and metastatic properties of mouse B16 melanoma sublines. Science. 1983;220:611–3.
17. Nakamori S, Kameyama M, Imaoka S, Furukawa H, Ishikawa O, Sasaki Y, Kabuto T, Iwanaga T, Matsushita Y, Irimura T. Increased expression of sialyl Lewisx antigen correlates with poor survival in patients with colorectal carcinoma: clinicopathological and immunohistochemical study. Cancer Res. 1993;53:3632–7.
18. Nicolson GL. Organ specificity of tumor metastasis: role of preferential adhesion, invasion and growth of malignant cells at specific secondary sites. Cancer Metastasis Rev. 1988;7:143–88.
19. Nicolson GL, Brunson KW, Fidler IJ. Specificity of arrest, survival, and growth of selected metastatic variant cell lines. Cancer Res. 1978;38:4105–11.
20. Paget S. The distribution of secondary growths in cancer of the breast. Lancet. 1889;133:571–3.
21. Rafii S, Lyden D. S100 chemokines mediate bookmarking of premetastatic niches. Nat Cell Biol. 2006;8:1321–3.
22. Rankin EB, Giaccia AJ. Hypoxic control of metastasis. Science. 2016;352:175–80.
23. Turajlic S, Sottoriva A, Graham T, Swanton C. Resolving genetic heterogeneity in cancer. Nat Rev Genet. 2019;20:404–16.
24. van der Kooij MK, Speetjens FM, van der Burg SH, Kapiteijn E. Uveal versus cutaneous melanoma; same origin, very distinct tumor types. Cancers (Basel). 2019;11:845.
25. Weis SM, Cheresh DA. Tumor angiogenesis: molecular pathways and therapeutic targets. Nat Med. 2011;17:1359–70.
26. Wortzel I, Dror S, Kenific CM, Lyden D. Exosome-mediated metastasis: communication from a distance. Dev Cell. 2019;49:347–60.

What Is Cancer? 3 Cancer Genetics

3

Ryoko Semba and Masami Arai

Abstract

Heredity means the transmission of some characteristics from parents to their children. And such a characteristic is called a trait. Traits include not only characteristics that we can see but also those that we cannot see, including predisposition or behavior.

Cancer develops by accumulating genetic abnormalities. Genes are preserved in the nucleus of each cell. This is information on the base sequence of DNA, a design for constructing proteins. If a congenital germline mutation in genes associated with cell proliferation, cell cycle, DNA repair, et al. is transmitted from the parents, it can cause a predisposition to cancer. This is called hereditary cancer syndrome.

The final diagnosis of hereditary tumor syndrome is performed by germline genetic testing. Germline genetic testing is also one kind of private information and should be handled with prudence. In principle, genetic testing should be carried out in the process of genetic counseling.

FAP and HBOC are outlined below as examples of hereditary tumors.

For people who are at high risk of cancer, the intervention of medical management, such as risk-reducing surgery or planned surveillance, can improve their outcome and quality of life.

Keywords

Heredity · Hereditary cancer syndrome · Mendel's laws of heredity · Gene · Tumor suppressor gene · DNA Hereditary breast and ovarian cancer (HBOC) · Familial adenomatous polyposis (FAP) · Genetic testing

3.1 What Is Heredity?

Children resemble their parents because they inherit various characteristics from them. The offspring of a koala is a koala, and that of a mouse is a mouse. This transmission of characteristics from parents to offspring is called "heredity." Heredity is a feature of not only animals but also of plants, as is exemplified by the transmission of phenotypes such as plant seed shape across generations (Fig. 3.1). In 1865, Gregor Johan Mendel (1822–1884) showed for the first time that visible characteristics, such as the shape of pea seeds and the color of their pods, were transmitted down to the next generation. These laws of heredity are known as Mendel's laws of inheritance and were published as "A Study of Hybrid Plants," which apply not only to plants and animals but also to humans. Parents and children are similar not only in terms of their appearance, such as hair color, facial features, and height, but also in terms of internal characteristics, such as inability to metabolize alcohol. The characteristics

R. Semba
Department of Breast Oncology, Graduate School of Medicine, Juntendo University, Bunkyo-ku, Tokyo, Japan

M. Arai (✉)
Department of Clinical Genetics, Juntendo University, Graduate School of Medicine, Bunkyo-ku, Tokyo, Japan
e-mail: ms-arai@juntendo.ac.jp

© The Author(s), under exclusive license to Springer Nature Singapore Pte Ltd. 2026
M. Endo et al. (eds.), *Cancer and Work in Asia Volume 2*, https://doi.org/10.1007/978-981-95-6537-5_3

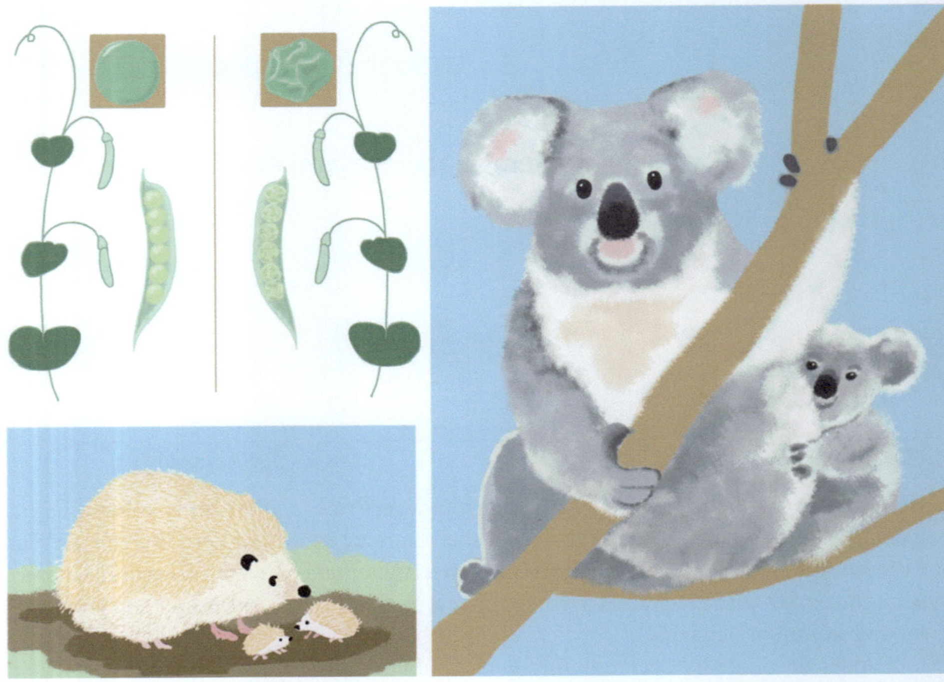

Fig. 3.1 What is heredity? As the Japanese proverb says, "A frog's child is a frog," i.e., the characteristics of a child are similar to those of the parents. (Original Figure)

that children inherit from parents are called "traits." However, all aspects of life are not determined by heredity, and much remains unexplained.

3.2 What Are Genes?

The human body consists of approximately 37 trillion cells. Genes, present in the nuclear DNA, are the basis of heredity. Nucleotides are the basic units of DNA, which consists of pentose, phosphate, and four types of bases, namely, adenine (A), guanine (G), cytosine (C), and thymine (T). The pentoses and phosphates are covalently linked to form the backbone of the DNA helix (Fig. 3.2), while the bases protrude from the helix inside the grooves of the helix. The two strands of DNA are paired via C-G and A-T bonds, leading to the formation of a double-stranded helix. The human DNA consists of two sets of 3×10^9 nucleotides (one set is from the father and the other from the mother).

The information in the DNA blueprint is transcribed into RNAs in the nucleus and subsequently into proteins in a small synthetic factory called the ribosome in the cytoplasm. In RNAs, C bonds with G and A with U (uracil) instead of T. The sequences of genes, and subsequently amino acids, are determined by the order of the three bases in the DNA. For example, ATG codes for methionine, and ATT codes for isoleucine. Termination codons such as TGA do not encode any amino acids and are present at the end of a protein (Fig. 3.3a). Therefore, assuming that genes constitute the "recipe of life" necessary to make a body, the bases of DNA can be considered to be the "letters written in the recipe." Genes constitute only a small part of the genomic DNA, while the function of the non-gene part of DNA still remains largely unknown. The basic flow of genetic information from DNA to protein via RNA is called the "central dogma" of life (Fig. 3.3b).

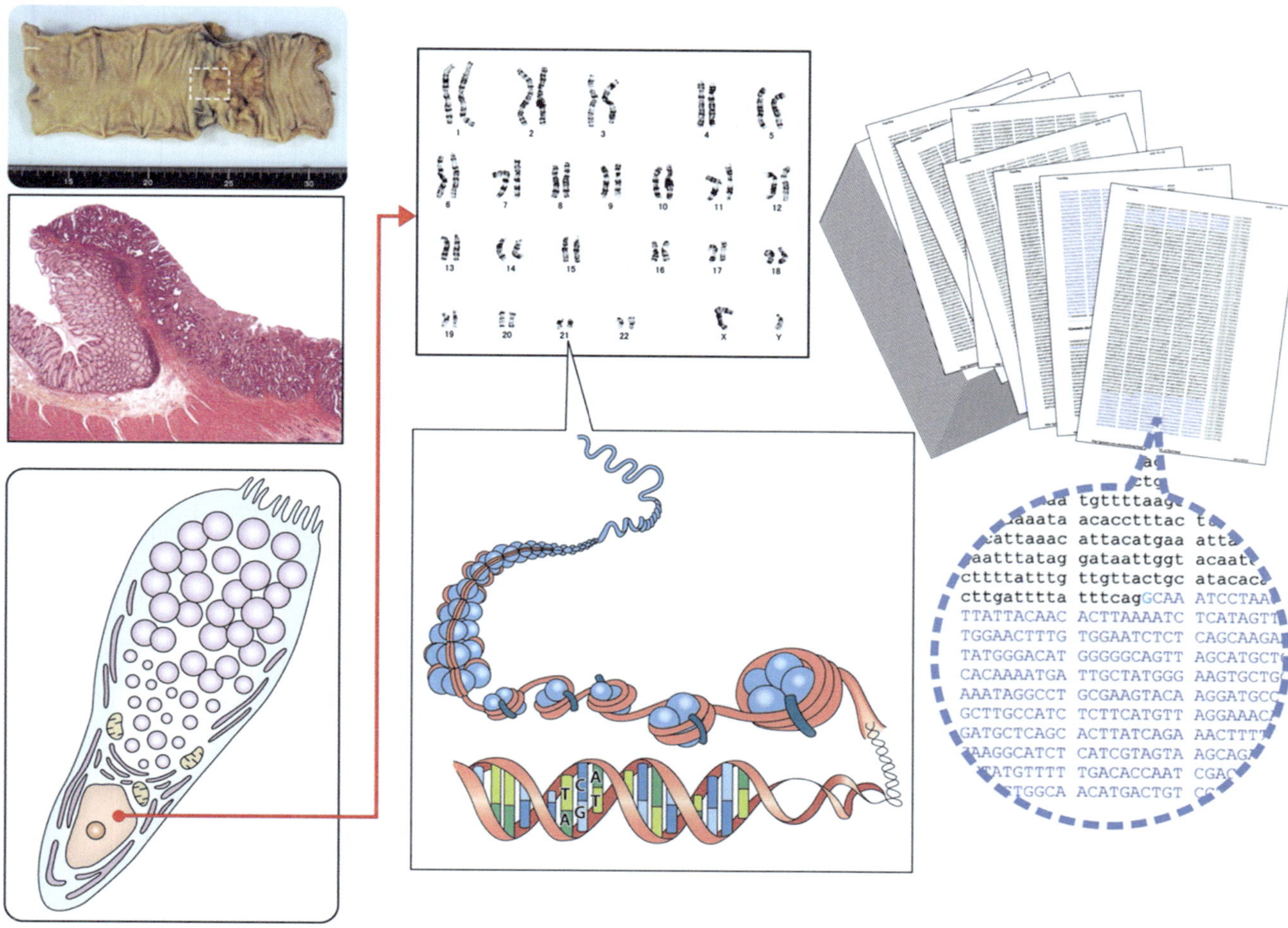

Fig. 3.2 What are genes? Our body is composed of many cells, and genetic information is stored in the nucleus of the cell. Chromosomes, present in the nucleus, contain DNA, which consists of four types of bases. The sequences of these four bases determine the arrangement of amino acids in the gene. (Quoted from Reference [1] with consent to reprint.)

Fig. 3.3 (**a**) Table showing the genetic code. Combinations of three bases determine one amino acid. The first ATG (methionine) acts as a signal for initiating protein synthesis. TAA, TAG, and TGA are termination codons, which signal the end of protein synthesis. Proteins consist of different combinations of amino acids. (**b**) The central dogma of life refers to the process via which information in the DNA is copied into RNA (transcription), which is then translated into amino acid sequences (translation) by ribosomes in the cytoplasm. (Original Figure)

a

first codon	second codon								third codon
	T		C		A		G		
T	TTT	Phenylalanine	TCT		TAT	Tyrosine	TGT	Cysteine	T
	TTC	(Phe)	TCC	Serine	TAC	(Tyr)	TGC	(Cys)	C
	TTA		TCA	(Ser)	TAA	Stop	TGA	Stop	A
	TTG		TCG		TAG		TGG	Tryptophan(Trp)	G
C	CTT	Leucine	CCT		CAT	Histidine	CGT		T
	CTC	(Leu)	CCC	Proline	CAC	(His)	CGC	Arginine	C
	CTA		CCA	(Pro)	CAA	Glutaminc acid	CGA	(Arg)	A
	CTG		CCG		CAG	(Glu)	CGG		G
A	ATT	Isoleucine	ACT		AAT	Asparagine	AGT	Serine	T
	ATC	(Ile)	ACC	Threonine	AAC	(Asn)	AGC	(Ser)	C
	ATA		ACA	(Thr)	AAA	Lysine	AGA	Arginine	A
	ATG	Methionine(Met)	ACG		AAG	(Lys)	AGG	(Arg)	G
G	GTT		GCT		GAT	Asparatic acid	GGT		T
	GTC	Valine	GCC	Alanine	GAC	(Asp)	GGC	Glycine	C
	GTA	(Val)	GCA	(Ala)	GAA	Glutamic acid	GGA	(Gly)	A
	GTG		GCG		GAG	(Glu)	GGG		G

b

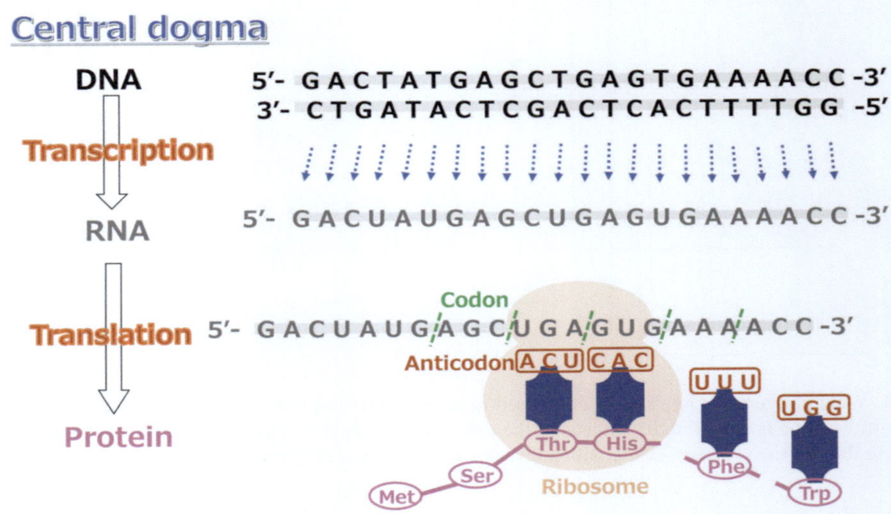

3.3 Genetic Mutations and Variations

Gene sequences vary among individuals of a species. These differences are of three types: those that do not affect gene function, those that do, and those that are currently unknown (uncertain). Among the first type are mainly single nucleotide polymorphisms (SNPs), in which only one base varies with individuals. (The frequency is one base per 1000 bases, i.e., approximately 0.1% of human genome.) Studies have shown that "constitution" or "individuality," such as susceptibility to disease, personality, and intelligence, is also related to SNPs. In addition, the number of repeats of monotonous repetitive sequences, called microsatellites (such as AAAAAAA· · ·), varies with individuals. Hence microsatellites can be used to distinguish among individuals; they are used in forensics to identify criminals and in medicine to assess the success rate of bone marrow transplantation.

Gene sequences vary even among apparently healthy individuals. However, genetic changes in a single gene that severely affect its function can cause diseases (the second type of difference in gene sequence). The term "mutation" has been used to describe such genetic changes; however, nowadays, a comprehensive term, "variation," is used instead of mutation, as it is sometimes difficult to evaluate the cause of diseases. They are also sometimes called pathogenic variants to indicate their role in pathogenicity. Severe changes within one gene or the accumulation of multiple mutations in moderate- to low-risk genes may cause diseases; however, the significance of multifactorial inheritance has not yet been established in clinical practice.

Determination of gene sequences has become easier with the development of testing technologies, such as next-generation sequencing. It is now known that the genome sequence of even healthy people differs from the standard gene sequence by approximately 76–190, and 20 genetic mutations have been shown to cause diseases [2]. Thus, all human beings carry some genetic mutations. In addition, it is unlikely that any two people will have the same gene set, as their facial contours and finger length differ slightly. In other words, every human being is unique, and the existence of various types of people is necessary for the survival of humans. Gene sequences have changed with human evolution, as the factors necessary for survival have changed. In the past, Africans were transported by ship to the United States and Europe as slaves. Among them, those who could thrive on the small amount of food/carbohydrates provided during the voyage eventually survived. However, because of lifestyle-induced obesity and diabetes nowadays, people of African origin in the United States and Europe are believed to be at higher risk of developing adult diseases.

The third case involves genes, changes in which are not known to affect their functions; hence, such genes are called variants of uncertain significance (VUS). For example, approximately 5% of all *BRCA* genetic testing harbors VUS in *BRCA*, which is currently the most common target of genetic tests for cancer.

3.4 Patterns of Inheritance (Autosomal Dominant, Autosomal Recessive, and X-Linked Recessive Inheritance)

Mendel crossbred peas with round and wrinkled seeds to investigate the patterns of transmission of genetic information and discovered dominant and recessive patterns of inheritance. In cases where the disease is caused by a pathogenic mutation in a single gene, the disease runs in the family according to Mendelian laws. In autosomal dominant inheritance, the disease develops when only one of the two alleles, either from the father or mother, severely influences the function of the gene (Fig. 3.4a). Basically, the probability that the next generation will have the same genetic change is 50%, and often, one or more than one person in each generation develops the disease. However, the disease may not develop even in the presence of a genetic change. The risk of developing a disease in the presence of a mutation is known as the penetrance rate. Familial adenomatous polyposis coli (FAP) and hereditary breast and ovarian cancer syndrome (HBOC) are representatives of hereditary cancer syndromes. As will be discussed in more detail later (in Sect. 3.8, "Hereditary cancer"), almost 100% of patients with FAP will eventually develop colorectal cancer. In contrast, patients with HBOC have a 60–70% risk of developing breast cancer in their lives.

In the case of autosomal recessive inheritance, the disease develops when a disease-causing gene is inherited from both parents (Fig. 3.4b). The characteristics of this inheritance pattern are that both parents must be carriers (have a mutation in one of the two chromosomes); thus, the child has a 25% probability of developing the disease, and the parents may sometimes be cousins or be in a consanguineous marriage. Examples of these diseases include hereditary deafness and phenylketonuria, caused by the dysfunction of enzymes involved in amino acid metabolism.

X-chromosome recessive inheritance occurs mainly in males (Fig. 3.4c). This is because, unlike women, men have one X chromosome. In other words, the X chromosome of a male is always derived from his mother. However, even if the mother does not develop the disease, the chances that her sons may develop the disease are 50%, while 50% of her daughters will be carriers. Color blindness and hemophilia are transmitted in an X-linked recessive manner.

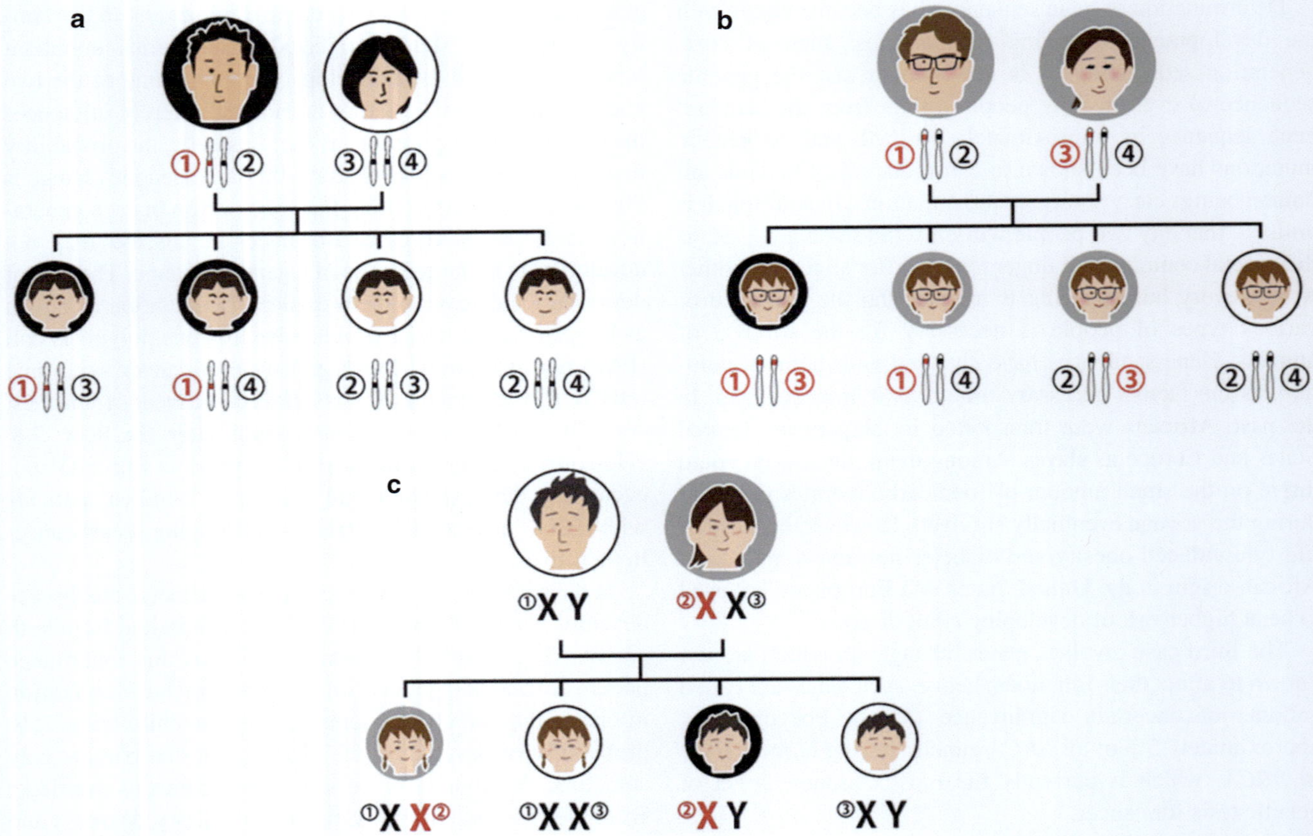

Fig. 3.4 Patterns of inheritance. (**a**) Autosomal dominant inheritance. If a pathological mutation is present in either the paternal or maternal chromosome, the chance that the child will inherit the mutation is 50%. (**b**) Autosomal recessive inheritance. Disease occurs when the disease-causing gene is inherited from both parents. If both parents are carriers of the disease, the child may develop the disease in 25% of cases. (**c**) X-linked recessive inheritance. If the mother harbors mutated genes, her sons have a 50% probability of developing the disease. Females only develop the disease if they inherit the mutated gene on the X chromosomes from both parents. ※ Black background indicates the affected person, grey background indicates the carrier of mutated genes (usually without onset of the hereditary disease), and white background indicates absence of mutations. (Quoted from Reference [3] with consent to reprint)

3.5 Cancer Is Caused by the Accumulation of Mutations in some Genes

Cancer is defined as the autonomous proliferation of tissues, invasion of surrounding tissues, and metastasis to distant organs. In addition, cancer is also known to be caused by the accumulation of genetic mutations in some genes. Here, we will briefly explain multistage carcinogenesis using the adenoma-carcinoma sequence. Colorectal cancer develops from the normal mucosa and progresses to malignant colorectal cancer via benign adenoma. The normal mucosa changes to adenoma because of inactivation of a cancer suppressor gene called *APC* in the first step, followed by worsening of the adenoma due to a mutation in *KRAS*; further, colorectal cancer is caused by inactivation of *P53*. Additionally, various other genetic abnormalities are related to causing invasion and metastasis (Fig. 3.5).

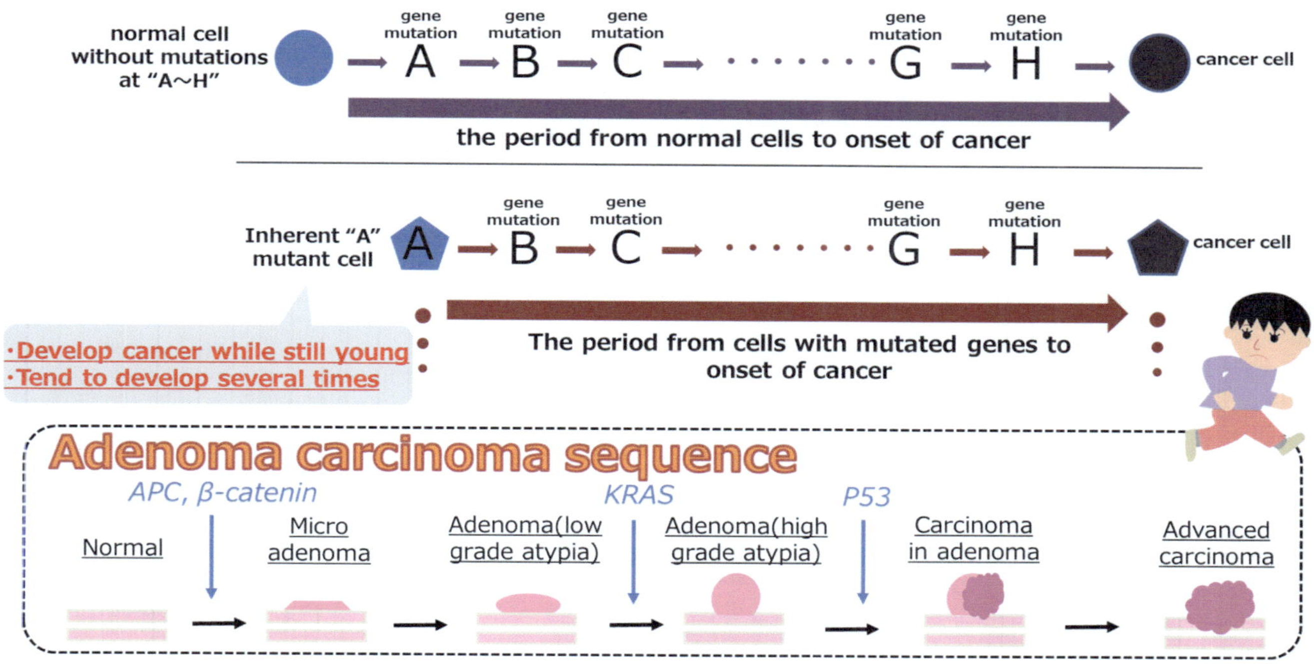

Fig. 3.5 Multistage carcinogenesis. Normal cells develop cancer cells as a result of the accumulation of mutations in cancer-related genes. Cells with mutations in genes originally related to the development of cancer will require fewer mutations before becoming cancerous, and the time until the onset of cancer will be shorter. The scheme illustrates the adenoma-carcinoma sequence of colorectal cancer, where the accumulation of genetic mutations in the normal mucosa first leads to adenoma and then to adenocarcinoma [4]. (Original Figure)

3.6 Inheritance of Cancer

Cancer itself cannot be inherited; however, the predisposition to cancer development can be. As mentioned previously, cancer can be inherited if there is a germline mutation in cancer-related genes. Cells can be classified into "somatic cells" and "germ cells." Somatic cells occupy most of the body, including the gastrointestinal mucosa, muscles, bones, nerves, and blood. Genetic mutations in these cells can cause cancer after birth; however, they are not passed on to the next generation. Many cancers belong to this category. In contrast, cancer-predisposing mutations in germ cells, which become sperm in men and eggs in women, may be passed on to the next generation (Fig. 3.6).

A few cancers are hereditary. In autosomal dominant manner, which is mainly in hereditary cancer syndromes, people with germline mutations in cancer-related genes already harbor mutations in one of the two alleles; therefore, a secondary mutation in the other allele can induce the development of cancer. Therefore, people who harbor mutations in cancer-related genes from birth are more likely to develop cancer than others, and it tends to occur at a younger age; cancer may develop in one or multiple organs. However, the remaining cancer-related genes may not be 100% mutated (see Sect. 3.4, "Penetration rate"). Not only germline mutations of cancer-related genes, but also interactions between mutations in moderate-risk genes and environmental factors such as lifestyle are believed to be associated with the development of cancer. This suggests that understanding the genetic constitution and adoption of appropriate measures may reduce the risk of developing cancer in even people with latent elevated risk of cancer.

Certain points regarding genetic information merit deliberation and exercise of caution. For example, germline genetic information, which does not change throughout life and is partially shared with relatives, must be handled with caution, as it belongs to private information, like name and date of birth, to name some. As this information can be used to possibly predict future diseases, a person known to harbor such critical mutations may be subjected to discrimination and prejudice, such as disadvantages when purchasing life insurance or searching for employment. Discrimination based on genetic information is a legal offense in the United States. Although similar legislation is not yet available in Japan, the rules to be followed when using genetic information in clinical practice and conducting genomic research have been summarized in certain guidelines. What is the situation in your country? Why don't you look up the regulations

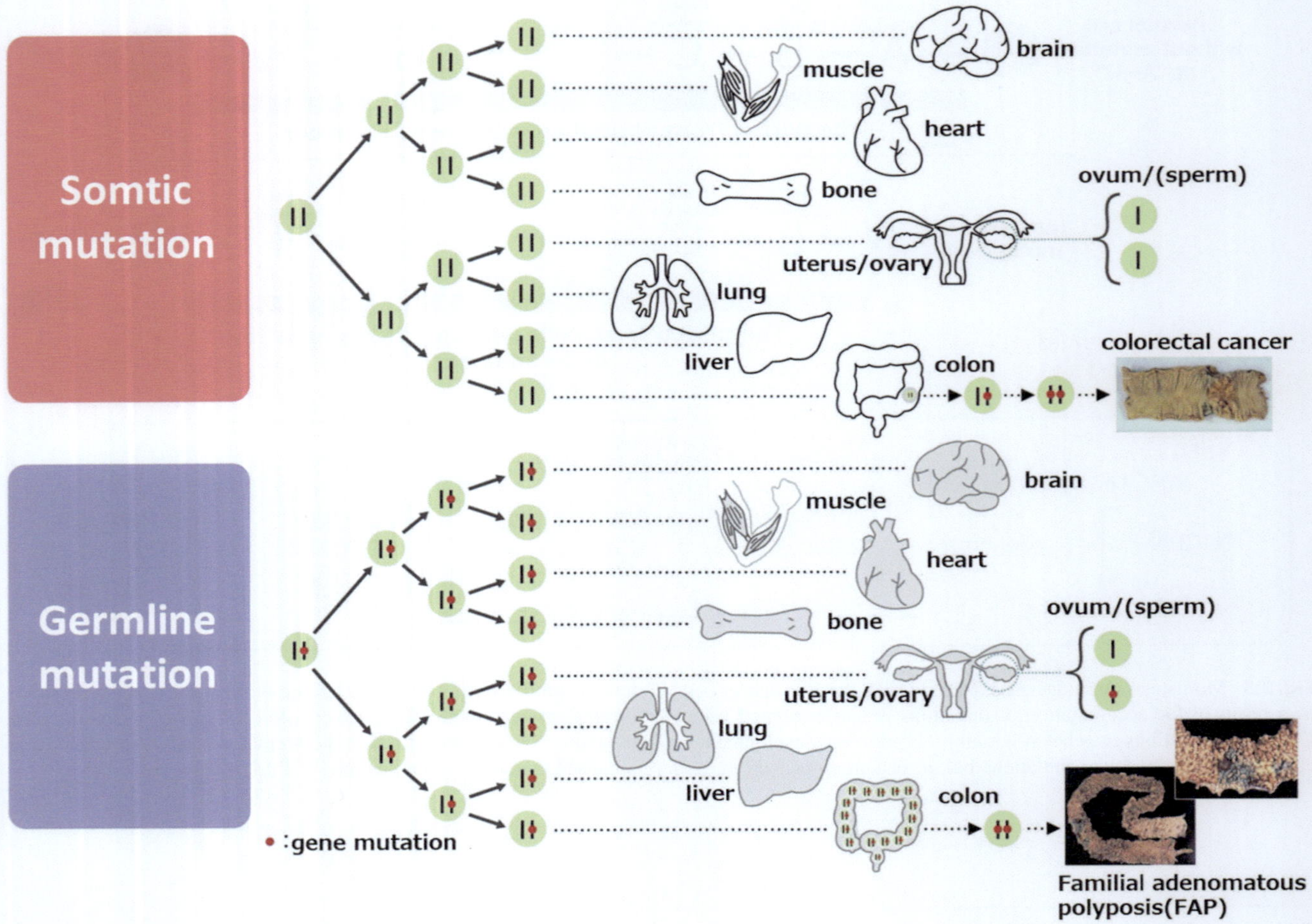

Fig. 3.6 Somatic and germline mutations. Sporadic cancer is caused by the accumulation of mutations after birth. However, if a cancer develops due to a mutation in a gene present in a germ cell, the mutation may be passed on to the next generation. Such cancers are called hereditary cancer. (Cited from reference with permission)

regarding the handling of genetic information in your own country?

3.7 Oncogenes and Tumor Suppressor Genes

We have previously explained that cancer is a genetic disease. However, the human genome comprises more than 20,000 genes, and cancer does not necessarily develop because of mutation in any gene. Cancer possibly develops due to mutations in genes involved in cell proliferation (oncogenes), regulation of the cell cycle (tumor suppressor genes), and repair of genetic damage (DNA repair genes), which perturb their expression (Fig. 3.7).

Regarding the development of cancer, oncogenes are often compared to the gas pedal and cancer suppressor genes to the brakes of a car. The probability of accidents increases if the gas pedal or brake malfunctions. *RET*, *KRAS*, *C-ERB2*, *N-MYC,* and *C-MYC* are some of the well-known oncogenes, while *P53*, *APC*, and *Rb* are the well-known cancer suppressor genes.

The DNA repair-related genes can be compared to the parts involved in car maintenance. Proliferation of cells with mutations in DNA repair genes leads to cancer, as these cells are unable to repair mutations arising in their genome. *BRCA1/2*, *MSH2*, and *MLH1* are the most common DNA repair genes.

Most abnormalities in these three types of genes are due to acquired factors, such as smoking, exposure to radiation, or genetic damage caused by biological activity. Thus, these mutations are somatic mutations. In contrast, people may be born with mutations in oncogenes, tumor suppressor genes, and repair genes, which are germline mutations. Thus,

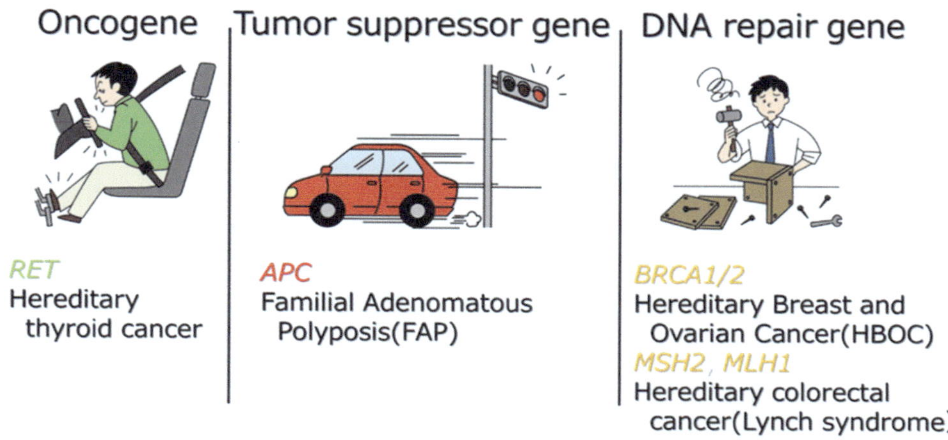

Fig. 3.7 Types of genes related to cancer. Typical genes related to the development of cancer are classified as oncogenes (similar to the accelerator of a car), cancer suppressor genes (the brakes of a car), and DNA repair genes (the mechanic who repairs car parts). Mutations in specific genes cause hereditary tumors(Original Figure)

although cancer itself is not inherited, the genetic characteristics that predispose individuals to the development of cancer may be inherited (Fig. 3.6).

The number of cells in the human body is regulated such that the total number of cells in an adult human remains almost unchanged. Cancer occurs when this regulatory mechanism is perturbed and cells proliferate in an uncontrolled manner.

3.8 Hereditary Cancer

In this section, we will introduce two typical hereditary cancers, FAP and HBOC. FAP is an autosomal dominant hereditary tumor caused by a germline mutation in *APC*, a cancer suppressor gene. Usually one hundred or more polyps form in the colon, which grow into cancer, resulting in colorectal cancer in about 50% of patients by their 40s and in almost 100% of patients by 60 years. In typical cases, the number of polyps is >1000 (Fig. 3.8a). Although total colorectal resection is the basic treatment for FAP, some patients with attenuated FAP (less than 100 polyps) can be followed up with endoscopic treatment once every 6 months. If a person might have inherited a mutation in *APC* and FAP is diagnosed for his/her relative, colonoscopy should be started from an early age (teen years), and polyps should be followed up regularly. An increase in genetic testing of *APC* genes has enabled the identification of variant carriers earlier, and patients commonly undergo prophylactic total colorectal resection at the early stage of colorectal cancer to prevent death from the disease. Moreover, there is an approximately 15% risk of developing adenomas or cancers in the duodenal papilla. Therefore, upper gastrointestinal endoscopy is performed every year, and treatment is provided if necessary. In the past, the average life expectancy of patients with FAP was approximately in their 40s. Currently, the life expectancy of patients with FAP has increased and is now close to the average life expectancy of the general population because of the ease of identification of blood relatives with *APC* mutations using genetic tests, advancements in surgical procedures, and elucidation of the natural history of FAP.

In contrast, HBOC is an autosomal dominant hereditary tumor caused by germline mutations in *BRCA1* or *BRCA2* DNA repair genes that account for 5% of all breast cancers. Mutations in these genes are known to predispose a person to breast and ovarian cancer at birth; the estimated cumulative risk of developing breast cancer by the age of 70 years is 60–65% in people harboring *BRCA1* or *BRCA2* mutations. Similarly, the risk of developing ovarian cancer is estimated to be 20–50% [6]. Women with HBOC are not only more likely to develop breast and ovarian cancer but also to develop "breast cancer at a younger age (average age of onset is in the early 40s)" and "multiple breast cancers (contralateral and ipsilateral)." The total incidence of contralateral breast cancer for individuals with *BRCA1* and *BRCA2* mutations 10 years after surgery for unilateral breast cancer is approximately 20%.

Men with HBOC are more likely to develop breast and prostate cancers than those without HBOC; therefore, continuous screening at intervals appropriate for HBOC patients is recommended for those evaluated with HBOC. In addition, mastectomy is presented as an option even if breast-conserving therapy is possible when she is a *BRCA1* or *BRCA2* mutation carrier. Ovarian and fallopian tube removal for risk reduction or mastectomy of breasts that have not developed breast cancer may be considered as an option after considering various situations. In Japan, risk-reducing salpingo-oophorectomy (RRSO) and risk-reducing mastectomy (RRM) have been under insurance coverage since 2020 (Fig. 3.8b). The total costs of RRSO and RRM are approximately 230,000 and 130,000 yen, respectively (Japan has a universal health insurance system, and as a general rule, one can receive medical care covered by insurance at 30% of the actual cost). In a genetic counseling session, a patient with

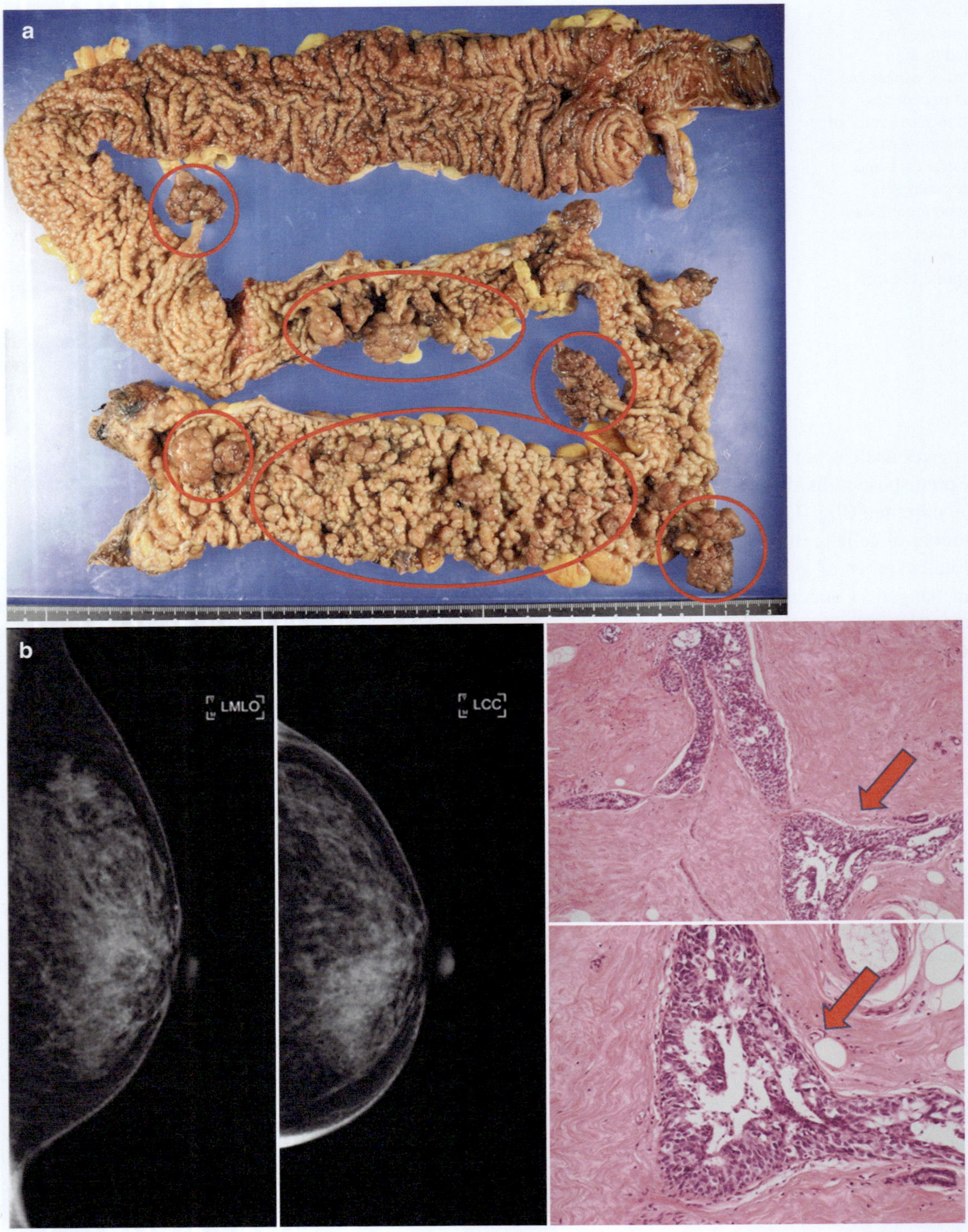

Fig. 3.8 Hereditary cancer. (**a**) Proctocolectomy was performed on a patient with FAP. Numerous adenomas (red circle) were evident in the colonic mucosa. These are highly likely to develop into cancers if left untreated. Indeed some adenomatous polyps had already become cancerous. (Provided by: Department of Coloproctological Surgery, Juntendo University). (Original Figure with permission of the patient). (**b**) Contralateral risk-reducing mastectomy was performed in a *BRCA2* mutation carrier with a history of unilateral breast cancer. The image is that of the preoperative breast. Malignant lesions were not detected. Unexpectedly, microscopic cancer was detected during the postoperative pathological examination of the resected specimen. (Quoted from Reference [5] with permission of the publishing company and the patient)

HBOC is provided a detailed explanation regarding the types of medical treatment available, from which the patient can select the suitable options.

3.9 Conclusion: Application of Information on Individual Genome to Diagnosis and Treatment of Cancer

Cancer is a multigene disease. Currently, methods for determining genetic variants have improved, and the genetic information of cancer cells can be analyzed using next-generation sequencing. In the cancer gene panel test, more than a hundred genes are analyzed to identify genetic variants associated with the disease. This cancer panel gene testing, which is now covered by medical insurance, aimed to analyze the characteristics of genetic mutations in cancer and identify suitable drugs for treating cancer (called molecule-targeted drugs) based on the characteristics of the mutations. Sometimes unanticipated congenital genetic abnormalities (called secondary findings) are detected while investigating genetic variants in cancer, which may affect the future health care of not only the patient but also of his or her family. In such cases, genetic counseling should be provided. Genetic counseling is a medical support system that provides clients with basic information regarding cancer genetics and psychosocial support. Currently, genetic counseling is a medical practice that is handled by physicians in Japan, although professional genetic counselors are also available nowadays. Currently, there are 318 registered genetic counselors in Japan (as of December 2021).

Genetic testing for cancer is critical for selecting appropriate treatment. It is noteworthy that the diagnosis and treatment of cancer do not vary with the nature of the oncogenic mutation, i.e., whether it is congenital or acquired.

In the future, predicting the relationship between an individual's genetic composition and the risk of developing cancer will become increasingly systematic, as the emerging methods will focus on not only the well-known genetic mutations but also on accumulated mutations in moderate- to low-risk genes and their relationship with environmental factors. Overall, cancer genetics will change from an era in which only a few people are involved to that in which everyone is involved.

References

1. Arai M, editor. Genetic medicine for cancer (in Japanese). Tokyo: Nanko-do; 2015.
2. 1000 Genome Project Consortium. An integrated map of genetic variation from 1,092 human genomes. Nature. 2012;491:56–65.
3. Arai M. The forefront of modern clinical genetics (in Japanese). In: Takeda Y, Ohtaki J, editors. Outline of medical science. Tokyo: Medical-friend co.; 2020. p. 90–4.
4. Kinzler KW, Vogelstein B. Cancer-susceptibility genes. Gatekeepers and caretakers. Nature. 1997;386:761–3.
5. Sasaki R, Horimoto Y, Semba R, et al. A patient with hereditary breast and ovarian cancer syndrome who underwent contralateral risk-reducing mastectomy at age 70s (In Japanese). J Hereditary Tumors. 2020;20:168–71.
6. Chen J, Bae E, Zhang L, et al. Penetrance of breast and ovarian cancer in women who carry a *BRCA1/2* mutation and do not use risk-reducing salpingo-oophorectomy: an updated meta-analysis. JNCI Cancer Spectr. 2020;4:pkaa029.

4 What Is Cancer? 4 Cancer Immunology

Tadashi Yokosuka, Wataru Nishi, Tetsuji Nishikawa, Ryohei Matsushima, Yosuke Yoshida, Hiroko Toyota, Masae Furuhata, Hitoshi Nishijima, Hiroaki Machiyama, Arata Takeuchi, and Ei Wakamatsu

Abstract

Tumor immunotherapy, which began with Coley's toxin, has long been tried by various therapeutic methods based on the concept of "immune surveillance" and has now become the fourth standard tumor therapy due to the success of "immune checkpoint inhibitors (ICI)." Some fundamental problems with tumor immunotherapy have been overcome by a new strategy improving the immunosuppressive state around the tumor, where inhibitory cytokines and negative receptor-ligand pairs suppress tumor immune responses in the so-called "tumor microenvironment." Immune checkpoint inhibitor therapy is also based on many advances in physicochemical research, such as antibody engineering technology and the evolution of drug delivery systems. Furthermore, new adoptive immunotherapies such as chimeric antigen receptor T (CAR-T) cells and bispecific antibodies have also been ready for use (Bargou R, et al. Science 321(5891):974–977, 2008). Tumor immunotherapy is being developed into a new stage, which is "combination therapy" with conventional golden standards: surgery, chemotherapy, and radiotherapy.

Keywords

Bispecific antibody · Chimeric antigen receptor (CAR) Cancer-immunity cycle · CTLA-4 · Immune checkpoint inhibitor (ICI) · Immune-related adverse event (irAE) Neoantigen · PD-1 · Tumor-infiltrating lymphocyte (TIL) · Tumor microenvironment

4.1 History of Tumor Immunotherapy

Inspired by the regression of a tumor in a patient after high fever with erysipelas, a purulent streptococcus infection, a surgeon in the United States, William Coley, intentionally administered killed bacteria of the species *Streptococcus pyogenes* and *Serratia marcescens* to a patient with a pharyngeal tumor in 1891 (Fig. 4.1) [2]. These events are known to be the beginning of tumor immunotherapy for malignant tumors. Thereafter, the toxins extracted by heat treatment to remove several side reactions were called "Coley toxin" and were clinically trialed just like a current immunostimulant therapy, but they could not clearly give us any stable effects on the tumor regression due to variations in the manufacturing methods of the toxin. Therefore, cancer immunotherapies have been replaced by other treatments, such as chemotherapy and radiotherapy, since 1900. The ideas of cancer immunotherapies result in the fundamental scientific research followed by the discovery of a variety of innate immune receptor ligands, which are known as immunostimulants or adjuvants.

In the 1940s, in an experiment in which drug-induced sarcoma was transplanted into inbred mice with a homogenous background in the genome, the concept of tumor-specific antigens was discovered from the results of repeated transplants of tumors to mice that were able to reject tumor

T. Yokosuka (✉) · H. Toyota · M. Furuhata · H. Nishijima · H. Machiyama · A. Takeuchi · E. Wakamatsu
Department of Immunology, Tokyo Medical University, Tokyo, Japan
e-mail: yokosuka@tokyo-med.ac.jp

W. Nishi · Y. Yoshida
Department of Immunology, Tokyo Medical University, Tokyo, Japan

Department of Nephrology, Tokyo Medical University, Tokyo, Japan

T. Nishikawa
Department of Immunology, Tokyo Medical University, Tokyo, Japan

Department of Dermatology, Tokyo Medical University, Tokyo, Japan

R. Matsushima
Department of Immunology, Tokyo Medical University, Tokyo, Japan

Department of Respiratory Surgery, Kumamoto University, Kumamoto, Japan

© The Author(s), under exclusive license to Springer Nature Singapore Pte Ltd. 2026
M. Endo et al. (eds.), *Cancer and Work in Asia Volume 2*, https://doi.org/10.1007/978-981-95-6537-5_4

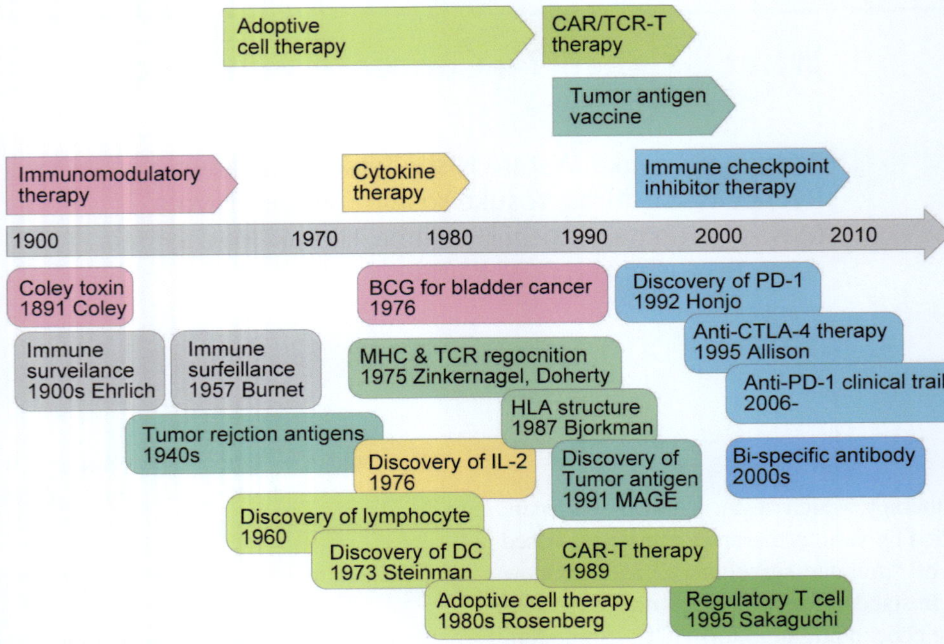

Fig. 4.1 History of cancer immunotherapy. Tumor immunotherapy was known to start by injection of Coley toxin as an "immunomodulatory therapy," which means overall stimulation of innate immunity, as we call it now. The discovery of lymphocytes in 1960 led to the therapy with the transfer of patients' lymphocytes as cell therapy, called "adoptive immunotherapy," and the discovery of tumor antigens in 1991 has developed such adoptive immunotherapy into more antigen-specific ones. With advances in the development of antibody drugs, antigen specificity has been passed down to "CAR-T cell therapy" and "bispecific antibodies." On the other hand, immunomodulatory therapy was developed into the "immune checkpoint inhibitory" drugs, which recover the exhaustion state of lymphocytes within tumors [2]

implantation and rejection through a stronger immune response. In humans, there was a disability in the use of tumor immunotherapy because of the heterogeneity of HLA. Because the peak of tumor development overlaps in both childhood and old age when immunity is downregulated, and tumors occur due to immunity decline, such as in patients receiving anticancer drugs or immunodeficiency patients, the concept that immunity monitors and prevents the development of cancer has been proposed without any doubt. This concept was proposed by Paul Ehrlich and is called "immune surveillance," which Frank Macfarlane Burnet revived in the 1950s [3].

In the 1970s, the discovery of MHC molecules by Ralph Zinkernagel and Peter Doherty gave us the concept of "tumor antigens." Therefore, in the 1980s, the variety of human tumor antigens was progressively identified, and the representative is melanoma-associated antigen, MAGE, cloned as the first antigen of melanoma recognized by human immunity [4]. Since then, technological innovation has succeeded in unveiling many pairs of HLA and a novel bound antigen, such as MART-1, gp100, tyrosinase, and NY-ESO-1 for melanomas [5]. These have been the basis for the development of cancer vaccine treatment using single-chain peptides with adjuvants, which were initially considered as immunostimulants but have been revealed as innate receptor ligands during the progress of innate immunology research, supporting current cancer vaccine research.

In the same period, many cytokines were actively identified and first used directly for cytocidal effect, while it also became possible to culture human lymphocytes in vitro with those cytokines. Steven Rosenberg transferred self-lymphocytes in melanoma patients and showed high response efficiencies in tumor reduction and established a foundation for adoptive immunotherapy [6]. In this strategy, tumor-infiltrating lymphocytes (TILs) were first transferred into the patients, and after many tumor-specific antigens were identified, lymphocytes were initially cultured in vitro with dendritic cells pulsed by those antigens for skewing their specificities against tumors. Such ideas are progressing toward new strategies in adoptive immunotherapies with gene transfer of an antigen-specific TCR pair or a chimeric antigen receptor (CAR) [7]. A CAR contains both a variable region of an antibody against a tumor protein and a cytoplasmic motif of T-cell signaling molecules.

Although a number of tumor antigens have been identified and methods of adoptive immunotherapy have progressed, anti-tumor effects comparable to chemotherapy and radiotherapy have not been achieved. The breakthrough that solved these issues was the introduction of the concept of "exhaustion of immune cells" into cancer immunotherapies.

In other words, unless tumor cells release an immunosuppressive state around the tumor, called "tumor microenvironment," tumor antigen-specific immune responses would actually be suppressed by T-cell exclusion, immune privilege, and the tumor microenvironment [8]. The idea that paid attention to the costimulatory or coinhibitory receptor signaling in T cells solved these issues. First, it was performed to enhance the signaling of the active costimulatory receptor, CD28, which is essential for the natural activation of a T cell by using anti-CD28 antibodies, in addition to the TCR signaling [9]. But, as a result of the excessive immune response, a cytokine storm was induced in the subject, and further clinical trials were canceled due to the approach of enhancing T cell costimulation. In 1995, James Allison had an idea to suppress T-cell coinhibitory signaling via CTLA-4, identified as the first T-cell coinhibitory receptor, on exhausted T cells in tumors expressing CTLA-4 by adding a neutralizing antibody to CTLA-4 [10]. This is the fundamental idea of immune checkpoint blocking therapy, which won the Nobel Prize in Physiology or Medicine in 2018. CTLA-4 originally functions as a negative feedback regulator to avoid excessive activation of T cells, but in the tumor microenvironment and chronic viral infections, the negative feedback mechanism precedes and falls into an immunosuppressive state via producing exhausted T cells expressing CTLA-4 and the second coinhibitory receptor, PD-1. Tasuku Honjo and his colleagues identified PD-1 [11] and found that the blocking effects on exhausted T cells suppressed by PD-1, whose ligands are expressed throughout the body to maintain the homeostasis of T cell activation. As with anti-CTAL-4 antibodies, the administration of anti-PD-1 enhances tumor immunity, which has recently been a breakthrough in cancer therapy.

The Japanese idea of releasing immunosuppression also extends to the control of regulatory T cells identified by Shimon Sakaguchi in 1995 [12]. Regulatory T cells are differentiated by the master transcription factor, Foxp3, and characterized by the expression of the IL-2 receptor α chain, CD25, and coinhibitory receptors, including CTLA-4 and PD-1 [13]. Regulatory T cells control the total immune system by suppressing $CD4^+$ helper T cells, which are the main players in acquired immunity. Although a trial to remove regulatory T cells by adding anti-CD25 antibodies was not successful from the viewpoint of adverse drug reactions, the anti-CTLA-4 antibody used as an immune checkpoint inhibitor (ICI) therapy could remove regulatory T cells, which is one of the mechanisms of the anti-CTLA-4 antibody as a recovery from immune suppression. In addition, various inhibitory cells that introduce immunosuppressive states in the cancer microenvironment by secreting inhibitory cytokines, such as IL-10 and TGF-β, were also regulatory T cells. Therefore, it is no exaggeration to say that regulatory T cells become the conceptual basis of such inhibitory immune cells.

4.2 Tumor Microenvironment and Cancer-Immunity Cycle

The vague idea that cancer reduces the host immune system has been established as the phenomenon that cancer cells are actively constructing a "tumor microenvironment" that causes the surroundings to enter an immunosuppressive state via inhibitory cytokines and coinhibitory receptor-ligand binding. The concept of "cancer-immunity cycle" is quite important to understand this phenomenon in an easy-to-understand manner [14]. The cancer immunity cycle includes the following seven steps (Fig. 4.2): (1) Tumor antigens are released and captured by antigen-presenting cells (APCs), dendritic cells (DCs), for antigen processing (2). DCs present those captured antigens on class I and class II MHC molecules to naïve T cells in draining lymph nodes (3). DCs initiate and activate effector T cell responses to tumor-specific antigens in lymph nodes (4). Activated tumor-specific effector T cells traffic from lymph nodes toward the tumors (5). These effector T cells infiltrate the tumor bed, (6) specifically recognize and bind to cancer cells through the interaction between the TCR and the cognate antigen bound to MHC class I, and (7) kill their target tumor cells. Killing of the tumor cells releases additional tumor-associated antigens in subsequent revolutions of the cancer-immunity cycle. If we try to improve tumor immunotherapy, we add inventives to tumor antigens in steps 1, 3, and 6; develop a renewed adjuvant that enhances the effect of tumor vaccines or improves engineered dendritic cells in step 3; enhance effector T cell activation by using ICI therapies in step 3; and increase cytotoxic activity by ICI-treated effector T cells in step 7. While this cycle is spinning on a good basis, a single cancer cell that spontaneously develops 3000 per day is excluded by immune cells, but for some reason, if the cycle collapses, a single tumor cell develops as a mass.

Various factors that disrupt the cancer-immunity cycle may occur at every step. In step 1, immune tolerance will occur in the form of cell death, like apoptosis, which is difficult to induce innate immune receptors. If it would be required for enhancing the innate immune response by adding adjuvants; those are now known as ligands for those receptors. In step 3, in situations where T cells are easily suppressed by coinhibitory receptors CTLA-4 and PD-1 in a negative feedback loop, anti-CTLA-4 and/or anti-PD-1/PD-L1 antibodies are required to release the immune checkpoint inhibition. In step 5, intratumor infiltration of T cells

Fig. 4.2 Cancer-immunity cycle. The cancer-immunity cycle involves the following seven steps [14]: (1) Release of tumor antigens (2). Presentation of tumor antigens by dendritic cells (DCs) (3). DCs prime and activate T cells in lymph nodes (4). Trafficking of activated T cells from lymph nodes to the tumors via the vessels (5). T cells infiltrate tumors (6). T cells recognize tumor antigens (7). T cells kill tumors

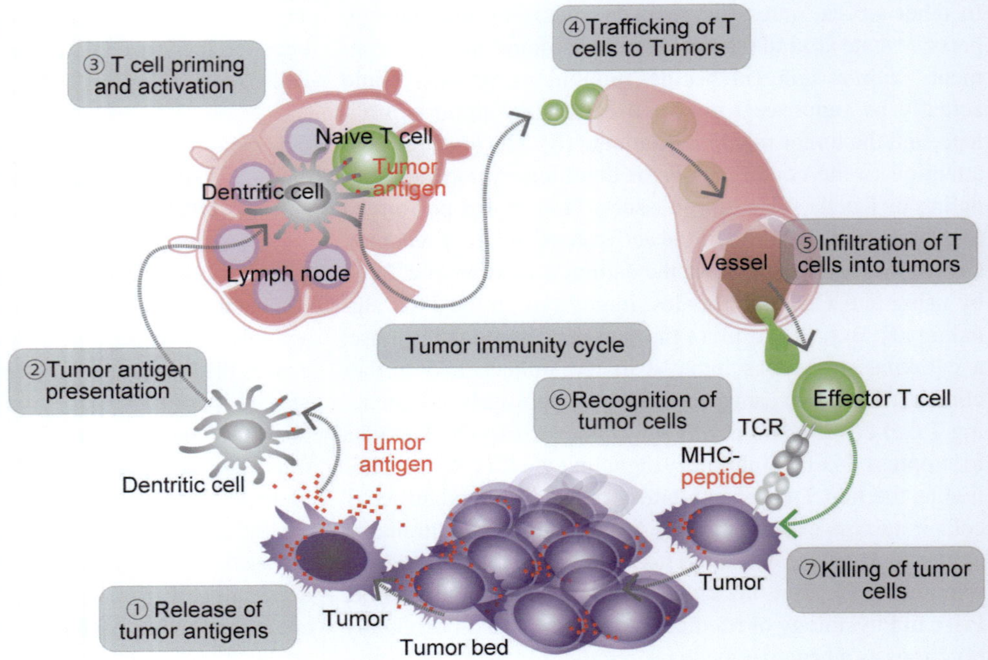

could be suppressed by the effect of VEGF produced from tumor cells. In step 6, tumors often reduce their expression of MHC Class I, which presents tumor antigens toward infiltrating effector T cells through the mechanism of defecting in β2 microglobulin or some basic proteins essential for processing antigens on MHC Class, like transporter associated with protein processing, TAP. In step 7, tumors express PD-L1 to escape from killing by cytotoxic T cells expressing PD-1, which transmits inhibitory signaling in these T cells.

Coinhibitory ligands and various inhibitory substances such as IL-10, TGFβ, indoleamine 2,3-dioxygenase (IDO), cooperatively introduce differentiation of regulatory T cells, which further promote the other subsets of immune-inhibitory cells, such as bone marrow-derived inhibitory cells (MDSC), tumor-related fibroblast (CAFs), and M2-type tumor-related macrophages (TAMs). These cells comprehensively create an area of the immunosuppressive state at the neighboring of a tumor, known as the tumor microenvironment [15].

4.3 Cancer Immunotherapy

Cancer immunotherapies can be divided into two types: a method that focuses more on antigen specificity and another that improves the overall immune response regardless of antigen specificity [16]. The former contains identification of tumor-specific antigens, development of cancer vaccines or dendritic cell therapy with those identified antigens, cloning of tumor-specific T cells, and adoptive transfer of TCR-T cells. These are introduced with tumor-specific TCRs and CAR-T cell therapies. On the other hand, the latter includes ICI therapies, improvement of adjuvants, selective removal of regulatory T cells, fecal transplantation with antitumor species of gut microbiota, and recovery of exhausted T cells by improving glucose metabolism. Although adoptive immunotherapies or tumor vaccines were not as effective as initially expected, if the concept of the tumor microenvironment is much more generalized due to the efficacy of the ICI, which has revealed that inactivating the entire immune system enables dominant antigen-specific tumor therapies, many tumor antigen-specific therapies are currently being revived by combination with ICIs.

4.4 Tumor Antigens and Vaccines

It has been easily shown by the term "tumor antigens," but we can classify them into several groups below [17] (Fig. 4.3).

1. Tissue differentiation antigens are those expressed by some specific cells during terminal differentiation into functional cells or tissues. It includes melanoma gp110, MART-1 tyrosinase, and the like [5].
2. Overexpressed antigens are those expressed in small amounts even in normal tissues but whose expression rises rapidly due to tumorigenesis. It includes WT-1 and CEA. This type of antigen generally possesses lower antigenicity and requires large differences in expression when comparing tumors and normal tissues.

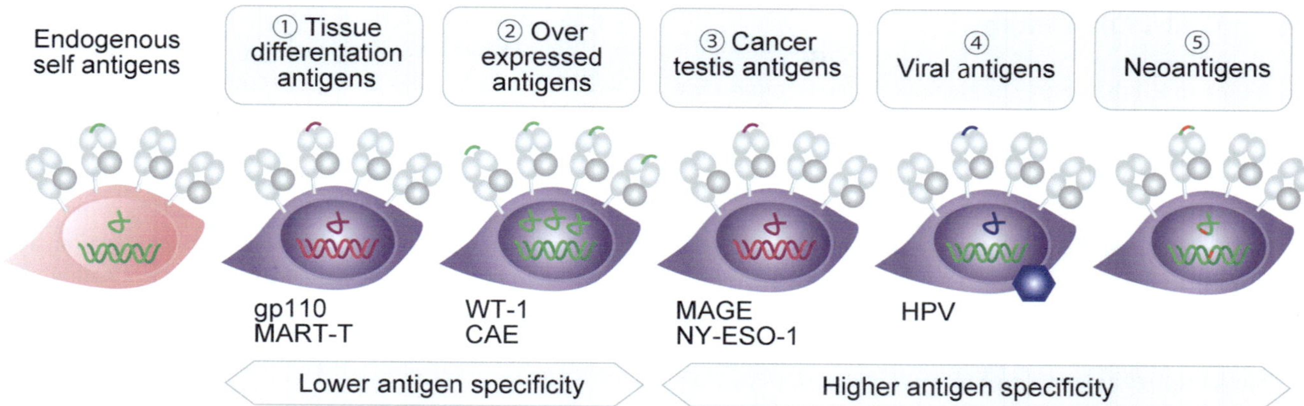

Fig. 4.3 Varieties of tumor antigens. MHC molecules generally load endogenous self-peptides and change these peptides to tumor antigens by tumorigenesis of the host cells [17]. There are the following classifications of tumor antigens depending on whether the sequence of the peptides loaded on MHC molecules includes amino acid mutation or not. While tumor antigens without any mutations form lower antigen specificity, those with any mutations have higher antigen specificity

3. Cancer testis antigens are antigens expressed only in the testis, placenta, and tumor, and can be used as a common antigen among patients and are often highly antigenic, such as MAGE and NY-ESO-1.
4. Viral antigens originate from peptides encoded in viral genomes. In the case of a virus linked to carcinogenesis, such as human papillomavirus, the gene products derived from the virus can be a tumor antigen peptide.
5. Neoantigens are endogenous peptides with somatic mutations [18]. As a result of the mutations, an endogenous peptide shows a tumor antigen peptide that is different from the amino acid sequence that we usually have. It is divided into "driver mutation," which directly contributes to tumorigenesis, and "passenger mutation," which is an unrelated simple mutation. Driver mutations are more critical for cancer itself, but passenger ones are much more likely to be neoantigens.

A simple inoculation of tumor antigen peptides would not induce an antitumoral immune response; therefore, they are injected with adjuvants. Tons of studies on innate immunity classified these adjuvants into two categories: (1) pathogen-associated molecular patterns (PAMPs) and (2) damage-associated molecular patterns (DAMPs), which are identified by distinct pattern-recognition receptors (PRRs) [19]. Much more detail of ligand-receptor pairs has been elucidated, and some of them have been theoretically used as adequate adjuvants for all cases of antitumor therapies. As immunostimulant adjuvants, so-called PRR ligands, like Toll-like receptor (TLR) ligands, are generally included here: poly I:C (TLR3 ligand), LPS-derivative monophosphoryl lipid A, MPLA (TLR4 ligand), imiquimod (TLR7 ligand), CpG-ODN (TLR9 ligand), cGAMP, c-di-GMP, and c-di-AMP (STING ligand). The other side is the particulate adjuvant, including a hydrated double sulfate salt of aluminum, alum, a solution of antigen emulsified in mineral oil, Freund's adjuvant, a liposome, and so on. In order to increase the antigen-specificity of T cells administered by adoptive immunotherapy, coculturing of T cells with dendritic cells pulsed with particular tumor antigens has been practiced for a long time. Administration of the entire dendritic cells with tumor peptides was also tested as a new vaccine with greater efficacy.

4.5 Cloning of a Tumor Antigen-Specific TCR and TCR-T Cell Therapy

In the 1990s, Steven Rosenberg and his colleagues performed an adoptive transfer therapy with T cells, which are tumor-infiltrating lymphocytes (TILs) that were cultured in vitro with cytokines after being collected from a tumor bed [6]. Because a polyclonal T-cell population was generated by such in vitro culture, it is very useful for avoiding a resistance to tumors that repeatedly mutate their own antigen peptides. In contrast, this method is often limited to some types of tumors whose mutations are frequently occurring, such as melanoma. Later, to increase the specificity of TCR against a tumor, it was attempted to stimulate these T cells by APCs with the targeted tumor antigens, but in 2000, TCRs isolated from tumor-specific T cells were retroviral gene transferred into T cells cultured in vitro as "TCR-T cell therapy." Recently, a single pair of TCR α-chain and β-chain can be isolated from a single cell, and many trials with these engineered T cells have been conducted on various cancer antigens and specific TCR combinations [20].

4.6 CAR-T Cell Therapy

In addition to ICI therapies, simple tumor-specific antibodies such as anti-CD20 and anti-HER2 showed good results in some malignant tumors via cytocidal effects by complements or antibody-dependent cellular cytotoxicity (ADCC). CAR-T cell therapy has now become an evolution of adoptive immunotherapy that takes advantage of characteristics of an antibody in specificity and high affinity; therefore, CARs have been frequently introduced into patients' T cells instead of TCRs [21]. CAR is structurally constructed by (1) an antigen recognition site (scFv), (2) a hinge derived from an antibody, (3) a transmembrane region such as CD8, (4) an intracellular signaling domain of a costimulatory receptor (4-1BB or CD28), and (5) a cytoplasmic region of CD3ζ (Fig. 4.4). It is a completely artificial chimeric protein in which the intracellular signaling domains are tandemly linked. The target protein for the original antibody must be a molecule expressed on the surface of tumor cells. If possible, they are not expressed in normal tissues, and even if they are expressed, it is preferred that the difference be large in expression between tumor and normal tissue, and if they are expressed in normal tissue, there should be no harmful effect on life support in the deletion of the targeted cells. CD19 CAR-T cell therapy has now been clinically applied for B-cell leukemia and malignant lymphoma, confirming that it will work at a high rate even in patients whose standard therapy is ineffective [7]. Cytokine release syndrome (CRS) initially developed in 1/3 of the cases, but can now be controlled with anti-IL-6 antibodies. Although encephalitis is sometimes caused by CAR-T cell therapy for CD19, which is mildly expressed in the central nervous system, and HER2, which is expressed at a low level in lung tissue, could be a target for HER2 CAR T cells to induce pneumonia. Useful improvements have been further tested in CAR T cell therapies; introduced into T cells by genes encoding some cytokines or chemokines to improve T cell exhaustion and migration to tumor beds, and deletion of TCRs in patients' T cells or the development of iPS cells of patients' tissues to avoid graft versus host disease, GVHD, and to efficiently produce CAR-T cells.

4.7 PD-1

PD-1 is a coinhibitory receptor expressed in immune cells, such as activated T and B cells. PD-1 is expressed from several hours after the activation of T cells to avoid excessive activation of T cells leading to auto-inflammation [22]. PD-1 possesses two ligands, PD-L1 (PD-1 ligand-1, H7-H1, CD274) and PD-L2 (B7-DC, CD273). While PD-L2 is expressed mainly in professional APCs, PD-L1 is constitutively and ubiquitously expressed, such as in endothelial cells and epithelial cells, and its expression rises further due to interferon stimulation, inflammatory cytokine signaling, and hypoxia. That is the reason why PD-1 ligands are highly expressed in any inflammatory sites. Therefore, immune cells, such as T cells, are in a natural suppressive state in a

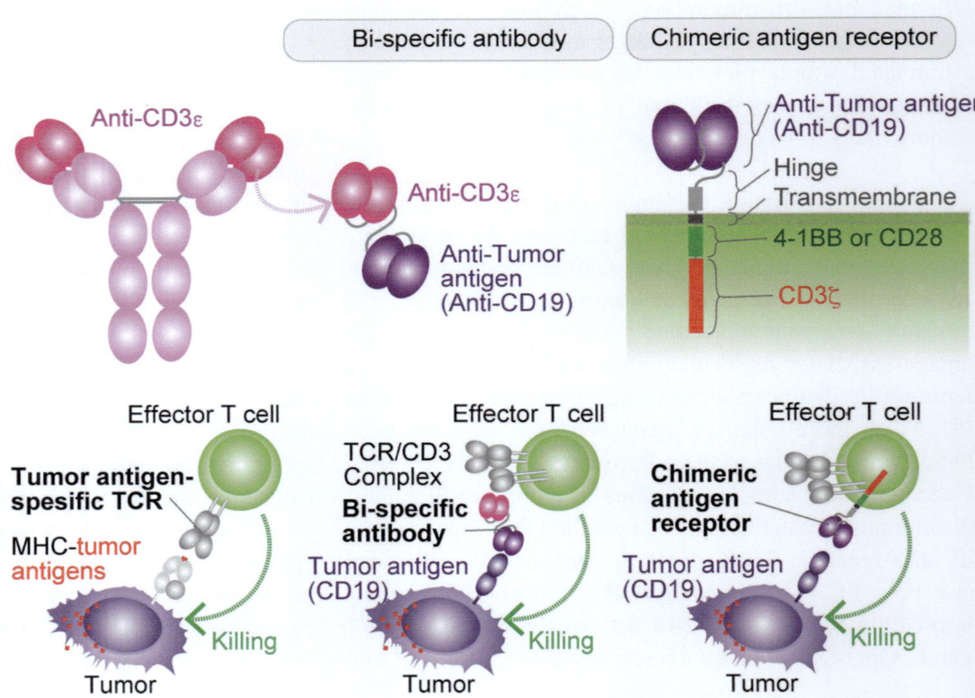

Fig. 4.4 Bispecific antibody and chimeric antigen receptor. A bispecific antibody is constructed by (1) an antigen recognition site (scFv) of anti-CD3, (2) a hinge, and (3) an scFv of anti-tumor antigen, such as CD19 [1]. Bi-specific antibodies link T cells and tumors to induce cytocidal effects by T cells. A chimeric antigen receptor (CAR) is constructed by (1) an scFv of anti-tumor antigen, (2) a hinge, (3) a transmembrane region, (4) a cytoplasmic region of a costimulatory receptor, 4-1BB or CD28, and (5) that of CD3ζ. CAR-introduced T cells (CAR-T cells) recognize and kill the tumors [1]

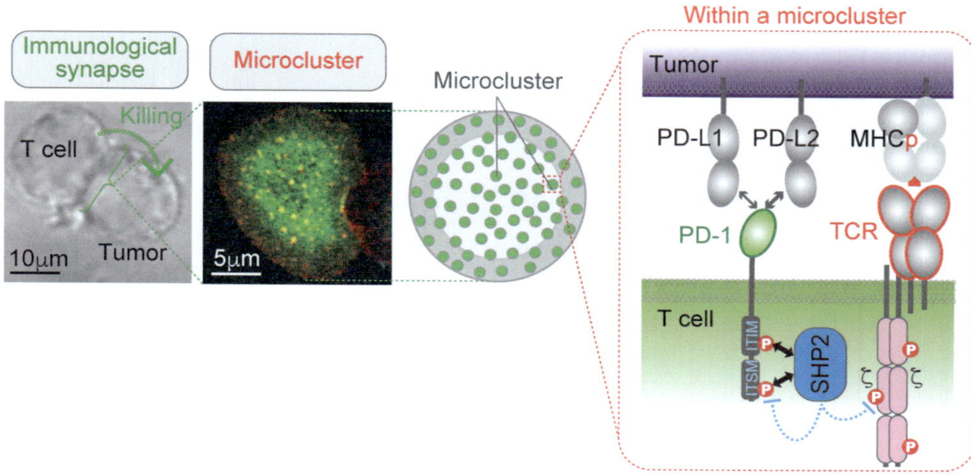

Fig. 4.5 PD-1-mediated coinhibitory signaling through microcluster formation. A T cell forms an "immunological synapse" at its interface with a tumor cell to recognize and kill a tumor antigen. At an immunological synapse, TCR (red) is gathering together to form "TCR microclusters" to recognize an antigen on an MHC and to introduce activation signaling [23]. When PD-1 (green) and PD-L1 or PD-L2 are expressed in a T cell and a tumor, respectively, PD-1 forms PD-1 microclusters at the same region of the TCR microcluster. By binding to PD-L1 or PD-L2, PD-1 recruits a phosphatase, SHP2, through two distinct motifs at the PD-1 cytoplasm and dephosphorylates the TCR/CD3 complexes and their downstream molecules [24]

tumor microenvironment. In the cytoplasmic region, PD-1 possesses two tyrosine motifs, the immunoreceptor tyrosine-based switch motif (ITSM) and the immunoreceptor tyrosine-based inhibitory motif (ITIM), which are important for signal transduction via recruitment of phosphatase and SH2-containing tyrosine phosphatase 2 (SHP2) (Fig. 4.5). SHP2 removes phosphates from cytoplasmic signaling molecules downstream of a TCR and CD28 to reduce T cell activation. For this purpose, T cells must adhere to APCs or target tumor cells, and the boundary interface of the two cells works as a communication site called "immunological synapse" (Fig. 4.5). Through super-resolution imaging analysis, we have succeeded in capturing the real signaling domain of suppression by discovering the independent aggregation of PD-1 or TCR, named "microclusters" [23]. When anti-PD-1 antibodies are added to the T cell-APC or tumor cell conjugates, PD-1 microclusters are disrupted, but TCR microclusters are still intact, indicating a recovery from T-cell exhaustion [24].

4.8 ICI Therapy

ICI therapy focuses on the recovery of exhausted tumor-specific T cells via the PD-1-PD-L1/PD-L2 axis by administration of anti-PD-1 or anti-PD-L1 antibodies [25, 26] (Fig. 4.6). In the case of ICI therapy with anti-CTLA-4, this antibody blocks the CTLA-4-CD80/86 binding to enhance active signaling through CD28 binding to CD80/86 instead. It was quite impressive to show that ICI therapy has demonstrated progressin-free survival in some lung cancer patients who were ineffective to standard therapies such as chemotherapy and radiotherapy. ICI therapy also showed more than 10% progress-free survival over a year-long survival period, and also dominance of overall survival compared to the control docetaxel group. It sounds like a revolutionary therapy in internal medicine for cancer. What should be noted is the characteristics of this therapy: we found initial tolerance in almost half of the patients, in which the survival rate temporarily worsened 3 months after the start of the treatment. But surprisingly, we found a long-term progression-free survival (PFS) and a tail plateau drawn in the survival curve.

Because of the basis of ICI as a blocker for negative feedback loops of the entire immunity, the patients suffer from side effects known as immune-related adverse events (irAE) [27]. Interestingly, such irAEs are not the same as the symptoms of systemic autoimmune diseases. The difference in antigenicity between anti-PD-1 and anti-CTLA-4 antibodies and as well as different isoforms of antibodies, out in various clinical symptoms. We generally find mild irAEs such as skin erosions and sometimes severe enteritis, pneumonia, or thyroid dysfunction due to autoantibody response. Corticosteroids and immunosuppressants are commonly used in clinical cases with irAEs, and anti-TNF and anti-IL-6 antibodies are administered in serious cases with cytokine storms.

Unfortunately, in some patients whose effects of ICI are not expected, a diagnosis that determines whether the drugs work effectively, so-called "companion diagnostic," has been devised by various factors [28]. Such diagnostics are now

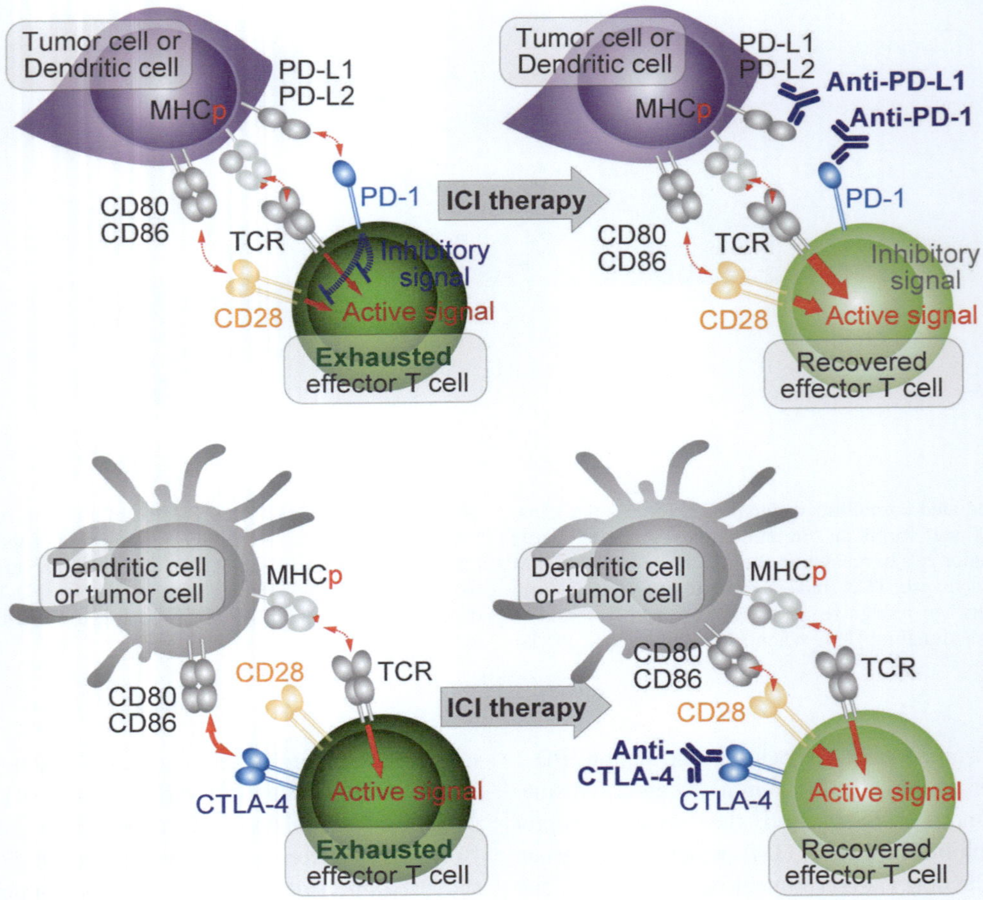

Fig. 4.6 Immune checkpoint inhibitor therapy. In the tumor microenvironment, exhausted T cells express coinhibitory receptors PD-1 and CTLA-4 (left) [25, 26]. PD-1 introduces inhibitory signaling by binding its ligands, PD-L1 and PD-L2, through recruiting a phosphatase, SHP-2, which removes phosphates from TCR- and CD28-associating signaling molecules (top left). The anti-PD-1 or anti-PD-L1 antibody blocks the PD-1-PD-L1 binding, resulting in the recovery of effector T-cell functions by cancelling inhibitory signals via PD-1 (top right). CTLA-4 expressed whose affinity toward CD80/CD86 is 50 times higher than that of CD28, can dominantly bind to its ligands and exclude CD28-mediated costimulatory signaling in exhausted T cells (bottom left). Since anti-CTLA-4 antibodies block the CTLA-4-CD80/CD86 binding, CD28 then introduces costimulatory signaling, indicating the recovery of the exhausted state. Both PD-1 and CTLA-4 suppress T cell activation, but anti-PD-1 preferentially recovers T-cell activation in the effector phase, in which cytotoxic T cells kill tumors, and anti-CTLA-4 doses in the priming phase, where naïve T cells are initially presented by antigen peptides at a draining lymph node.

used to extract patients with high therapeutic effects [29]. First, PD-L1 is highly expressed in the tumor tissue itself to directly inhibit PD-1$^+$ T cells bearing tumor antigen-specific TCRs, and the rate of PD-L1$^+$ cells in the tumor mass is statistically correlated with the PFS; therefore, histological staining of PD-L1 expression of the tumor mass is routinely performed for every patient as the first choice of companion diagnostics [30]. On the other hand, since PD-1 also functions as a suppressor molecule for the initial activation of T cells in a draining lymph node, the expression of PD-L1 on APCs in the lymph nodes is also involved in developing T cell exhaustion. Next, the number of infiltrating immune cells in the tumor bed, so-called TILs, is another companion diagnostic factor. Depending on the number of TILs, tumors can be divided into two states relating to immune responsiveness, in which tumors with poor TILs are called "cold tumors" and those with rich TILs are called "hot tumors." The number of CD8 T cells that directly kill the tumor may actually be important for eliciting the effect of ICI, while Th1-like CD4 T cells are also important for helper functions in ICI treatment. Therefore, some reports have recently recommended that the number of CD4 T cells among TILs should be suitable for a companion diagnostic [31]. In addition, it is considered that it is easier to activate TILs if there are many targets presented on tumors as neoantigens, because the probability of endogenous TCRs adapting to a certain neoantigen will be increased. Focusing on the frequency of neoantigens, the other indicators are suitable for a companion diagnostic. Solid tumors with high-frequency microsatellite instability (MSI) caused by functional deficiencies during mismatch repair (MMR) of the genome and cancer with high genetic mutations are generally defined as high scoring of tumor burden (TMB) [32]. High TMB tumors are known to be correlated with higher therapeutic effects by ICIs, and melanoma and lung cancer are generally known as high TMB tumors. Recent return-translational studies that provide a lot of clinical evidence will give a new epidemiological advantage to the mechanisms [33].

4.9 Development of Immunotherapy in the Future

The advent of ICI is an evolutionary treatment that can cure patients with malignant tumors that have not achieved sufficient therapeutic effects. However, if we can select the patients in each step of the cancer-immunity cycle, which indicates the relationship between the tumor invasion and the host defense, we can expect more effective results than randomly sorting the adapted patients. The existence of the tumor microenvironment, which had been hidden for more than 50 years as a reason for the unsuccessful tumor immunotherapy, can be unveiled by the evolution with ICI therapy. Recovery from the immune exhaustion by ICI therapy will bring unsatisfied tumor peptide vaccines targeting neoantigens into the sun. Many clinical trials currently being conducted for cancer immunotherapy are based on the combination with anti-PD-1/PD-L1 antibodies (1). A combination of anti-PD-1/PD-L with other ICIs, (2) with conventional cytocidal therapies such as chemotherapy and radiotherapy that induce necrosis of tumors and release tumor antigens. Especially, the phenomenon that the tumor shrinks at the other region against the irradiated area has been known as the "abscopal effect." (3) With new tumor therapy that can be expected to enhance tumor antigens, such as oncolytic virus therapy, (4) with a tumor vaccine by using neoantigens, and (5) with CAR-T or TCR-T therapy, which further strengthens antigen specificity. All tumor therapies are being developed now, and research is underway after understanding both local and systemic immune systems, which can be judged from histopathological findings and peripheral blood analyses.

Acknowledgement We thank H. Toyoda, M. Furuhata, M. Kozuka, and the former members of the laboratory. T. Yokosuka was supported by JSPS KAKENHI (JP25113725, JP15H01194, JP16H06501, JP17H03600, JP19K22545, and JP20H03536), JST PRESTO, the Takeda Science Foundation, and the Naito Foundation.

References

1. Bargou R, Leo E, Zugmaier G, Klinger M, Goebeler M, Knop S, et al. Tumor regression in cancer patients by very low doses of a T cell-engaging antibody. Science. 2008;321(5891):974–7.
2. Galon J, Bruni D. Tumor immunology and tumor evolution: intertwined histories. Immunity. 2020;52(1):55–81.
3. Burnet FM. Immunological surveillance in neoplasia. Transplant Rev. 1971;7:3–25.
4. van der Bruggen P, Traversari C, Chomez P, Lurquin C, De Plaen E, Van den Eynde B, et al. A gene encoding an antigen recognized by cytolytic T lymphocytes on a human melanoma. Science. 1991;254(5038):1643–7.
5. Kawakami Y, Eliyahu S, Sakaguchi K, Robbins PF, Rivoltini L, Yannelli JR, et al. Identification of the immunodominant peptides of the MART-1 human melanoma antigen recognized by the majority of HLA-A2-restricted tumor infiltrating lymphocytes. J Exp Med. 1994;180(1):347–52.
6. Yang JC, Rosenberg SA. Adoptive T-cell therapy for cancer. Adv Immunol. 2016;130:279–94.
7. June CH, O'Connor RS, Kawalekar OU, Ghassemi S, Milone MC. CAR T cell immunotherapy for human cancer. Science. 2018;359(6382):1361–5.
8. Joyce JA, Fearon DT. T cell exclusion, immune privilege, and the tumor microenvironment. Science. 2015;348(6230):74–80.
9. Suntharalingam G, Perry MR, Ward S, Brett SJ, Castello-Cortes A, Brunner MD, et al. Cytokine storm in a phase 1 trial of the anti-CD28 monoclonal antibody TGN1412. N Engl J Med. 2006;355(10):1018–28.
10. Leach DR, Krummel MF, Allison JP. Enhancement of antitumor immunity by CTLA-4 blockade. Science. 1996;271(5256):1734–6.
11. Ishida Y, Agata Y, Shibahara K, Honjo T. Induced expression of PD-1, a novel member of the immunoglobulin gene superfamily, upon programmed cell death. EMBO J. 1992;11(11):3887–95.
12. Sakaguchi S, Yamaguchi T, Nomura T, Ono M. Regulatory T cells and immune tolerance. Cell. 2008;133(5):775–87.
13. Hori S, Nomura T, Sakaguchi S. Control of regulatory T cell development by the transcription factor Foxp3. Science. 2003;299(5609):1057–61.
14. Chen DS, Mellman I. Oncology meets immunology: the cancer-immunity cycle. Immunity. 2013;39(1):1–10.
15. Chen DS, Mellman I. Elements of cancer immunity and the cancer-immune set point. Nature. 2017;541(7637):321–30.
16. Sharma P, Hu-Lieskovan S, Wargo JA, Ribas A. Primary, adaptive, and acquired resistance to cancer immunotherapy. Cell. 2017;168(4):707–23.
17. Schumacher TN, Schreiber RD. Neoantigens in cancer immunotherapy. Science. 2015;348(6230):69–74.
18. Matsushita H, Vesely MD, Koboldt DC, Rickert CG, Uppaluri R, Magrini VJ, et al. Cancer exome analysis reveals a T-cell-dependent mechanism of cancer immunoediting. Nature. 2012;482(7385):400–4.
19. Demaria O, Cornen S, Daeron M, Morel Y, Medzhitov R, Vivier E. Harnessing innate immunity in cancer therapy. Nature. 2019;574(7776):45–56.
20. MacKay M, Afshinnekoo E, Rub J, Hassan C, Khunte M, Baskaran N, et al. The therapeutic landscape for cells engineered with chimeric antigen receptors. Nat Biotechnol. 2020;38(2):233–44.

21. Yang W, Bai Y, Xiong Y, Zhang J, Chen S, Zheng X, et al. Potentiating the antitumour response of CD8(+) T cells by modulating cholesterol metabolism. Nature. 2016;531(7596):651–5.
22. Francisco LM, Sage PT, Sharpe AH. The PD-1 pathway in tolerance and autoimmunity. Immunol Rev. 2010;236:219–42.
23. Yokosuka T, Sakata-Sogawa K, Kobayashi W, Hiroshima M, Hashimoto-Tane A, Tokunaga M, et al. Newly generated T cell receptor microclusters initiate and sustain T cell activation by recruitment of Zap70 and SLP-76. Nat Immunol. 2005;6(12):1253–62.
24. Yokosuka T, Takamatsu M, Kobayashi-Imanishi W, Hashimoto-Tane A, Azuma M, Saito T. Programmed cell death 1 forms negative costimulatory microclusters that directly inhibit T cell receptor signaling by recruiting phosphatase SHP2. J Exp Med. 2012;209(6):1201–17.
25. Pardoll DM. The blockade of immune checkpoints in cancer immunotherapy. Nat Rev Cancer. 2012;12(4):252–64.
26. Ribas A, Wolchok JD. Cancer immunotherapy using checkpoint blockade. Science. 2018;359(6382):1350–5.
27. Weber JS, Kähler KC, Hauschild A. Management of immune-related adverse events and kinetics of response with ipilimumab. J Clin Oncol. 2012;30(21):2691–7.
28. Seymour L, Bogaerts J, Perrone A, Ford R, Schwartz LH, Mandrekar S, et al. iRECIST: guidelines for response criteria for use in trials testing immunotherapeutics. Lancet Oncol. 2017;18(3):e143–e52.
29. Topalian SL, Taube JM, Anders RA, Pardoll DM. Mechanism-driven biomarkers to guide immune checkpoint blockade in cancer therapy. Nat Rev Cancer. 2016;16(5):275–87.
30. Garon EB, Rizvi NA, Hui R, Leighl N, Balmanoukian AS, Eder JP, et al. Pembrolizumab for the treatment of non-small-cell lung cancer. N Engl J Med. 2015;372(21):2018–28.
31. Tumeh PC, Harview CL, Yearley JH, Shintaku IP, Taylor EJ, Robert L, et al. PD-1 blockade induces responses by inhibiting adaptive immune resistance. Nature. 2014;515(7528):568–71.
32. Rizvi NA, Hellmann MD, Snyder A, Kvistborg P, Makarov V, Havel JJ, et al. Cancer immunology. Mutational landscape determines sensitivity to PD-1 blockade in non-small cell lung cancer. Science. 2015;348(6230):124–8.
33. Le DT, Uram JN, Wang H, Bartlett BR, Kemberling H, Eyring AD, et al. PD-1 blockade in tumors with mismatch-repair deficiency. N Engl J Med. 2015;372(26):2509–20.

Cancer Pathology

5

Yoshiya Horimoto

Abstract

Pathological assessment is a microscopic examination of cells and tissues to determine whether it is a malignant disease. Without a pathological diagnosis, the patient cannot start the treatment for a malignant disease. Pathological diagnosis also plays an important role in evaluating the nature of cancers. Basic pathological assessment is conducted by the human eye, employing hematoxylin and eosin staining. Immunohistochemistry may support the diagnosis by evaluating some protein expressions to provide useful information about the tumor. In this chapter, the flow of a pathological diagnosis was also mentioned. To ensure the quality of medical care, an accurate pathological diagnosis is essential.

Keywords

Cancer · Breast cancer · Pathological diagnosis · Biopsy · Immunohistochemistry

5.1 What Is a Pathological Diagnosis?

A pathological diagnosis is a diagnosis based on the pathological assessment made by specialized pathologists. Pathological assessment is a microscopic examination of cells and tissues taken from a suspected lesion to determine whether it is benign or malignant. If the lesion is malignant, it can be examined in detail to determine the nature of the cancer.

5.2 Necessity for Obtaining a Pathological Diagnosis

In order to start the treatment for a malignant disease, it is necessary to first obtain a definitive diagnosis based on pathological assessment. It is not possible to diagnose cancer or choose a treatment based only on the symptoms and imaging diagnosis. Without a pathological diagnosis, the patient might end up receiving unnecessary and harmful treatment if the disease is not cancer. Moreover, treatments of cancer in the same organ can vary depending on the nature of the individual cancer. Pathological diagnosis plays an important role in evaluating the nature of such cancers.

5.3 Examples of Histopathological Images

Examples of histopathological images of normal breast tissue and breast cancer are shown below. Figure 5.1 shows "structural" differences between normal breast ducts, non-invasive breast cancer, and invasive breast cancer. Breast cancer generally arises from epithelial cells composed of ducts whose original function is to transport breast milk to the nipple. Figure 5.2 shows the appearance of cancer cells at the cellular level. Since cancer cells proliferate in an

Y. Horimoto (✉)
Department of Breast Oncology, Juntendo University, Tokyo, Japan

Department of Human Pathology, Juntendo University, Tokyo, Japan

Department of Breast Surgery and Oncology, Tokyo Medical University, Tokyo, Japan
e-mail: horimoto@juntendo.ac.jp

© The Author(s), under exclusive license to Springer Nature Singapore Pte Ltd. 2026
M. Endo et al. (eds.), *Cancer and Work in Asia Volume 2*, https://doi.org/10.1007/978-981-95-6537-5_5

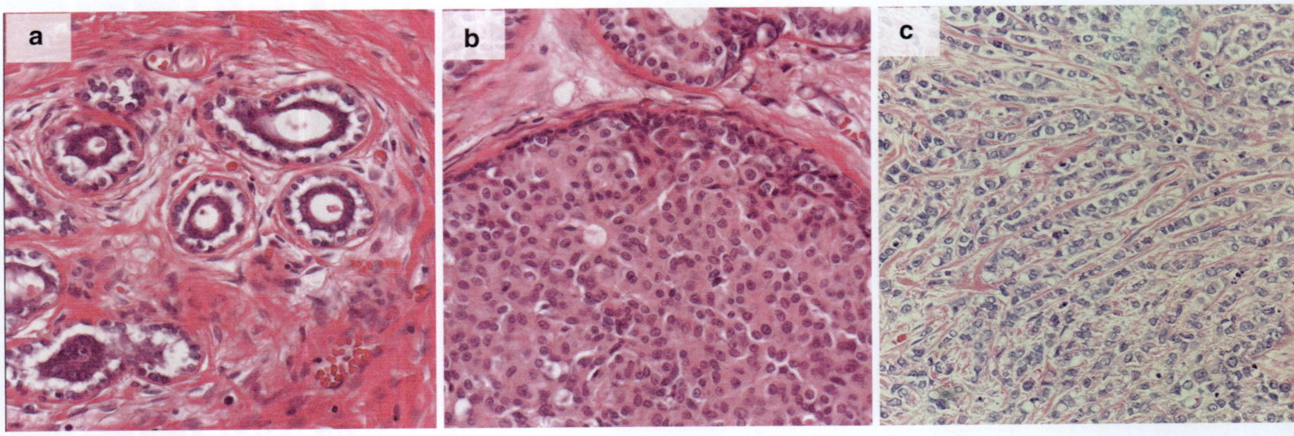

Fig. 5.1 Histopathologic findings of normal breast ducts, non-invasive breast cancer, and invasive breast cancer. Hematoxylin/Eosin-stained tissue specimens. (**a**) Normal breast ducts are composed of two layers of cells, epithelial and myoepithelial cells. (**b**) Ductal carcinoma in situ (non-invasive) is an early stage of breast cancer. Atypical cells proliferate densely but remain within the duct space surrounded by a layer of myoepithelial cells. (**c**) Invasive carcinoma. Atypical cells diffusely infiltrate the breast tissue. Duct structures are no longer observed

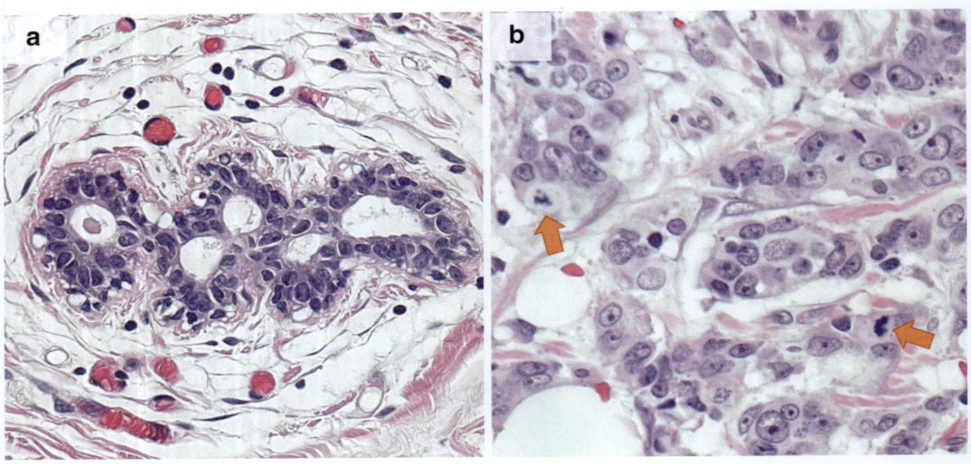

Fig. 5.2 Abnormal appearance of cancer cells. Hematoxylin/Eosin-stained tissue specimens. (**a**) Normal breast ducts and (**b**) invasive breast cancer. The size and shape of individual cancer cells are different compared to normal cells. Cancer cells frequently have larger, polygonal nuclei and line up irregularly. Such an abnormal appearance of cells is called "atypia." Orange arrows indicate mitotic cells that are in the process of undergoing cell division from one to two cells

uncontrolled manner, cancer nests lose their function as an organ.

5.4 Immunohistochemistry

Hematoxylin and Eosin (HE) staining is the most basic method for pathological diagnosis, which is assessed by the human eye. Immunohistochemistry (IHC) is a tool used to support pathological diagnosis based on HE. Pathologists determine the proteins needed for diagnosis, and IHC will be conducted to evaluate the protein expression. IHC alone cannot determine whether a tumor is cancerous or not; however, it can evaluate the nature of the tumor. For example, Ki67 protein expression, which serves as a marker for cell proliferation, can be used to quantify how much the tumor tends to grow (Fig. 5.3) [1]. Such an examination will provide useful information to help physicians select the most appropriate treatment for their patients.

In addition, IHC can also be used to make assumptions about the tumor origin. Figure 5.4 shows the differential diagnosis of lung tumors. In HE sections obtained from a very small biopsy sample, it is often difficult to tell which organ the cancer originated from. In this case (Fig. 5.4c),

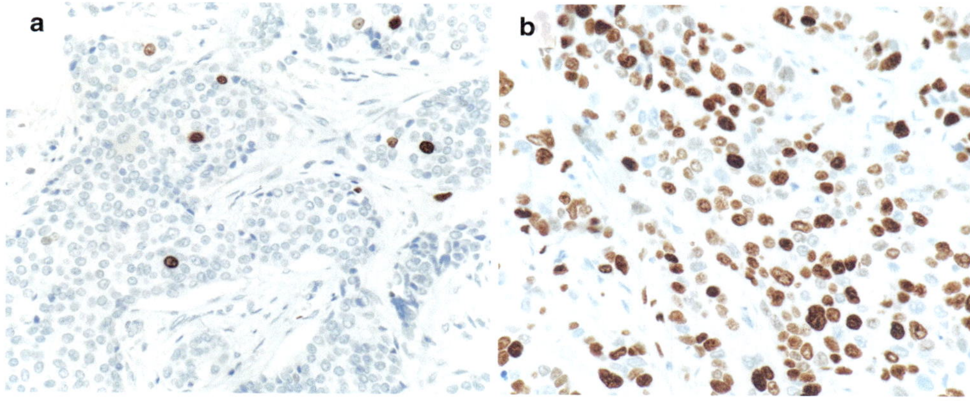

Fig. 5.3 Immunohistochemistry of Ki67. Tumors with (**a**) low and (**b**) high Ki67 protein expression (indicated by brown color). A tumor with a high Ki67 labeling index is generally considered to be aggressive in nature

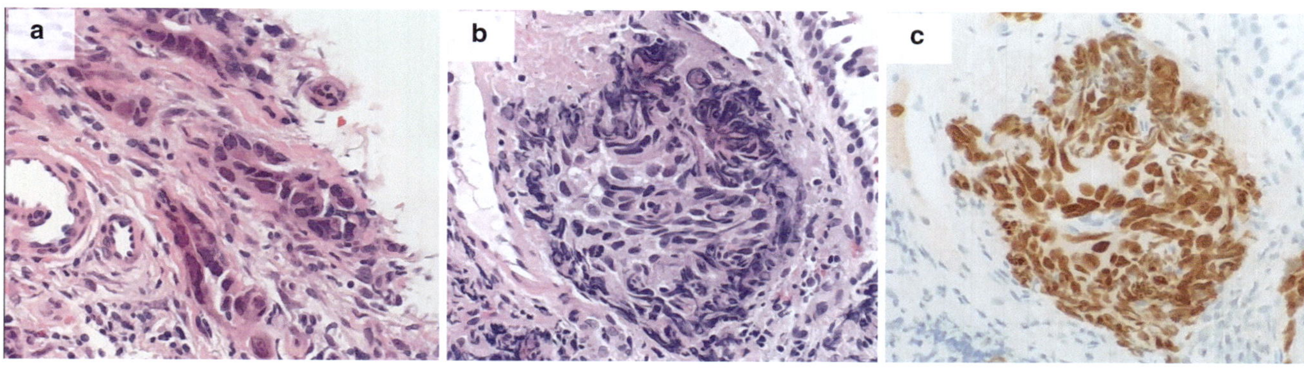

Fig. 5.4 Differential diagnosis of lung tumors. Histological findings of transbronchial needle biopsies from lung tumors. (**a**) Primary lung cancer (HE). (**b**, **c**) Breast cancer metastasis in the lung, as diagnosed by HE (**b**) and IHC of GATA-3 (**c**)

staining of GATA-3, a nuclear marker for epithelial neoplasms and specific to some organs, including the breast [2], was positive in IHC and thus useful to diagnose that this metastatic tumor originated from breast cancer.

Once again, IHC alone cannot be a replacement for a histopathological diagnosis, but it will often be very helpful by providing useful information.

5.5 Typical Flow of a Pathological Diagnosis

5.5.1 Biopsy

A biopsy is a procedure that is often performed at an outpatient clinic. When a suspicious cancerous lesion is detected by imaging tests, a needle biopsy will be performed in order to obtain a definitive diagnosis. For example, in the case of a breast tumor, a needle is carefully advanced to the lesion under local anesthesia while the location of the target lesion is monitored using ultrasound or mammography. The collected tissue is then immediately fixed in formalin and stored in paraffin blocks. The tissue block is then cut into thin slices and processed for observation under a microscope. Examples of HE-stained biopsy specimens are shown in Fig. 5.5. It usually takes several days, sometimes up to 1 week, from the initial tissue collection to the pathological diagnosis.

5.5.2 Intraoperative Diagnosis

In some cases, a small piece of tissue is taken during surgery, and pathologists quickly diagnose whether the tumor was completely removed or not, or how much the cancer has spread to the lymph nodes. Based on the results, surgeons can decide on the appropriate surgical procedure. Moreover, in cases where performing a biopsy is difficult at the outpatient clinic (e.g., brain tumors), a surgical biopsy may be performed to obtain a definitive diagnosis. Figure 5.6 shows a brain tumor that appeared during the treatment of a stage IV breast cancer (liver and pleural metastases), as we previously reported [3]. Although the image findings were consistent with breast cancer metastasis, the intraoperative pathological assessment revealed that this tumor was a primary malignant lymphoma arising from the central nervous system.

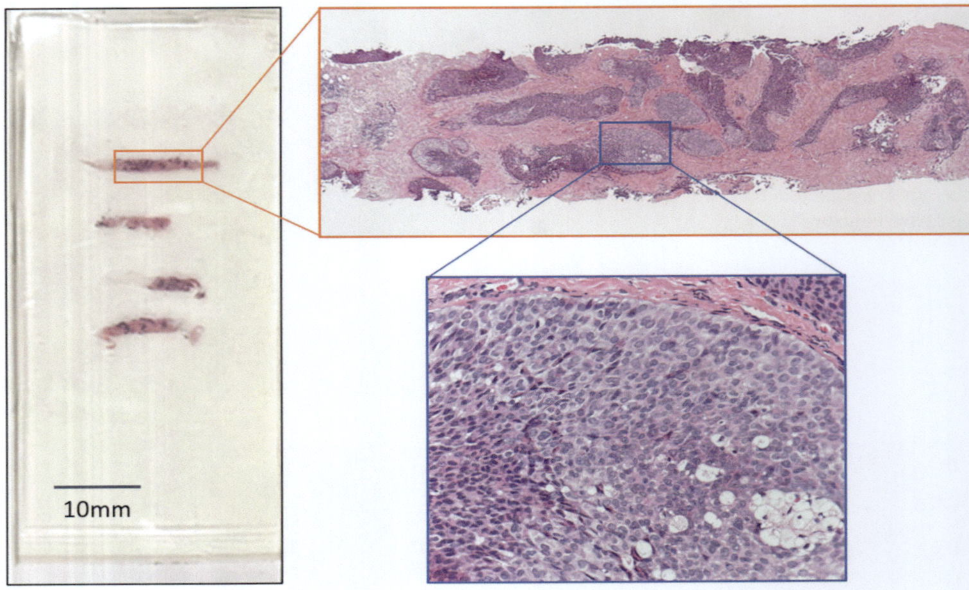

Fig. 5.5 Macro- and micro-images of a breast tumor needle biopsy. Hematoxylin/eosin-stained tissue specimen of needle biopsy. The left image shows four pieces of needle biopsies taken from a breast tumor. The orange and blue rectangles on the right indicate enlarged views (×40 and ×400, respectively). This case was a ductal carcinoma in situ (non-invasive)

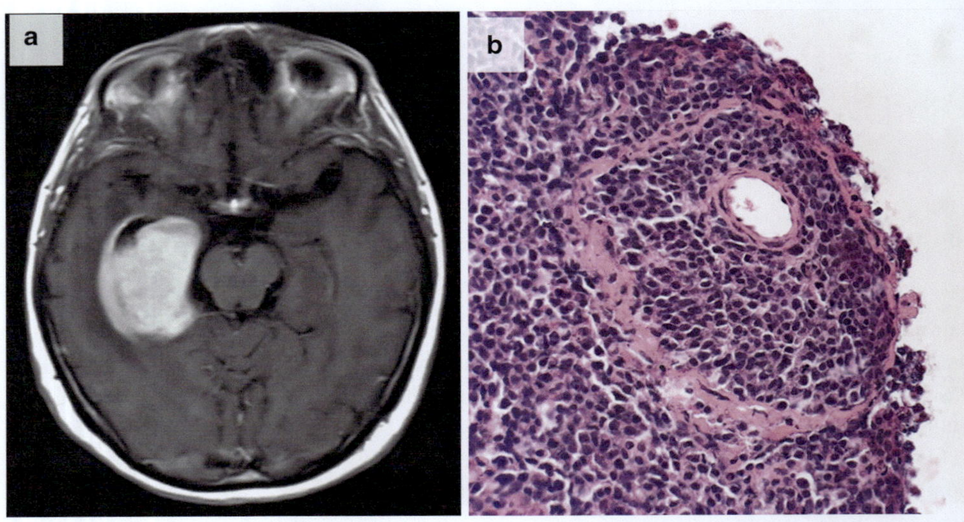

Fig. 5.6 A brain tumor was found during the treatment of metastatic breast cancer. (**a**) Brain magnetic resonance imaging (MRI) examination (T1-weighted) revealed a 30-mm mass lesion in the right temporal lobe. (**b**) Intraoperative pathological assessment (HE) revealed that this tumor was a primary malignant lymphoma, not a breast cancer metastasis. (This figure has been adopted from reference [3])

5.5.3 Surgical Specimen

After curative surgery for cancer, a detailed pathological diagnosis of the surgical specimen will be performed. This allows for an accurate staging of the tumor, including determining the size of the tumor and obtaining a more detailed assessment of the nature of the cancer. It can generally provide more information than a needle biopsy and will be useful in determining the treatment after surgery.

5.6 Pathological Diagnosis Is Not Absolute

Since pathological diagnosis is a static evaluation, it is not suitable for capturing the dynamic aspects of the disease. For example, cancer cells often spread via blood/lymphatic vessels, but this cannot always be captured by pathological assessment because these cells are moving. Figure 5.7 illustrates how lymphatic vessel invasion by cancer cells can occasionally be observed in an HE tissue section. For evaluating such dynamic aspects, liquid biopsy, which evaluates cancer cells and cancer-derived factors in the blood, plays a significant role.

Equalization of diagnosis has been a major challenge in the field of cancer pathology [4]. First, there are some diseases that are diagnosed differently among pathologists,

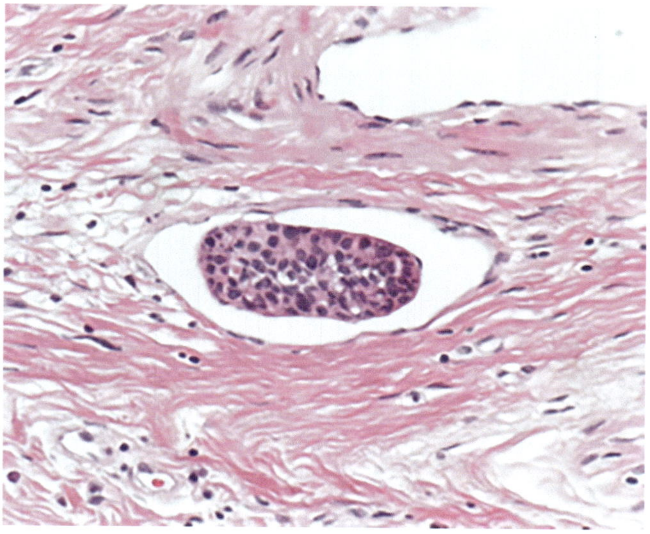

Fig. 5.7 Lymphatic vessel invasion. Hematoxylin/eosin-stained tissue specimen. A cluster of breast cancer cells is observed in a dilated lymph duct

regardless of diagnostic abilities. In general, this affects lesions that are somewhere between benign and malignant. Second, not all diseases equally occur in every region or country. Thus, there will be differences in the level of diagnostic experience among pathologists. To overcome this problem, a tremendous amount of effort is being made, for example, by establishing diagnostic guidelines for each organ so that the same diagnosis can be made in any hospital and in any country.

5.7 Concluding Remarks

Pathological diagnosis is based on the enormous knowledge that has been established through longstanding research and experience. New knowledge is continuously being added. Therefore, even for the same lesion, the name of the diagnosis may change over time, and there are some diseases for which the judgment is still divided among pathologists. There will even be lesions for which no diagnostic name exists. AI (artificial intelligence) tools for pathological diagnosis have been developed all over the world. Although these tools will probably be able to assist human diagnosis in the very near future, all the data on which they are based is gathered by pathologists. In other words, pathological diagnosis is changing and advancing day by day through the continuous effort of human beings.

Since the beginning of the 2000s, the molecules and genes that define the characteristics of various cancers have been elucidated. In addition to the aforementioned IHC, it has become possible to examine cancer-related mutations in a large number of genes at once by so-called gene panel tests, which can lead to the development of "molecular targeted drugs" that work on specific molecules or genes. Although the genes that can be tested vary among cancers and the drugs available are also different among countries, offering individualized treatment is the current trend in clinical practice, and it will continue to accelerate, as will the technology for testing and developing new drugs. Nevertheless, without an accurate pathological diagnosis, the quality of such individualized medical care cannot be ensured.

Acknowledgement The author sincerely appreciates Dr. Katrin Beate Ishii-Schrade (Juntendo University) for language editing.

References

1. Querzoli P, Albonico G, Ferretti S, Rinaldi R, Magri E, Indelli M, Nenci I. MIB-1 proliferative activity in invasive breast cancer measured by image analysis. J Clin Pathol. 1996;49(11):926–30.
2. Ordóñez NG. Value of GATA3 immunostaining in tumor diagnosis: a review. Adv Anat Pathol. 2013;20(5):352–60.
3. Semba R, Horimoto Y, Arakawa A, Edahiro Y, Takaku T, Iijima K, et al. Difficulty diagnosing a brain tumor during clinical maintenance of a complete response to anti-HER2 treatments for metastatic breast cancer: a case report. Case Rep Oncol. 2020;13(3):1311–6.
4. Cazap E, Magrath I, Kingham TP, Elzawawy A. Structural barriers to diagnosis and treatment of cancer in low- and middle-income countries: the urgent need for scaling up. J Clin Oncol. 2016;34(1):14–9.

Part II

Cancer Treatment and Supportive Care in Asia

Diagnosis of Cancer

6

Katsuya Nakai

Abstract

A cancer diagnosis is made after a comprehensive diagnostic process, which includes recording the medical history and current symptoms of the patient and performing diagnostic imaging of affected organs and pathology of affected tissues and cells, as well as a range of laboratory tests. Based on the combined results, the location and the stage of the cancer is determined and an appropriate treatment plan is conceived. Further testing is performed during and after the treatment to monitor the efficacy of the treatment and any tumor recurrence or side effects. This chapter is intended to give a brief overview of the steps and the technology and tests currently used in cancer diagnostics.

Keywords

Computed Tomography · Sentinel Lymph Node Biopsy
Positron Emission Tomography · Endoscopy ·
Mammography

6.1 Introduction

When cancer is suspected, the doctor will interview and examine the patient. In addition to inspecting the physical condition and symptoms, the doctor will interview the patient to collect detailed information about past illnesses, current illnesses, and the medical history of family members and blood relatives, in order to obtain clues to the diagnosis. Lifestyle habits (smoking, drinking, occupation, etc.) should also be checked. In order to obtain more detailed information, blood tests, pathological tests, imaging tests (X-ray, computed tomography (CT), magnetic resonance imaging (MRI), positron emission tomography (PET), ultrasonography, endoscopy, etc.), and various other tests are performed. Although the tests performed depend on the type of cancer and the organ affected, it is common to combine several tests. The physical and financial burden and complications associated with the tests are taken into consideration. The purpose of tests performed before diagnosis is to confirm the presence of cancer. If multiple tests confirm a suspicious lesion, cells and tissues are collected from the site and examined under a microscope to confirm the presence of cancer. In some organs, it is not possible to collect cells or tissues, thus a definitive diagnosis may not be made until after surgery. The purpose of the examination after the definitive diagnosis is to confirm the spread and the depth of the cancer. The cancer stage is determined by checking not only the location of the cancer, but also whether it has metastasized to the surrounding lymph nodes or other organs. Based on this information, a treatment plan appropriate to the stage is formulated. At the same time, the patient's general condition, including the function of vital organs (heart, lungs, liver, kidneys, etc.), is examined to evaluate whether the patient is able to withstand surgery, drug therapy, and radiation therapy. This examination is performed not only before but also during the treatment to monitor the effect of the treatment and to check for any side effects and complications. After the main treatment is completed, follow-up examinations should be performed to check for continued treatment effects, metastasis, or recurrence.

6.2 Diagnostic Imaging

Doctors use imaging tests to take pictures of the inside of your body. Imaging tests can be used to look for cancer, find out how far it has spread, and to judge if cancer treatment is working. Generally, the report is presented to the attending physician about a week after being double-checked by a diagnostic imaging specialist.

K. Nakai (✉)
Department of Breast Oncology, Graduate School of Medicine, Juntendo University, Bunkyo-ku, Tokyo, Japan
e-mail: nakai@juntendo.ac.jp

© The Author(s), under exclusive license to Springer Nature Singapore Pte Ltd. 2026

M. Endo et al. (eds.), *Cancer and Work in Asia Volume 2*, https://doi.org/10.1007/978-981-95-6537-5_6

6.2.1 CT (Computed Tomography)

CT is an examination to detect morphological abnormalities of organs by X-ray irradiation. 360-degree X-ray irradiation from all directions produces images of the human body cut into a circle. It is possible to obtain a three-dimensional image of the inside of the body by layering several X-ray images. It is a powerful tool for examining large areas of the body and for examining the lungs and bones, which are difficult to visualize with MRI. The use of contrast media makes it possible to clarify the location of lesions such as tumors, and to understand the extent and the pattern of vascularization near the tumor. 3D images, arbitrary cross-sectional images, and vascular images can be created from the imaging data, allowing a three-dimensional observation and diagnosis. However, due to the radiation exposure, a CT may not be performed in the early stages of pregnancy or when there is a possibility of pregnancy.

6.2.2 MRI (Magnetic Resonance Imaging)

Magnetic resonance imaging (MRI) uses a powerful magnetic field, radio waves, and a computer to produce detailed pictures of the inside of your body. The contrast between lesions and normal tissues is excellent, and cross-sectional images of various parts of the body can be taken from any angle, including vertically, horizontally and obliquely, without changing posture. Since there is no radiation exposure, it is suitable for repeated examinations and examinations of children and pregnant women. It is not suitable for examining moving organs, such as the stomach or the intestine, because of the long imaging time. Because of the strong magnetic field that hits the body, patients with internal metal devices such as cardiac pacemakers or those who are claustrophobic may not be able to undergo this examination.

6.2.3 PET (Positron Emission Tomography)

In contrast to CT and MRI, which detect abnormalities based on the morphology of the lesion, PET detects abnormalities based on the function of glucose metabolism and other factors. Observing the metabolic activity of the lesion can be used to improve the accuracy of a diagnosis in cases where the morphology of the lesion alone is insufficient. PET-CT is a combination of PET and CT systems, which enables highly accurate positioning and clear images of the location and size of the tumor. Since the whole body can be examined in a single examination, it is used to diagnose unknown primary cancers that are suspected to be cancerous but whose lesions cannot be detected by other examinations, to stage the disease, and to check for metastasis or recurrence. However, FDG (fluorodeoxyglucose, a radioactive tracer) accumulates strongly in the brain and the heart, where glucose metabolism is active, and is excreted in urine, making it difficult to diagnose cancer in the kidney, the ureter, and the bladder.

6.2.4 Ultrasound

Ultrasound is an examination in which an ultrasound probe (an instrument that emits ultrasound waves) is placed on the surface of the body and the ultrasound waves rebounding from organs in the body are projected as images. It is possible to check the location of the cancer, the shape and size of the cancer, and the relationship between the cancer and the surrounding organs. There is no pain, no radiation exposure, and little burden on the body. Ultrasonography is used to diagnose cancers of various organs, including the liver, gallbladder, pancreas, kidney, bladder, ovary, uterus, prostate, thyroid, and mammary gland. On the other hand, ultrasound cannot be used to examine lesions in the brain and lungs because air, bone, and thick fat do not allow ultrasound to pass through.

6.2.5 Endoscopy

In endoscopy, a tube about 1 cm thick with a small camera (CCD) or lens built into the tip is inserted through the mouth or anus, and the lumen of the esophagus, stomach, duodenum, or colon can be directly observed. A biopsy of a suspected cancerous site can be performed to obtain a definitive diagnosis. Endoscopic treatment, including hemostasis and resection of polyps and tumors, can also be performed.

6.2.6 Mammography

Mammography is used to detect and diagnose breast diseases and breast cancer in women who have breast problems, such as a lump, pain, or nipple discharge, as well as in women who have no breast complaints. It usually involves taking two X-ray images of each breast. In addition, regular breast cancer screening using mammography has been reported to reduce mortality in randomized controlled trials conducted in Europe and the United States [1].

6.3 Pathology

Pathology is a microscopic examination of the properties of cells and tissues from a suspected cancer site and is used for the definitive diagnosis of cancer.

6.3.1 Cytopathology

Cytopathology is the practice of collecting cells and making a diagnosis using a microscope. Cytopathology involves the collection of cells from the mucous membranes of the oral cavity, trachea, bladder, uterus, etc., by scraping with a brush-like object, aspiration with a needle through the skin, or collection of cells suspended in liquids such as sputum or urine.

6.3.2 Histopathology

Histopathology is a pathological examination performed in the diagnosis of cancer, in which a piece of tissue from a lesion is taken and examined under a microscope. Histopathology provides information on structural abnormalities in addition to cellular atypia and is used for the definitive diagnosis of cancer with a higher diagnostic yield than cytopathology.

6.3.3 Lymph Node Biopsy

Lymph node biopsy is a procedure in which a swollen lymph node that appears to be diseased is taken for detailed examination under a microscope. The biopsy is performed to confirm the diagnosis when the cause of the lymph node swelling is unknown. There are various histological types of malignant lymphoma, and a biopsy can help to select the appropriate treatment and to estimate the prognosis. In principle, excisional biopsy is used for lymph node biopsy, and, in most cases, it is performed under local anesthesia.

6.3.4 Bone Marrow Aspiration and Biopsy

Bone marrow aspiration and biopsy is a procedure in which a needle is inserted into the iliac bone to obtain bone marrow tissue from the bone. There are two types of biopsy: bone marrow aspiration, in which bone marrow fluid is aspirated with a syringe, and bone marrow biopsy, in which a portion of bone marrow tissue is extracted with a special thick needle. By observing the tissue under a microscope, the function of blood production, causes of blood diseases, and the presence of tumor cells can be determined. It is an important test for the diagnosis of hematological cancers, selection of treatment methods, and evaluation of treatment effects.

6.3.5 Intraoperative Rapid Diagnosis

During surgery, some cells and tissues of the lesion are collected, and a pathologist quickly determines whether the tumor is benign or has lymph node metastasis. Based on the results, it is possible to determine the excision range and change to an appropriate surgical method.

6.3.6 Sentinel Lymph Node Biopsy (SLNB)

A sentinel lymph node is defined as the first lymph node to which cancer cells are most likely to spread from a primary tumor. A negative SLNB result suggests that cancer has not yet spread to nearby lymph nodes or other organs. A positive SLNB result indicates that cancer is present in the sentinel lymph node and that it may have spread to other nearby lymph nodes (called regional lymph nodes) and, possibly, to other organs. This information can help a doctor determine the stage of the cancer (extent of the disease within the body) and develop an appropriate treatment plan. It is commonly used in evaluating breast cancer and melanoma [2].

6.4 Laboratory Tests

Laboratory tests are tests that analyze various components present in blood and urine to determine if there are any abnormalities in the body, which part of the body is diseased, if there is inflammation, and to evaluate the nutritional status. It is useful not only for diagnosing cancer but also for detecting a wide range of diseases. Biochemical tests useful in the diagnosis of cancer include tumor marker tests and endocrine tests.

6.4.1 Tumor Markers

Tumor markers are used in a variety of cancers to aid in the diagnosis of cancer, as well as to determine the effectiveness of treatment and whether or not the cancer has recurred or metastasized. Tumor markers measure proteins and carbohydrate antigens that are uniquely produced by different types of cancer (Table 6.1). Tumor marker values alone do not lead to a definitive diagnosis, but in combination with the results

Table 6.1 Tumor markers

Thyroid cancer	Tg, CEA
Non-small cell lung cancer	CYFRA21-1, CEA, SLX, CA125, SCC
Small cell carcinoma	NSE, ProGRP
Esophageal cancer	SCC, CEA
Gastric cancer	CEA, CA19-9
Colon cancer	CEA, CA19-9, p53 antibody
Hepatocellular carcinoma	AFP, PIVKA-II, AFP-L3
Biliary tract cancer	CA19-9, CEA
Pancreatic cancer	CA19-9, Span-1, DUPAN-2, CEA, CA50
Bladder cancer	NMP22, BTA
Breast cancer	CEA, CA15-3
Cervical cancer	SCC, CA125, CEA
Ovarian cancer	CA125
Prostate cancer	PSA

of other tests, such as imaging tests, the doctor can make a comprehensive judgment. The burden on the body is minimal, as it is performed mainly by measuring the components of body fluids such as blood and urine. However, hepatic and renal disorders, lifestyle factors such as alcohol consumption and smoking, and comorbidities may cause high tumor marker values regardless of the presence or absence of cancer. On the other hand, a tumor marker value may not be high even in the presence of cancer.

6.4.2 Endocrine Tests

Endocrine organs, such as the thyroid gland and the pancreas, secrete hormones as needed, but the presence of tumors can cause hyperactivity of the endocrine glands or hypofunction due to an atrophy of the glands. By examining the amount of hormone secretion, lesions in the pituitary gland, thyroid gland, and adrenal glands can be identified.

6.5 Biomarker Testing for Cancer

A biomarker is a substance in the body, such as a protein or gene, that is an indicator of changes in disease status or treatment effects.

6.5.1 Genetic Testing for Cancer

In hematological and other cancers, oncogene testing is used to determine the definitive diagnosis of the disease, to make a prognosis, to select therapies, such as molecularly targeted drugs and hematopoietic stem cell transplantation, and to determine the efficacy of the therapy. For example, chronic myelogenous leukemia can be confirmed by the presence of a specific gene (BCR-ABL fusion gene) that is responsible for the disease.

6.5.2 Multigene Panel Testing

The oncogene panel test is a test that examines mutations in several cancer-related genes that are involved in the development of cancer at once. A new technology using a machine called a "next-generation sequencer" is used. In the cancer gene panel test, DNA and other materials are extracted from the cancerous tissue and blood of the patient and analyzed for mutations in a panel of cancer-related genes. By examining a large number of genes at once, it is possible to find mutations that cannot be detected by conventional tests, which focus on only one type of gene.

6.5.3 Tumor Cell Surface Antigen Analysis

Tumor cell surface antigen analysis is a method for analyzing markers on the surface of cells that indicate the origin and character of the cell, using an instrument called a flow cytometer. It can be performed on cells collected from blood, bone marrow, or lymph nodes. This test makes it possible to distinguish tumor cell types that cannot be determined by microscopic observation. It can also be used to check for the presence of remaining cancer cells after treatment.

6.5.4 Chromosome Analysis

Chromosome analysis is a test to search for chromosome numbers and morphological abnormalities. In G-banding, chromosomes are stained appropriately, and the band patterns can be compared to identify individual chromosomes. Recently, spectral karyotyping has been developed, in which all chromosomes are color-coded for accurate testing.

6.5.5 Companion Diagnostics

Companion diagnostics are clinical tests used to predict the effects and side effects of drugs before they are administered. Companion diagnostics are used to promote personalized medicine by testing the response of individual patients to drugs prior to treatment and are distinguished from ordinary clinical tests. In companion diagnostics, mutations and expression levels of genes encoding drug-targeted proteins and drug-metabolizing enzymes are examined to understand individual differences in the efficacy of specific drugs and the occurrence of side effects and to assist physicians in determining the appropriateness of medication.

6.6 Clinical Practice Guidelines

Clinical practice guidelines are defined as documents that evaluate evidence through systematic reviews and provide recommendations that are considered optimal, taking into account the balance of benefits and harms, in order to support the decision-making of health care users and providers on important health-related issues. Of course, the final decision in clinical practice needs to be made in collaboration between the patient and the attending physician. When a patient is suspected of having cancer and visits a medical institution, the patient is examined, tested, and treated. In the course of such a series of medical treatments, multiple options arise. For example, it is necessary to choose a test method or a treatment method (surgery, drug therapy, etc.). A medical guideline is a document that provides a "recommendation" of the most appropriate method, taking into consideration the evidence of multiple testing and treatment methods, the balance of benefits and harms associated with testing and treatment, the patient's values and wishes, and the economic perspective.

The ESMO (European Society for Medical Oncology) guidelines [3] are based on expert literature searches and recommendations. They are published on the Web and in print in the *Annals of Oncology*. The American Society of Clinical Oncology (ASCO) guidelines [4] are in the form of recommendations and explanations for clinical questions and are published on the web and in print in the *Journal of Clinical Oncology*. The NCCN (National Comprehensive Cancer Network) guideline [5] is based on a search of articles in PubMed, with explanations provided by experts and data presented as a basis. The guidelines are somewhat different from the usual guidelines in that they are not written in the form of an answer to a clinical question. There is no description of the level of evidence, but the content is in the form agreed upon by the committee. It is published only on the web, not in print. Since the guidelines are not formulated in a strict manner, they can be revised frequently on the web.

References

1. Duffy SW, Vulkan D, Cuckle H, Parmar D, Sheikh S, Smith RA, Evans A, Blyuss O, Johns L, Ellis IO, et al. Effect of mammographic screening from age 40 years on breast cancer mortality (UK Age trial): final results of a randomised, controlled trial. Lancet Oncol. 2020;21:1165–72. https://doi.org/10.1016/S1470-2045(20)30398-3.
2. Krag DN, Anderson SJ, Julian TB, Brown AM, Harlow SP, Costantino JP, Ashikaga T, Weaver DL, Mamounas EP, Jalovec LM, et al. Sentinel-lymph-node resection compared with conventional axillary-lymph-node dissection in clinically node-negative patients with breast cancer: overall survival findings from the NSABP B-32 randomised phase 3 trial. Lancet Oncol. 2010;11:927–33. https://doi.org/10.1016/S1470-2045(10)70207-2.
3. The European Society for Medical Oncology (ESMO). The European Society for Medical Oncology (ESMO) guidelines. Available online: http://www.esmo.org/Guidelines. Accessed 22 Apr 2022.
4. The American Society of Clinical Oncology (ASCO). The American Society of Clinical Oncology (ASCO) guidelines. Available online: https://www.asco.org/practice-patients/guidelines. Accessed 22 Apr 2022.
5. The National Comprehensive Cancer Network (NCCN). The National Comprehensive Cancer Network (NCCN) guidelines. Available online: https://www.nccn.org/guidelines. Accessed 22 Apr 2022.

7 Diagnosis and Treatment for Gynecological Cancer

Yasuhisa Terao

Abstract

Gynecological cancer is specific to females and refers to cancer of the female reproductive organs. The female reproductive organs include the vulva, vagina, uterus, fallopian tubes, and ovaries. The uterus is an important organ for pregnancy and childbirth. It is characterized by a younger age of onset than cancers of other organs. Therefore, uterine or ovarian cancers at a fertile age may affect future fertility. Cancer and its treatment may affect marriage, childbirth, and sexual life. Cervical cancer can be prevented through vaccination against HPV or early detection through screening. Hereditary cancer syndromes predispose to the uterine body and the ovary. Understanding the risk factors for gynecologic cancer can help prevent cancer and detect it early. Molecular targeted therapy and immune checkpoint inhibitors have been shown to be effective for treatment. Therefore, the treatment of gynecological cancers is expected to change dramatically in the future.

Keywords

Cervical cancer · Uterine cancer · Ovarian cancer
HBOC · *BRCA1/2* · Treatment · Compilations

Gynecological cancer is specific to females and refers to cancer of the female reproductive organs. The female reproductive organs include the vulva, vagina, uterus, fallopian tubes, and ovaries. Although cancers can occur in any of these areas, cancers of the uterus and ovaries are the most common. Thus, this chapter focuses on cancers of the uterus and ovaries. The uterus is shaped like a pear with a cavity (uterine cavity) and consists of a body (upper part) where the fetus resides and a cervix (lower part) that connects to the vagina. The ovaries are 3–4 cm oval-shaped organs, with one on each side of the uterus. Together, the ovaries and fallopian tubes are called the uterine adnexa. The functions of the ovaries include the maturation and ovulation of oocytes, as well as the secretion of female sex hormones to create and maintain a feminine body. The uterus is an important organ for pregnancy and childbirth. Therefore, uterine or ovarian cancers at a fertile age compromise future fertility. Cancer and its treatment may affect marriage, childbirth, and sexual health. If you require help, you may consult with your doctor, nurses, pharmacists, and social workers.

Y. Terao (✉)
Department of Obstetrics and Gynecology, School of Medicine, Juntendo University, Bunkyo-ku, Tokyo, Japan
e-mail: yterao@juntendo.ac.jp

7.1 Uterine Cancer

There are two types of uterine cancers: cervical cancer is a cancer of the cervix, and corpus uteri cancer (uterine cancer) is a cancer of the uterine body. Cervical cancer and uterine cancer differ in terms of causes, diagnosis, treatment, and prognosis; thus, they will be explained separately.

7.2 Cervical Cancer

7.2.1 Cervical Cancer Basics

Cervical cancer develops in the cervix, most commonly in the transformation zone near the squamocolumnar junction, which is the entrance to the uterus. In particular, it occurs near the border between squamous cells and columnar epithelial cells that cover the surface of the cervix (SCJ) and can be broadly classified into squamous cell carcinoma and adenocarcinoma. Cervical cancer can affect any woman, and it is most common in women in their late 30s and 40s. The most common cause of the disease is the human papillomavirus (HPV). Approximately 80% of women are infected with this virus at least once in their lifetime through sexual intercourse. It is usually eliminated naturally by the immune

© The Author(s), under exclusive license to Springer Nature Singapore Pte Ltd. 2026
M. Endo et al. (eds.), *Cancer and Work in Asia Volume 2*, https://doi.org/10.1007/978-981-95-6537-5_7

system. There are about 15 types of high-risk HPV that are thought to be closely related to the development of cervical cancer. Some of them become dysplastic (pre-cancer lesions) due to persistent HPV infection, and some of them go through mild, moderate, and severe dysplasia over a period of 5–10 years and then develop cancer. Low-grade squamous intraepithelial lesion (LSIL) refers to mild dysplasia, while high-grade squamous intraepithelial lesion (HSIL) refers to moderate dysplasia to severe dysplasia. In addition to persistent HPV infection, risk factors for developing cervical cancer include a history of smoking, high parity, oral contraceptive pill use, being sexually active at an early age, a high number of sexual partners, and a history of sexually transmitted infection, autoimmune disease, and human immunodeficiency virus (HIV). There are a few symptoms in the early stages, and as it progresses, symptoms include irregular bleeding (intercourse or other than during menstruation), bloody discharge with odor, lower abdominal and back pain, and swelling of the lower extremities.

7.2.2 Diagnostic Examination for Cervical Cancer

In cancer screening, cells from the cervix are scraped off with a brush and observed under a microscope. As a result, if cervical cancer is suspected, a detailed examination is performed. The cytological diagnosis is made according to the Bethesda System. In women over 30 years of age, an HPV test is performed at the same time as a cytological examination to check for high-risk HPV infection. In women under 30 years of age, HPV testing is performed only when abnormalities are found in the cytological examination, because the HPV positivity rate is high. However, there is a high possibility that HPV will disappear spontaneously. For a detailed examination, a magnifying glass called a colposcope is used to magnify the surface of the cervix, observe the fine details, and collect tissue from the suspected cancerous area. Cervical cancer undergoes a clear process of carcinogenesis, and cancer screening can detect it at the stage of dysplasia (precancerous lesion) before it becomes cancer. The risk of dysplasia progressing to cancer is approximately 3% for mild dysplasia, 10% for moderate dysplasia, and 21% for severe dysplasia. In case of mild or moderate dysplasia, the patient is followed up periodically without treatment, and in the case of severe dysplasia or more, a cervical conical resection is performed.

7.2.3 Staging of Cervical Cancer

The cervix is composed of epithelial cells (squamous cells and glandular cells) that cover the surface and stromal cells inside the epithelial cells, which are separated from each other by the basement membrane. Cervical cancer develops in the epithelial cells through the squamous intraepithelial lesion and remains in the epithelium for a while, but gradually breaks through the basement membrane and enters the stroma. As the cancer progresses, it can spread beyond the cervix into the vaginal wall, parietal tissues of the uterus, pelvic wall, bladder, and rectum, and spread distantly to the lungs and other organs. When cervical cancer is diagnosed, the stage of the cancer is determined based on the depth and spread of the cancer. The stage is important for a treatment plan and is comprehensively determined by referring to the clinical findings obtained from internal examination and ultrasonography, as well as the results of tests, such as colposcopy, cystoscopy, colonoscopy, and urography, as well as rectal and bladder mucosal biopsy. In addition, CT (computed tomography), MRI (magnetic resonance imaging), and PET (positron emission tomography) are used to evaluate the size of the cancer, lymph node metastasis, and distant metastasis when determining the stage. Currently, the International Federation of Gynecology and Obstetrics (FIGO) "FIGO system (2018)" is used for staging [1]. There are four stages: I, II, III, and IV.

7.2.4 Treatment for the Early Stages of Cervical Cancer

The early stages of cervical cancer include intraepithelial carcinoma, where the cancer is confined within the epithelial cells, and microinvasive carcinoma (stage IA), where the cancer is confined to the cervix but has invaded the stroma on a millimeter scale. Most intraepithelial cancers can be cured by cone-shaped resection of the cervix (conization). Hysterectomy is necessary in principle for stage IA cancer that has spread beyond the epithelial cells. In stage IA1, a simple hysterectomy is recommended to remove only the uterus, and in stage IA2, a semi-radical hysterectomy plus pelvic lymph node dissection is recommended to remove a slightly larger area. However, if there is a strong desire for pregnancy in stage IA, cervical conization can be performed in stage IA1. In stage IA2, this surgery can be considered if the conditions are met. If you have a strong desire for pregnancy at another stage, consult your doctor.

7.2.5 Treatment for Advanced Stages of Cervical Cancer

For stage IB, where the cancer has invaded the cervical stroma, and stage II, where the cancer has spread beyond the cervix but has not reached the lower one-third of the vaginal wall or pelvic wall, radical hysterectomy is recommended to

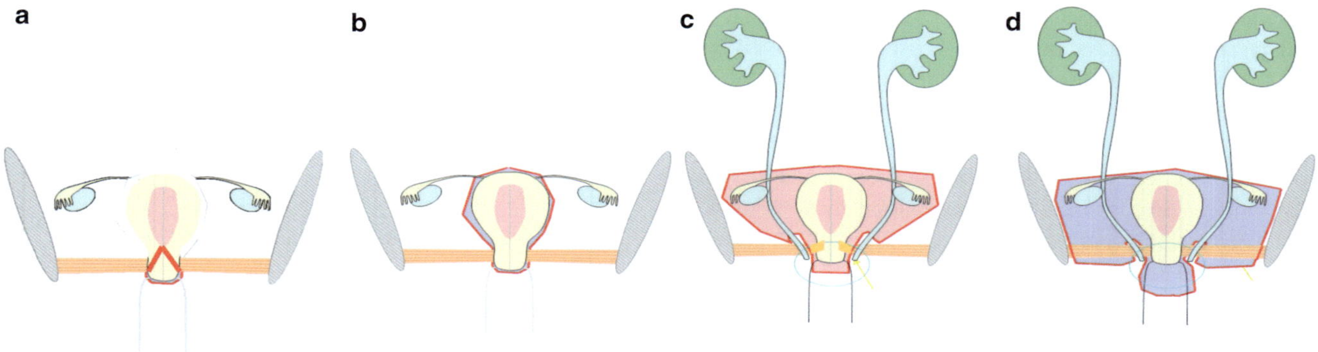

Fig. 7.1 There are four main types of surgery. The procedure chosen depends on the stage. (**a**) Cervical conization is a procedure in which only tissue of the cervix where the cancer is located is removed in a conical shape. In addition to intraepithelial lesions, stage IA1 can be treated. It is also a treatment method for those who wish to become pregnant, and fertility preservation is possible. (**b**) simple hysterectomy is a procedure in which only the uterus is removed by abdominal, vaginal, or laparoscopic resection at the end of the cervical side, between the cervix and surrounding organs such as the bladder, rectum, and ureters. (**c**) Semi-radical or (**d**) radical hysterectomy removes more of the cervix and vagina than a simple hysterectomy. In this method, the ureter is detached up to the point where it enters the bladder, and the uterus as well as the surrounding tissues of the cervix, such as a part of the vagina and the basal ligament that supports the uterus, are widely removed. A lymph node dissection is also performed to check for metastasis. Mainly indicated for stage IB and stage II. Ovaries are decided to be removed based on stage, histology, and age

remove the uterus, surrounding tissue, ovaries, part of the vagina, and lymph nodes. If there is a high risk of postoperative recurrence, or if surgery is not performed, radiation therapy or concurrent chemoradiation may be used. Stage III, where the cancer reaches the lower one-third of the vaginal wall or pelvic wall, can be treated with concurrent chemoradiation or radiation therapy alone. Stage IVB with distant metastasis is treated with chemotherapy.

There are four main types of surgery (Fig. 7.1), and the procedure chosen depends on the stage. In addition to the advanced stage of the cancer, the selection is based on the presence or absence of cancer cells in the conical resection specimen (margins), the presence or absence of vascular invasion (cancer has entered blood vessels or lymph vessels) or metastasis (cancer has spread), and whether the patient wishes to become pregnant.

Cervical conization is a procedure in which only the tissue of the cervix where the cancer is located is removed in a conical shape. In addition to intraepithelial lesions, stage IA1 can be treated. It is also a treatment method for those who wish to become pregnant, and fertility preservation is possible. A simple hysterectomy is a procedure in which only the uterus is removes only the uterus by abdominal, vaginal, or laparoscopic resection, while preserving surrounding organs such as the bladder, rectum, and ureters. A semiradical or radical hysterectomy removes more of the cervix and vagina than a simple hysterectomy. In this method, the ureter is detached up to the point where it enters the bladder, and the uterus, as well as the surrounding tissues of the cervix, such as a part of the vagina and the cardinal/uterosacral ligaments that supports the uterus, are widely removed. A lymph node dissection is also performed to check for metastasis. These procedures are mainly indicated for stage IB and stage II disease. Ovaries are decided to be removed based on stage, histology, and age.

7.2.6 Postoperative Complications

After a radical hysterectomy, disorders related to defecation and urination (constipation, urinary retention, leakage) may occur due to damage to the nerves that regulate rectal and bladder elimination. Edema of the legs and vulva may occur after lymph node dissection. If the bilateral ovaries are removed before menopause, symptoms similar to those seen in menopause, such as hot flashes, sweating, irritability, and headaches, may occur. A decrease in vaginal discharge may also cause problems with intercourse. Please do not hesitate to share any worries or discomfort. Talking with your care team can help.

7.2.7 Radiation Therapy for Cervical Cancer

Radiation can damage the DNA in the nucleus of a cell and stop cell growth. Radiation therapy utilizes this effect to reduce the size of the cancer cells by damaging their DNA. Radiation therapy is an effective treatment for cervical cancer. With the aim of achieving a cure without surgery, radiation therapy is used for stage IB1 and stage IIA1, and concurrent chemoradiation therapy is used for stages IB2 and IIA2, in which chemotherapy (cisplatin administered intravenously once a week, 5–6 times in total) is administered simultaneously with radiation therapy. In addition, if there is a high risk of recurrence after hysterectomy in stage IB and II, radiation therapy or concurrent chemoradiation may be used as postoperative adjuvant therapy. In stage III and IVA, concurrent chemoradiotherapy is the first choice of treatment.

There are two types of irradiation methods: external irradiation, in which radiation is delivered from outside the body through the skin, and intracavitary irradiation, in which an applicator is inserted into the uterus and vagina to deliver a device that gently delivers radiation from inside the uterus or vagina. The combination of both is standard treatment. It is important to complete the treatment within 8 weeks without interruption. Compared to surgery, radiation therapy is less likely to cause complications such as dysuria and sexual dysfunction, but it does not preserve ovarian function and may cause side effects such as dermatitis, mucositis, fatigue, nausea and vomiting, colitis, and cystitis. In stage IB and II, the curative rates of surgery and radiation therapy are almost the same; thus, one should consult with their doctor regarding which to choose.

7.2.8 Chemotherapy for Cervical Cancer

Chemotherapy kills cancer cells by acting on them as they repeatedly divide and multiply. Chemotherapy is used in cases of distant metastasis, when the cancer has recurred in the pelvis and has been treated with radiation therapy in the past, or when the cancer has recurred outside the pelvis. Cisplatin is the most effective treatment for cervical cancer. Currently, the combination of cisplatin and paclitaxel is the standard treatment; however, the combination of carboplatin and paclitaxel is also being used. Since chemotherapy drugs affect healthy cells, they cause a variety of side effects. Hair, mucous membranes of the mouth and gastrointestinal tract, and the bone marrow, which are metabolically active cells, are particularly susceptible to chemotherapeutic damage, resulting in hair loss, mouth ulcers, diarrhea, and bone marrow suppression. If the side effects are severe, a change in the treatment drug or suspension of treatment may be considered. It is important to know the side effects of the treatment and how to deal with them appropriately. If you know in advance what side effects will occur, you can often deal with them and avoid interruption or discontinuation of the treatment. Myelosuppression is a decrease in the number of white blood cells, neutrophils, and platelets. It appears within 1–2 weeks of starting anticancer drugs and requires attention because it increases the risk of infection and anemia. If you have any concerns, consult with your doctor, nurse, or pharmacist. Especially, if you are undergoing outpatient chemotherapy, make sure you have emergency contact information in case your health changes.

7.2.9 Recurrence of Cervical Cancer

Cervical cancer is considered to have recurred when (1) it reappears in the uterus after the cervical cancer has disappeared visually with treatment, or (2) it is confirmed that the cervical cancer cells have spread to other organs and have grown in size. In the case of cervical cancer, 80–90% of recurrences occur within 5 years after treatment. The majority of recurrences are localized in the pelvis; however, it is known that it tends to spread distantly to lymph nodes, lungs, liver, and bones. Therefore, patients should undergo regular checkups and examinations every 1–3 months from the first to third year after treatment, every 6 months until the fifth year, and every year after the sixth year. In case of local recurrence in the pelvis, radiation therapy is performed if the patient has not received radiation therapy. Recurrence of cancer is very hard to cure, and the emphasis is on maintaining a good quality of life. Therefore, systemic chemotherapy and palliative care are provided to alleviate the symptoms of cancer. If you have any concerns or problems, consult with your doctor, nurses, pharmacists, and social workers.

7.2.10 HPV Vaccine

The HPV vaccine prevents infection with the human papillomavirus (HPV) and can prevent the development of cervical cancer. The younger the person, the more likely he or she is to be infected with HPV. Thus, getting the vaccine before having sexual intercourse for the first time is more effective in preventing the development of cervical cancer.

Different HPV vaccines protect against different HPV types.

The bivalent vaccine (16, 18) and quadrivalent vaccine (6, 11, 16, 18) both prevent about 70% of cervical cancer, and the 9-valent vaccine (6, 11, 16, 18, 31, 33, 45, 52, 58) prevents about 90% of cervical cancer. The quadrivalent vaccine and 9-valent vaccine can also prevent condyloma acuminatum.

7.2.11 HPV Vaccination for Males

Since HPV infection is transmitted between men and women, vaccination of both men and women can reduce the spread of the infection. The purpose of vaccination for men is to prevent diseases caused by HPV infection in men themselves, as well as to protect their future partners from developing cervical cancer and other HPV infections by preventing them from becoming the source of infection.

7.2.12 WHO's Approach for the Elimination of Cervical Cancer

WHO has released a global strategy for the elimination of cervical cancer, which outlines three key steps: vaccination, screening, and treatment. If all three steps are successful, the incidence of the disease could be reduced by more than 40% by 2050, resulting in 5 million fewer deaths. The goals by 2030 are (1) to vaccinate 90% of girls up to 15 years old and increase the number of girls vaccinated, (2) to undergo screening for 70% of women by age 35 and again by age 45, and (3) to ensure that 90% of women identified with cervical disease have access to treatment. Cervical cancer is the fourth most common cancer among women in the world, but it is a preventable disease. It is also curable if detected early and treated properly. However, without these steps, the number of new cervical cancer cases per year is projected to increase from 570,000 to 700,000, and the number of deaths is expected to increase from 311,000 to 400,000 between 2018 and 2030. In middle-income countries, the incidence is two times higher, and the mortality rate is three times higher than in high-income countries.

7.3 Cancer of the Uterine Body

7.3.1 Uterine Cancer Basics

It is a cancer that develops in the lining of the uterine body and differs in nature from cervical cancer.

Uterine cancer begins to increase during the late 40s at around menopause and is most common in women in their 50s and 60s. Risk factors for uterine cancer include obesity, excessive estrogen, tamoxifen use, nulliparity, early menarche, late menopause, and Lynch syndrome.

7.3.2 Diagnostic Examination for Uterine Cancer

Symptoms that may raise suspicion of cancer include irregular bleeding that is not during menstruation, disturbance in the cycle or duration of menstruation, increased menstrual flow, postmenopausal bleeding, and watery discharge. At that time, internal examination, palpation, and ultrasonography are used to check the uterus, surrounding swelling, and thickness of the endometrium. First, an examination of the endometrial cells (cytology) is performed. If abnormal cells are found, the endometrium is collected with a special instrument, and the tissue is extracted. If cancer is diagnosed, a pelvic MRI or CT scan will be performed. Tumor markers such as CA125, CA19-9, and CEA are tested.

7.3.3 Staging of Uterine Cancer

The uterine body (uterine wall) is made up of three layers: the endometrium, the myometrium, and the serosa (peritoneum). Cancer of the uterine body originates from the endometrium and gradually penetrates into the myometrium. This is called myometrial invasion. As the myometrial invasion becomes deeper, the probability of metastasis outside the uterus via lymph vessels and blood vessels increases. As the disease progresses, it can spread to the lymph nodes, liver, and lungs. The cancer may also spread from the uterine body to the cervix or vagina and invade the surrounding organs, such as the adnexa (ovaries and fallopian tubes), rectum, and bladder. It can also spread to the bones and brain.

Since it is difficult to accurately diagnose uterine cancer, the pre-surgical stage is estimated by preoperative imaging. Regardless of the stage, surgery is the first choice of treatment for uterine cancer. However, the type of surgery depends on the stage. After the surgery, the cancer stage will be decided again according to the surgical stage. The surgical stage is based on the spread and lymph node metastasis. In addition, the possibility of "risk of postoperative recurrence" is examined. Based on the surgical staging and the risk of postoperative recurrence, we will decide whether additional treatment is needed after the surgery. The surgical stage classification is based on the International Federation of Gynecology and Obstetrics (FIGO) surgical stage classification, which was revised in 2008 [2]. This classification divides the disease into four stages: I, II, III, and IV.

7.3.4 Treatments for Uterine Cancer

Regardless of the stage, surgery is the first choice of treatment for uterine cancer. However, the type of surgery depends on the stage. If the risk of surgery is too high due to old age, serious diabetes or heart disease, severe obesity, or if the cancer has already spread throughout the body and surgery is not expected to be effective, chemotherapy, radiation therapy, or palliative care is recommended. In stage IA and low-risk groups, the patient is observed without any additional treatment, while in stage IB or higher, intermediate-risk, and high-risk groups, chemotherapy and radiation therapy are the standard postoperative treatments.

7.3.5 Surgical Treatment for Uterine Cancer

For early-stage uterine cancer, the uterus, ovaries, and fallopian tubes are removed. In advanced cases, the extent of removal is determined according to the condition of the disease.

In cases with stage I, the standard procedure is a "simple hysterectomy," in which the entire uterus is removed, and a "bilateral adnexal resection," in which both ovaries and fallopian tubes are removed simultaneously. The ovaries and fallopian tubes are removed because uterine cancer tends to metastasize to the ovaries and is often associated with ovarian cancer. For patients who wish to become pregnant, if the cancer is a well-differentiated type of endometrial cancer that is confined to the endometrium among stage IA cancers, the ovaries and fallopian tubes can be left in place, and progestin therapy can be performed. If the cancer is presumed to be a well-differentiated type of endometrial cancer and does not invade the myometrium, the lymph nodes will not be removed, since the possibility of recurrence is low. However, if it is diagnosed as a highly malignant type (serous carcinoma, clear cell carcinoma, or poorly differentiated carcinoma), the pelvic and para-aortic lymph nodes will most likely be removed.

In stage II, where the cancer is presumed to have spread to the cervix, the patient may choose between simple hysterectomy, semi-radical hysterectomy, or radical hysterectomy, depending on the institution. In stage III, where the cancer has spread outside the uterus, and stage IV, where the cancer has invaded or metastasized to other organs and not only the uterus, ovaries, fallopian tubes, and pelvic lymph nodes, but also organs such as the bladder and colon, the connective tissues are removed depending on the location and spread of the cancer. The extent of the surgery is determined according to each patient's condition.

7.3.6 Postoperative Complications

If the ovaries are removed before menopause, the ovaries will no longer produce female hormones, and menopause-like symptoms such as hot flashes, sweating, headaches, palpitations, irritability, osteoporosis, itching, and painful intercourse may occur. If lymph nodes are removed, swelling of the legs and lymphedema may occur. If you notice any of these symptoms, tell your doctor or nurse as soon as possible.

7.3.7 Nonsurgical Treatment for Uterine Cancer

For uterine cancer, chemotherapy and radiation therapy are used as adjuvant therapy after surgery. Patients who are unable to undergo surgery due to old age or chronic illness, or those who are diagnosed as being in the intermediate or high-risk groups, are given chemotherapy or radiation therapy. Progestin therapy is also an option for patients who wish to preserve fertility.

Chemotherapy is used as an adjuvant therapy after surgery for patients diagnosed in the intermediate or high-risk group in the "postoperative recurrence risk," or as treatment for patients who have had a recurrence. Previously, radiation therapy was the main treatment option following surgery; however, in recent years, chemotherapy has become the mainstay of treatment. Currently, the standard treatment is AP therapy, which is a combination of doxorubicin and cisplatin. Paclitaxel and carboplatin are also used as TC therapy.

The side effects of chemotherapy include hypersensitivity reactions (redness and itching of the skin, hives, abdominal pain, breathlessness, coughing, chest pain, back pain, lower back pain, palpitations, irregular heartbeat, changes in blood pressure, and loss of consciousness, among others) that appear within a short time; nausea and vomiting that appear immediately after use to about a week; myelosuppression (decrease in white blood cells, red blood cells, and platelets) that appears within a week to several weeks; fever; decreased kidney and liver function; and hair loss. It is important to discuss these issues with your doctor, nurse, or pharmacist, as they can help reduce the pain by having knowledge and preventive medicines.

Radiation can be delivered externally to the entire pelvis or para-aortic area or vaginally through an instrument.

There are two types of irradiation: intracavitary and external. Intracavitary irradiation is used for early-stage cancer, while external irradiation is mainly used when the cancer has progressed beyond the uterus. Both intracavitary and external beam radiation therapy have a lower pelvic recurrence rate when used as postoperative radiation therapy. The main side effects of radiation therapy include fatigue, lethargy, itching and redness of the skin, and diarrhea. Late side effects, such as gastrointestinal problems, urinary problems, and vaginal problems, may occur years to decades after irradiation.

7.3.8 Recurrence of Uterine Cancer

Recurrence is when the cancer that appeared to be gone returns to a size that can be seen.

Regular checkups are required for at least 5 years. However, even if the cancer appears to be gone, it may recur in the organs or abdominal cavity near the surgically removed uterus, ovaries, or fallopian tubes, or it may spread distantly to distant organs. In most cases, recurrence occurs within 2 years, but there have been cases of recurrence after 5 years or more. Thus, you should discuss the duration of follow-up with your doctor and have regular check-ups for at least 5 years: every 1–3 months until the third year, every 6 months until the fourth or fifth year, and once a year after the sixth year. During follow-up, you will be interviewed and have an internal examination, rectal examination, vaginal cytology, imaging tests, and blood tests. If you experience symptoms such as genital bleeding or lower abdominal pain during the follow-up, please do not wait for the next visit. If recurrence or metastasis is found, the treatment will focus on maintaining the quality of life. In addition to tumor reduction surgery to remove the cancer and alleviate the symptoms, chemotherapy and radiation therapy are used.

7.4 Ovarian Cancer

7.4.1 Ovarian Tumor Basics

Ovaries are organs about the size of a thumb located in the female pelvis. They are located on both sides (left and right) of the uterus and are supported by ligaments in the uterine body. The ovaries are connected to the uterus by the fallopian tubes. Ovarian cancer develops in the epithelium covering the surface of the ovaries and has few symptoms in the early stages. The entirety of the organs below the diaphragm, including the uterus, ovaries, stomach, intestines, and liver, is covered by the peritoneum. Ovarian cancer is similar to cancers that occur in the fallopian tubes and peritoneum, and these cancers are now treated based on the same category. A variety of tumors can develop in the ovaries. Ovarian tumors are classified into three main categories according to the location of the tumor: (1) epithelial tumors, (2) sex cord stromal tumors, and (3) germ cell tumors. The tumors are further divided into (1) benign, (2) borderline malignant (between benign and malignant), and (3) malignant. Epithelial tumors occur most frequently, and about 90% of malignant ovarian tumors are of this type. In general, the term "ovarian cancer" refers to epithelial malignant tumors.

Ovarian cancer is also classified by the "histological type." The four main types are serous carcinoma, endometrioid carcinoma, mucinous carcinoma, and clear cell carcinoma. Serous carcinoma, which is the most common type of ovarian cancer, is divided into high-grade serous carcinoma and less common low-grade serous carcinoma according to cell morphology. Most of the high-grade serous carcinomas start in the fallopian tubes and spread to the ovaries. Peritoneal carcinoma is also a high-grade serous carcinoma and is treated in the same way as ovarian cancer. Clear cell carcinoma and endometrioid carcinomas have been shown to arise from endometriosis.

Chemotherapy is effective for high-grade serous carcinoma, while it is less effective for low-grade serous carcinoma, clear cell carcinoma, and mucinous carcinoma. It is important to know the histological type of your cancer. Genetic factors are strongly associated with about 10% of ovarian cancers. Pathological variants in the *BRCA1* or *BRCA2* genes are more likely to cause ovarian or breast cancer. In addition, there is a high rate of homologous recombination deficiency (HRD) in ovarian cancer. HRD means that one of the main DNA repair systems is not working properly and is sometimes tested for to select chemotherapy agents.

7.4.2 Diagnostic Examination for Ovarian Cancer

Ovarian cancer is difficult to differentiate from benign tumors, so it is diagnosed through laparotomy to remove the tumor, as well as through pathological examination. In general, cancer is suspected when there is a tumor in the ovary. The doctor will also perform an internal examination and blood tests such as CA125. In addition, imaging such as ultrasonography, CT, and MRI are used to check the tumor, how it has spread to the surrounding organs, and whether or not it has metastasized. The stage and histological type of ovarian cancer can only be determined by performing surgery.

7.4.3 Hereditary Breast and Ovarian Cancer Syndrome (HBOC)

The *BRCA1/2* gene pathogenic variant is associated with ovarian cancer. If the presence of this pathological variant is suspected based on past or family history, a blood-based genetic test is performed. Prior counseling is important because it may reveal information that the patient does not want to know.

7.4.4 Staging of Ovarian Cancer

Ovarian cancer is classified into four stages, from stage I to stage IV, depending on how it has spread. Depending on the stage, there are differences in the treatment plan. Therefore, it is very important to know the stage of progression to check the results and effectiveness of treatment (what kind of treatment is given to patients with the same stage of progression and histological type, and how effective it is) and to predict prognosis. In the case of ovarian cancer, the stage of the cancer is determined after surgery and pathological examination of the removed tumor. The International Classification of Stages by the FIGO system is often used to evaluate the spread of ovarian cancer [3]. The stage is assessed from the perspective of (1) whether the cancer has spread to both ovaries, (2) whether the cancer is scattered in the abdomen, and (3) whether the cancer has spread to lymph nodes or other organs. Ovarian cancer is one of the most difficult cancers to detect at an early stage due to the lack of symptoms and the lack of appropriate screening methods. For this reason, more than 40% of ovarian cancers are found in the advanced stages of III and IV.

7.4.5 Treatment for Ovarian Cancer

When ovarian cancer is suspected, surgery is the first step at any stage. This is because it cannot determine whether the ovarian tumor is benign or malignant without pathological examination of the surgically removed tumor. As a result of the intraoperative pathological examination and ascites cytology, if the tumor is benign, the surgery is completed with the removal of the ovary. If the tumor is borderline malignant or malignant, both ovaries and the uterus are removed, as well as the greater omentum, where the spread of ovarian cancer (dissemination) is most likely to occur, which is excised. If the cancer has spread in the abdomen (peritoneal dissemination), tumor reduction surgery is performed to remove as much of the cancer as possible. Ovarian cancer has a better prognosis if less cancer remains. The standard treatment for ovarian cancer is to perform this type of surgery and then add chemotherapy. In the case of stage IA and IB without clear cell carcinoma, the patient will be followed up, but in other cases, chemotherapy will be given. If the cancer is spread in the abdomen and is expected to be left, preoperative chemotherapy (neoadjuvant chemotherapy) is often used to reduce the size of the cancer. Even in cases where neoadjuvant chemotherapy is chosen, tissue samples may be taken through a small incision or by laparoscopic observation of the abdominal cavity to confirm the histological type.

7.4.6 Postoperative Complications

One of the complications after surgery is intestinal obstruction. There is no specific way to prevent or deal with it, but dietary guidance is provided. In contrast, when the ovaries are removed in premenopausal women, estrogen may decrease, causing menopause-like symptoms. Hormone replacement therapy is available. If tumor reduction surgery is performed, a colostomy may be required along with bowel resection. Furthermore, lymph node dissection may cause lymphedema, which is a swelling of the legs. Before the surgery, it is important to check what kind of complications may appear after the surgery.

7.4.7 Adjuvant Therapy After Surgery

Ovarian cancer responds well to chemotherapy and molecular targeted agents. The standard of care for initial chemotherapy is TC therapy, which consists of intravenous injection of two anticancer drugs, namely, paclitaxel and carboplatin, every 3 weeks for 3–6 cycles after surgery, except during the early stages. Dose-dense TC therapy, in which paclitaxel is administered weekly, and carboplatin is infused every 3 weeks for 6–9 cycles, is also a promising option. The combination of TC therapy and bevacizumab, which is a molecular targeted therapy, has been shown to reduce relapse more than TC therapy alone.

Bevacizumab is a molecularly targeted therapy called an angiogenesis inhibitor that suppresses cancer growth by interfering with the formation of new blood vessels that deliver oxygen and nutrients to cancer cells. Bevacizumab is infused once every 3 weeks. Bevacizumab alone should be continued for 16 cycles or longer to reduce recurrence.

If TC therapy is not available, DC therapy, which is a combination of docetaxel and carboplatin, is a candidate. The frequency of chemotherapy, duration of treatment, cost, and side effects that are likely to occur vary depending on the type of therapy, with every treatment method having its own advantages and disadvantages. Depending on your lifestyle, you should consult with your doctor to decide which one to choose. TC therapy is also used for clear cell carcinoma and mucinous carcinoma.

7.4.8 Recurrence and Metastasis of Ovarian Cancer

Stage III and IV ovarian cancer have a high recurrence rate. Even after treatment is completed, follow-up is necessary, and within 2 years, when recurrence is likely, it is done at short intervals of about 1–3 months. In a recurrent or metastasized state, the goal of treatment changes from complete cure to living with the cancer. In the case of recurrence, chemotherapy is used, but the effects are often shorter in duration than the initial chemotherapy, and the side effects tend to be stronger. If you have pain or discomfort in the abdomen or other parts of the body, or if you feel anxious or uncomfortable, tell your doctor or nurse. In recent years, some patients have survived for a long time after recurrence by treatment with bevacizumab and PARP inhibitors.

7.4.9 Chemotherapy After Recurrence or Relapse

Chemotherapy is recommended for the treatment of recurrent ovarian cancer. The treatment depends on the time between the end of the initial treatment and whether the recurrence occurred in less than 6 months or after more than 6 months. If this period is more than 6 months, the chemotherapy is effective, and administration of multidrug chemotherapy, including platinum drugs (such as carboplatin), is recommended. If the side effects of TC therapy are very severe or still strong, the dosage of chemotherapy may be reduced, or the chemotherapy may be switched to another type. If the chemotherapy is effective, PARP inhibitors (olaparib and niraparib) are administered. On the other hand, if the time between the end of the initial chemotherapy and the recurrence is less than 6 months, it is expected that the chemotherapy will not be effective. Since the side effects tend to be more severe with multi-drug chemotherapy, chemotherapy with a single agent is recommended. Candidate agents include liposomal doxorubicin, irinotecan, and gemcitabine. How long to continue chemotherapy after a relapse depends on the effectiveness of the chemotherapy, the patient's age, physical and mental condition, and side effects.

7.4.10 Side Effects of Chemotherapy

Nausea and allergic reactions are more likely to occur during or within 24 h of the chemotherapy, and a decrease in white blood cells and platelets is expected to occur after 1–2 weeks. There are also side effects that appear after 2–4 weeks, such as hair loss and numbness in the hands and legs. The types of side effects, the intensity of symptoms, and the timing of their appearance depend on the agent used and vary from patient to patient. Some people have almost no side effects at all. The development of treatment for the side effects of chemotherapy has been progressing, and they are now much easier to control than before. Do not stop treatment on your own for fear of side effects. The most important things to be aware of in chemotherapy for ovarian cancer are allergic reactions such as rash, shortness of breath, chest tightness, or dizziness, which tend to occur during and immediately after the infusion, and myelosuppression, which is a decrease in white blood cells, red blood cells, and platelets starting 1–2 weeks later. In addition, there is a tendency for peripheral neurological symptoms, such as numbness in the hands and legs, to occur, especially with taxanes such as paclitaxel and docetaxel. If you feel difficulty in buttoning clothes or keep dropping things easily, tell your doctor as soon as possible. Bevacizumab is associated with bleeding from the gums or nose, perforation of the gastrointestinal tract, and thromboembolism. Perforation of the gastrointestinal tract may cause severe abdominal pain and bloody or tarry stools. Olaparib and niraparib often cause gastrointestinal side effects, myelosuppression, and vomiting. There are some side effects that you can handle on your own and some that you should not tolerate, for which you should contact a hospital immediately. If you have any concerns, do not hesitate to ask your doctor, pharmacist, or nurse, and make sure you know how to deal with side effects and when to call the hospital.

Cervical cancer can be eliminated with the combination of the HPV vaccine and screening. Hereditary cancers also exist in the uterine body, and molecular targeted therapy and immune checkpoint inhibitors have been shown to be effective for treatment. Therefore, the treatment of gynecological cancers will change dramatically in the future. Cancer in the uterus and ovaries at a fertile age may prevent pregnancy. Cancer and its treatment may affect marriage, childbirth, and sexual life. If you need help, you can consult with your doctor, nurses, pharmacists, and social workers.

References

1. WHO guideline for screening and treatment of cervical pre-cancer lesions for cervical cancer prevention, second edition. World Health Organization.
2. FIGO staging for carcinoma of the vulva, cervix, and corpus uteri. FIGO committee on gynecologic oncology. Int J Gynaecol Obstet. 2014;125(2):97–8. https://doi.org/10.1016/j.ijgo.2014.02.003. PMID: 24630859.
3. Prat J, FIGO Committee on Gynecologic Oncology. Staging classification for cancer of the ovary, fallopian tube, and peritoneum. Int J Gynaecol Obstet. 2014;124(1):1–5. https://doi.org/10.1016/j.ijgo.2013.10.001. PMID: 24219974.

Breast Cancer

8

Mitsue Saito

Abstract

This chapter delineates the challenges women and men face after being diagnosed with breast cancer. Current knowledge on breast cancer epidemiology, pathology, and types of diagnostic imaging techniques is reviewed, and the types of breast cancer treatment for different subtypes are presented. Special attention is given to introducing what progress has recently been made in the fields of supportive care, palliative care, and survivorship care, including what supportive measures are available in Japan to facilitate cancer patients' continued employment while undergoing treatment and a smooth return to work.

Keywords

Breast cancer · Screening mammography · Supportive care · Survivorship

8.1 Introduction

Breast cancer is the most common cancer among women worldwide. The incidence of this cancer is highest among postmenopausal women in Western countries; however, there is another peak among premenopausal women in Japan (Fig. 8.1). Therefore, balancing cancer treatment and social activities such as work is a challenging issue for women with breast cancer.

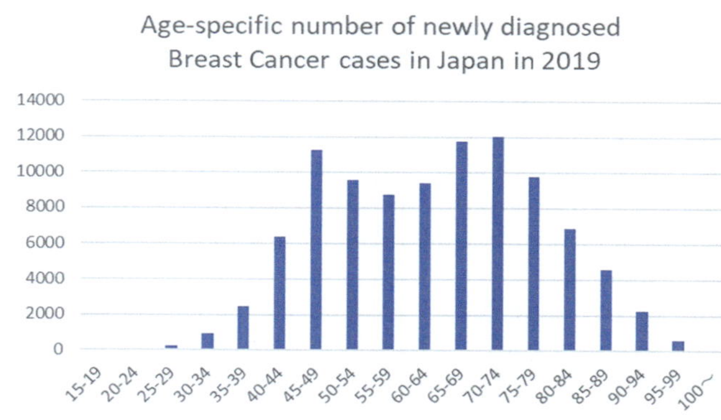

Fig. 8.1 Incidence of breast cancer in 2019 in Japan. (Data shown are from the open database of the National Cancer Center Japan [5]. Note the peak of newly diagnosed cases in the age group 45–49)

8.2 Epidemiology

Not only women but also men might suffer from this disease, although the ratio is about 100 to 1. Risk factors for breast cancer include a family history of breast or ovarian cancer, obesity in postmenopausal women, tall height in premenopausal women, no breastfeeding experience before age 30, habitual alcohol intake, and a history of any benign breast tumor. About 10% of breast cancer patients are diagnosed with hereditary breast and ovarian cancer syndrome (HBOC). (Please see Chap. 3 for more information about HBOC.) The incidence of breast cancer among the

M. Saito (✉)
Department of Breast Oncology, Graduate School of Medicine, Juntendo University Hospital, Bunkyo-ku, Tokyo, Japan
e-mail: mitsue@juntendo.ac.jp

© The Author(s), under exclusive license to Springer Nature Singapore Pte Ltd. 2026
M. Endo et al. (eds.), *Cancer and Work in Asia Volume 2*, https://doi.org/10.1007/978-981-95-6537-5_8

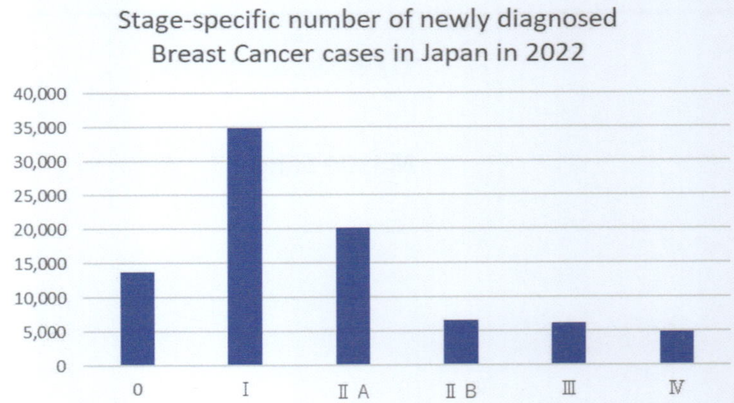

Fig. 8.2 Number of stage-specific newly diagnosed breast cancer cases in 2022 in Japan. (Data shown are from the open database of the National Cancer Center Japan [5])

Ashkenazi Jewish population is reported to be the highest in the world [1]. Among Western women, the incidence of breast cancer is almost 1 in 8; however, it is decreasing gradually. On the other hand, the incidence among Japanese women, which used to be 1 in 25 about 20 years ago, is now 1 in 12 and shows an increasing tendency [2–4]. In fact, 97,142 women were newly diagnosed with breast cancer in 2019 in Japan [5].

Mammography (MMG) is the most common breast cancer screening test among Western countries, where over 65% of women are reported to be actively utilizing MMG for early detection of breast cancer [6]. On the other hand, the level of breast cancer screening awareness has been low in Asia. Recently, things are changing gradually, and the most common newly diagnosed breast cancer has become stage I in Japan (Fig. 8.2).

8.3 Anatomy and Cancer

Most women have two mammary glands in their breasts; however, some of them have one more tiny pair in their axillae or more in their abdomen, including the inguinal lesions, called accessory mammary glands. In each mammary gland in the female breast, there are about 15 ducts open at the nipple, and each duct leads to lobules, which can produce milk associated with pregnancy. The areola is the colored area around the nipple. Fat and connective fibrous tissue is contained in between each lobule and duct. Between the skin and lobules there is a strong fibrous connective tissue called the Cooper ligament. Behind the mammary glands, there are pectoral muscles, each covered with their fascia. The anatomy of the breast is schematically depicted in Fig. 8.3.

The majority of breast cancers arise from a duct-epithelial cell, which is part of the inner wall of the milk duct. The damage imposed by inflammation or trauma on such a duct-epithelial cell could trigger the initiation of cell proliferation, although cell growth in terms of organogenesis is completed in adults, except for the period of pregnancy. Usually, self-repair systems are in place to recover from those damages; however, in the case of cancer, the self-repair cell proliferation continues as long as the host is alive. This proliferation continues inside the milk duct until the duct wall becomes ruptured and some cells invade into the interstitial connective tissues via the joints of the external wall of the milk duct, which consists of myoepithelial cells. Before this rupture, the diagnosis of this pathology is ductal carcinoma in situ and stage 0, from which metastasis does not occur theoretically if the whole structure of proliferated cells can be removed completely. Once cancer cells invade the tissue outside of the milk duct, the pathological diagnosis becomes invasive cancer and the stage changes to I, II, or III depending on the tumor size and the nodal status. Further, there is a possibility that metastasis has already started via lymphatic vessels or blood vessels, therefore systemic drug therapy is recommended to prevent macroscopical distant metastasis to other organs, such as bone, lung, and liver. Before distant metastasis, most of the breast cancer cells metastasize to the nearest axillary lymph nodes first; therefore, the nodal status is included for staging.

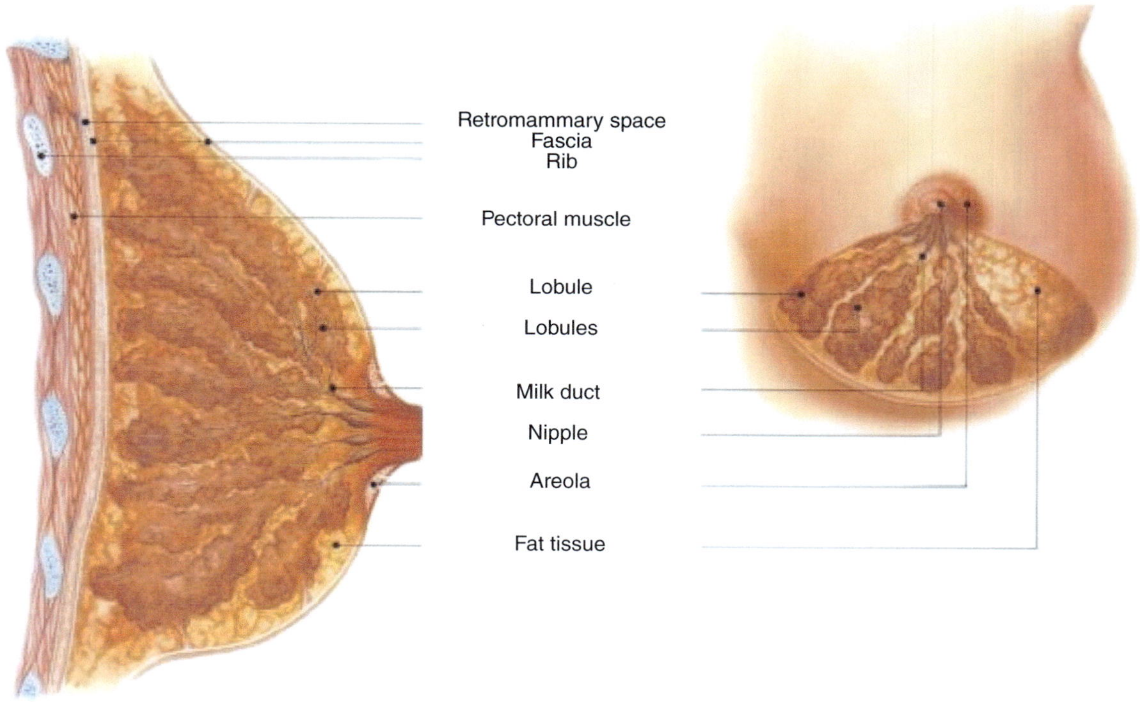

Fig. 8.3 Anatomy of the breast and mammary glands. (Permission to reuse this scheme was obtained from AstraZeneca and from Dr. Fujio Kasumi, who created the original schema)

8.4 Diagnostic Imaging

For breast cancer screening, MMG is recommended for women aged 50 or older. However, cancer incidence between ages 40 and 50 is very high, especially among Japanese women, so the combination of MMG with ultrasound (US) examination is common among Japanese for screening based on a nationwide study called J-START [7]. Under the age of 50, the breast is denser than in aged women because it contains more glands than fat tissue. Glands appear white in MMG, and cancer also appears white (Fig. 8.4). Therefore, contrast between the cancer and the background is not evident if the breast is dense. On the other hand, the cancer's white appearance is easier to be identified against a background of more fat tissue, which appears black in MMG. In contrast to MMG, most cancers look black in US, and glands appear white, so that even among young women or women with dense breasts, cancer is easily detectable by US (Fig. 8.4). However, the reason why screening MMG is more often recommended is the high detection capability of fine calcifications, which could be the only early sign of highly malignant cancer necrotic tissues, mainly in the cancer nest within the milk duct. In MMG the calcifications always appear as bright white spots, providing a good contrast even in the dense breast. On the contrary, they are usually masked by the background noise of US, which appears as white spots on ultrasound.

Once cancer is diagnosed by biopsy, enhanced magnetic resonance imaging (MRI) is useful to identify the area of cancer more precisely than is possible by MMG and US. However, the shortcomings of MRI are false positivity, possible allergic reaction to contrast agents, and a higher cost compared to MMG and US, depending on regional reimbursement policies.

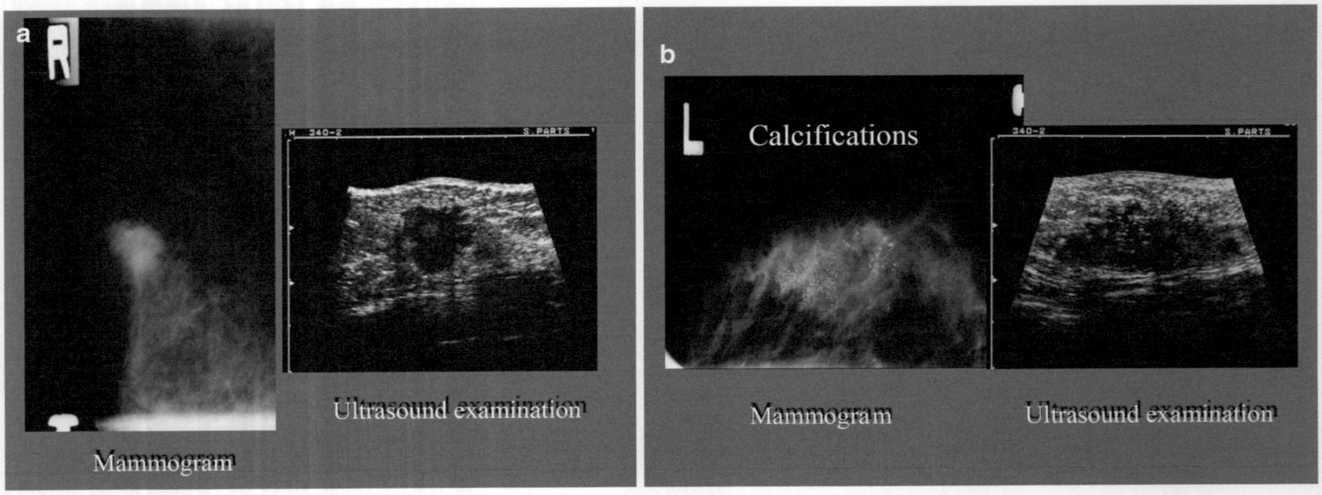

Fig. 8.4 Imaging techniques used in breast cancer screening. (**a**) Images of a breast tumor as visualized by mammography and ultrasound examination. In the mammogram the tumor appears white, while on ultrasound it appears black. (**b**) Images of calcifications in the breast as visualized by mammography and ultrasound examination. In the mammogram calcifications appear as bright white dots; they appear white also on ultrasound. Permission to publish the images used in this figure was obtained from the patient

8.5 Pathology

A definite diagnosis is obtained by pathological examination of a tissue specimen. Core needle biopsy (CNB) is commonly performed for a lump or abnormal findings detected by US under local anesthesia. If the lesion is too small to do CNB, vacuum-assisted biopsy (VAB) is recommended. Stereotactic VAB under MMG is performed if calcifications by MMG are the only abnormal finding. Pathology allows not only to make a differential diagnosis between cancer and a benign tumor but also to diagnose the subtype of cancer, which is required for determining the most suitable drug therapy regimen. For swollen axillary lymph nodes, fine needle aspiration biopsy cytology (FNA) is recommended. FNA cannot be used to make a definite diagnosis for any breast lump; however, the accuracy of FNA diagnosis for lymph nodes is almost as high as CNB. The samples from FNA look like several small pieces of a jigsaw puzzle. It is very difficult to tell a whole picture by such small pieces of breast cancer since the background of breast tissues consists of fibrous tissues, fat tissues, and the normal breast epithelium the cancer cell originated from, and each normal epithelial cell sometimes looks similar to malignant epithelial cells. In contrast, cancer cells in lymph nodes are easily identifiable because they are so different from the bulk of lymphocytes present in lymph nodes.

After breast surgery, the specimen is extensively examined by pathologists, and the results are reported to the attending surgeons, usually within a month. Diagnosis, pathological staging, cancer subtype according to immunohistochemical findings, and chemotherapeutic efficacy, if the patient underwent chemotherapy prior to surgery, are described in a report.

Sometimes immediate pathological diagnosis is required during surgery for surgical margin and sentinel node biopsy, which is a useful procedure to avoid overinvasiveness for breast or axilla. Examples of tumor specimens that have been prepared for pathological examination are shown in Fig. 8.5.

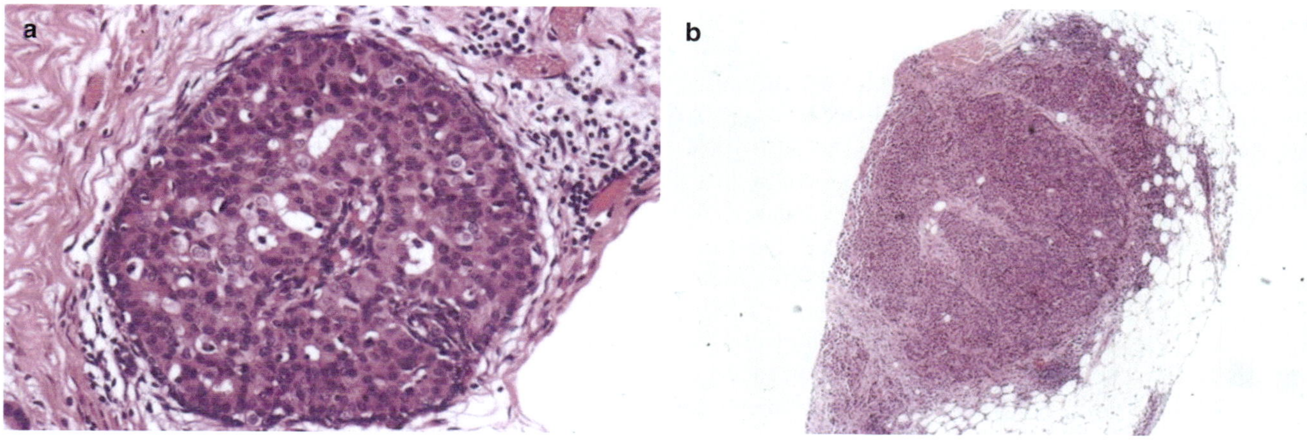

Fig. 8.5 Pathological examination of core needle biopsy specimens stained with hematoxylin-eosin. (**a**) Microscopical findings of ductal carcinoma in situ (DCIS). A cross-section of a duct with DCIS. Blue dots outside of the duct are lymphatic cells infiltrating the tissue surrounding the tumor. (**b**) Microscopical findings of invasive ductal carcinoma. Cancer cells invade in between fat cells whose color is white. Permission to publish the images used in this figure was obtained from the patient

8.6 Treatment

8.6.1 Surgery

If the area of cancer seems to be localized within a quarter of the whole breast by diagnostic imaging, partial mastectomy can be selected. On the other hand, if the area seems to be larger than a quadrant, mastectomy is recommended. After partial mastectomy, radiation for residual ipsilateral breast is highly recommended to prevent local recurrence. After mastectomy, if four or more axillary lymph nodes are positive for cancer, radiation for the chest wall with supraclavicular lymph nodes is highly recommended to prevent not only local recurrence but also distant metastasis. This irradiation is called postmastectomy radiation therapy (PMRT). For partial mastectomy, the breast is repaired by using residual own breast tissue. In the case of mastectomy, reconstruction surgery using an implant, which is only indicated for the non-irradiated area, or autologous tissues, whether or not the overlayed skin of the breast is irradiated, such as the latissimus dorsi muscle flap or the free transverse rectus abdominis myocutaneous flap (TRAM), could be considered with the plastic surgeons' advice. The type of reconstruction surgery ultimately depends on the patient's physical conditions, life plans, and preferences, such as comorbidities, allergies, and the desire for having children.

Mastectomy does not reduce the patient's activities of daily living (ADL). On the other hand, axillary dissection limits ADL and induces lymphedema of the ipsilateral arm. Therefore, modification of axillary dissection has been promoted. Sentinel node biopsy navigated by a locally injected radioisotope with or without blue dye for macroscopically node-negative cases is indicated to avoid axillary dissection. If the sentinel node is negative for cancer or positive, but with very limited volume or number, such as 2 mm or less according to immediate pathology during operation or prior to breast surgery, axillary dissection is not recommended.

Surgery for breast cancer takes less than 2 h, and tissue expander placement, which is the preparation for reconstruction surgery by implant, also takes less than 2 h. TRAM takes several hours. Surgeries for breast cancer require general anesthesia and hospitalization, which can range from a couple of days for minimal ones, such as partial mastectomy with or without sentinel lymph node biopsy, to a 1-week hospitalization for surgeries requiring drains, such as mastectomy or axillary dissection, plus one additional hospitalization if reconstruction surgery is performed simultaneously.

8.6.2 Radiation

As described above, after partial mastectomy and mastectomy for locally advanced cancer, irradiation to the breast or chest wall plus supraclavicular lymph nodes (PMRT) is highly recommended. For partial mastectomy cases, axillary dissection is avoidable if the irradiation field is extended to the axillary area, even if the sentinel node is positive for cancer, as the residual breast is scheduled to be irradiated at the same time. Each irradiation procedure takes less than 2 min, and between 16 and 25 irradiation procedures are required in total. The major side effects are a sunburn-like dermatitis in the acute phase and radiation pneumonitis, characterized by a dry cough after several months. The former one is very common but not severe, and moisturizer is recommended. The latter one occurs in around 5% of patients, and some need to be treated with medication, including steroids.

8.6.3 Drug Therapies

For stage II, III, and partially stage I with an indication of chemotherapy, preoperative chemotherapy (NAC: neoadjuvant chemotherapy) is usually recommended because of several reasons. One reason is that there is a possibility that a less invasive surgery can be performed if the response to the drug is good. Another reason is that the response to chemotherapy can be evaluated objectively only before surgery according to the changes in the size of the tumor or swollen lymph nodes and the final assessment by pathology of a surgical specimen. The latter leads to a new strategy called response-adapted postoperative drug therapy, whereby the postoperative drug therapy regimen is determined based on the pathological response to NAC, such as capecitabine or TS-1 added to standard treatment. For most of stage I and the biologically moderate stage II, surgery is the first line of treatment. Then, according to the pathological diagnosis of the surgical specimen, the drug therapy regimen is proposed based upon clinical guidelines; however, the final decision is made after shared discussion among the physician, other medical staffs, and the patient together with the family or caregiver.

The classically recommended chemotherapy regimen for stage I, II, and III is once per 3 weeks, repeated for a total of 4 times, with an anthracycline-containing regimen such as EC (epirubicin plus cyclophosphamide) followed by taxane, which includes 4 times 3 weekly docetaxel or once a week for 12 weeks with paclitaxel. All of them are administered by intravenous drip infusion. The chemotherapy regimen for NAC used to be the same as that for chemotherapy after surgery, and the overall survival rate has been the same irrespective of the timing, such as before or after surgery. However, in order to improve the complete response rate of NAC, dose-dense EC, which is an every-other-week EC administered 4 times together with G-CSF to avoid bone marrow suppression, followed by an every-other-week paclitaxel administered 4 times together with G-CSF, has become the standard therapy regimen. This type of NAC has an influence on postoperative chemotherapy, so biweekly chemotherapy is becoming common recently.

For HER2-type breast cancer, taxane is administered with anti-HER2 therapy such as trastuzumab when the lymph node was negative, and trastuzumab plus pertuzumab when the lymph node was positive for cancer. After those combination drug therapies and after surgery, only anti-HER2 therapy is recommended to be continued until the total administration duration reaches one year. Only when preoperative drug therapy is not effective, trastuzumab emtansine (T-DM1), which is an antibody-drug conjugate, is another option for adjuvant therapy.

Triple-negative breast cancer (TNBC) is an aggressive breast cancer with historically poor outcomes, primarily due to the lack of effectively targeted therapies. Neoadjuvant anthracycline and taxane-based chemotherapy remain the standard of care for early-stage TNBC. The addition of carboplatin to an anthracycline, cyclophosphamide, and taxane (ACT) regimen is associated with improved complete pathologic response (pCR) for advanced cancer. Immune checkpoint inhibitor (ICI) combinations with carboplatin and paclitaxel followed by AC significantly increase pCR also in advanced TNBC. Other targets, such as poly-ADP-ribosyl polymerase inhibitors (PARPi), are being evaluated in the neoadjuvant setting if the patient has BRCA1/2 germline mutations.

On the other hand, for luminal-type endocrine therapy using tamoxifen, if the patient is a premenopausal woman or a man, an aromatase inhibitor (AI) is used if the female patient is 5 or 10 years past menopause, depending on the recurrence risk. Recently, a combination of endocrine therapy and 2-year abemaciclib, which is a CDK4/6 inhibitor, has been approved for advanced luminal breast cancer as an adjuvant.

Medicines prescribed for endocrine therapy come in the form of tablets. The cure rate for stage 0 is theoretically 100%; even stage II shows almost 90%, while stage III goes down to less than 70%. A summary of indications for drug therapy and surgery depending on the breast cancer stage is shown in Table 8.1. Indications for drug therapies depending on the breast cancer subtype are summarized in Table 8.2.

If the patient has distant metastasis after surgery or the stage of the patient is stage IV, meaning the patient was diagnosed with breast cancer that metastasized to distant organs, such as bone, lung, or liver, the recommended treatment is basically continuous drug therapy according to subtype until the cancer becomes resistant, where the therapy will be continued for as long as the side effects are acceptable. Surgery for stage IV breast cancer is not necessary, because the most lethal site is not the breast but the distant organ, and a drug therapy that is effective for the metastatic lesion works for the primary cancer in the breast as well. Surgery for breast

Table 8.1 Indications for drug therapy and surgery depending on breast cancer stage

Stage	Stage 0	Stage I, II, III	Stage IV
Characteristics	Non-invasive carcinoma	Invasive carcinoma (Stage I: tumor smaller than 2 cm; Stage II: tumor 2–5 cm or presence of lymph node metastasis; Stage III: tumor larger than 5 cm)	With metastasis (bone/lung/liver)
Drug therapy	No	Yes	Yes
Surgery (+/− radiation)	Yes	Yes	No

Table 8.2 Indications for drug therapy regimens depending on breast cancer subtype

Subtype	Luminal	Luminal HER2	HER2	Triple-negative
ER	+	+	–	–
HER2	–	+	+	–
Drug therapy	Endocrine	Endocrine Anti-HER2 Chemotherapy	Anti-HER2 Chemotherapy	Chemotherapy (immune checkpoint inhibitor)

Drug therapy is administered to stage I, II, or III patients before or after surgery
ER estrogen receptor, *HER2* human epidermal growth factor receptor 2

cancer is indicated only for locally advanced cancer, which may cause symptoms like pain, bleeding, or infection sooner or later. However, if the tumor invades deeper into the chest wall or skin invasion is too extensive to be safely resected, surgery is not an option, but drug therapy is indicated, and irradiation is an option. Since, unfortunately, the cure rate for metastatic breast cancer is somewhere around 5%, the purpose of the treatment is extending the patient's life span and/or reducing the volume of cancer to relieve symptoms such as pain and dyspnea.

Owing to the development of new medicines, including molecular-targeted therapies such as mTOR inhibitors and CDK4/6 inhibitors for luminal-type breast cancer, trastuzumab deruxtecan (T-DXd), an antibody-drug conjugate for HER2-type breast cancer, PARP inhibitors for HBOC, and immune checkpoint inhibitors for a subgroup of triple-negative breast cancer, the overall survival rate for metastatic breast cancer is continuously getting better. As of the year 2000, the 5-year survival rate was almost 50% at MD Anderson Cancer Center.

8.7 Supportive Care

During anticancer therapy, patients are suffering not only from cancer but also from the side effects of anticancer therapies. Supportive care is aimed at relieving those side effects and the symptoms of cancer. There can be numerous side effects, and each patient's experience is different from others. They include nausea, vomiting, mucositis, dermatitis, diarrhea, constipation, loss of appetite, neuropathy, bone marrow suppression, pneumonitis, lymphedema, osteoporosis or bone fracture, cognitive dysfunction, fatigue, loss of fertility, hand and foot syndrome, dysguesia, delirium, asthenia, appearance changes such as alopecia, pigmentation, distortion of body image, and financial difficulties.

In the past, the improvement of cancer therapy to reduce the tumor size or extend the survival time used to be the top priority for oncologists, and supportive care trailed behind as the second priority, receiving insufficient attention. Fortunately, the mindset is changing, and it is increasingly being recognized that supportive care needs to be included in cancer therapy, as cancer treatment cannot be successful without considering the patients' quality of life. Recently, international and domestic guidelines for supportive care in cancer are being developed and updated accordingly [8–10], so that patients who are suffering from the side effects of cancer therapy or people who are worried about cancer therapy can be sure to receive guideline-based support and care from doctors, nurses, and pharmacists.

8.8 Palliative Care

The definition of palliative care is similar to supportive care; however, usually palliative care means the care for symptoms of cancer itself, such as pain, dyspnea, palpitation, fatigue, loss of appetite, insomnia, anxiety, numbness, dysesthesia, dizziness, edema, and so on. Although palliative care used to be provided after a series of chemotherapy was finished in the terminal stage of cancer, nowadays seamless palliative care is recommended for the period from the diagnosis of cancer through the end of life. Cancer pain is called "total pain," which consists of physical, mental, social, and spiritual pain, according to Cicely Saunders [11, 12]. Not only physical pain, but also all other pains need to be assessed and cared for.

Currently, cancer can be cured if the stage is early and/or cancer cells are vulnerable to the anticancer drugs applied. Particularly, the prognosis of breast cancer is getting better and better due to early detection by screening and the development of tailor-made drug therapy. However, once distant metastasis in bone, lung, or liver has developed, most patients have to live their lives with cancer until the end. Should you encounter a patient who is not only suffering from cancer but also from total pain without receiving sufficient palliative care, please advise her/him/them to ask the nearest medical professionals who are willing to help at the help desk of a hub hospital of cancer treatment. Physicians, nurses, pharmacists, medical social workers, psychologists, psychiatrists, and other professionals are ready to be involved with those patients.

8.9 Cancer Board

It is not an easy task to help decision-making to select the best treatment for each patient when the balance between benefit and harm is uncertain. Nevertheless, the diversity of patient preferences, conditions, ages, stages, comorbidities, family backgrounds, and socioeconomical situations are all important for medical professionals. Recommended treatment according to clinical practice guidelines sometimes needs to be modified, considering the patient's preferences and circumstances. Most physicians working in the division of oncology in a university hospital, cancer center, or general hospital have their own cancer board, which holds multidisciplinary meetings to discuss treatment recommendations for every patient. The goal of having a cancer board is to realize shared decision-making with every patient.

8.10 Survivorship

8.10.1 Appearance Care

Breast cancer patients are concerned about the changes in their appearance during and after cancer treatments. Therefore, appearance care is very important after mastectomy, and new knowledge and skills need to be acquired to lessen the burden of hair loss, changes in nails, skin texture, or complexion. Not only female patients but also male patients care about cosmesis, because they also lose their nipples, hair, eyelashes, and eyebrows without having adequate skills to utilize makeup techniques. Socioestheticians, nurses, plastic surgeons, and dermatologists are the professionals who are specialized in appearance care, and they are ready to support every patient.

8.10.2 Return to Work

The distress cancer sufferers feel when they lose their role in society or at home and the difficulties they experience when they lose their job and income are categorized into social pain, which is one of the 4 elements of "total pain" advocated by Cicely Saunders [12]. Securing employment while undergoing breast cancer treatment and returning to work after breast cancer treatment, including surgery and chemotherapy, are important components of cancer survivorship for individual rehabilitation and economic development. Particularly for premenopausal breast cancer survivors, a successful return to work is highly desirable, but it requires adequate support both from the healthcare sector and the workplace. Research on the factors that affect rehabilitation and the effectiveness of return-to-work interventions is beginning to gain momentum also in Asia [13–15]. It has been recognized that effective communication between the patient, the workplace, and the healthcare provider is the cornerstone of a successful rehabilitation and return to work [16]. In line with this, the Japanese government developed a guideline called "Guidelines for Balancing Treatment and Work Support in the Workplace" for companies to support cancer patients in 2016 [17] and started a financial support scheme for hospitals under which information can be exchanged with each patient's workplace with the permission of the patient. Also, the Japanese national health insurance started to cover the cost of such communications between physicians and companies in 2021 [18]. It is hoped that these supportive measures will facilitate cancer patients' continued employment while undergoing cancer treatment.

Fertility

Please refer to Chap. 23.

Genetics

In this textbook, please see Chap. 3.

Acknowledgement We would like to express our sincere appreciation to Dr. Katrin Ishii Shrade.

References

1. Dafni U, Tsourti Z, Alatsathianos I. Breast cancer statistics in the European Union: incidence and survival across European countries. Breast Care (Basel). 2019;14(6):344–53. https://doi.org/10.1159/000503219.
2. Liu L, Zhang J, Wu AH, Pike MC, Deapen D. Invasive breast cancer incidence trends by detailed race/ethnicity and age. Int J Cancer. 2012;130(2):395–404. https://doi.org/10.1002/ijc.26004.
3. Sung H, Rosenberg PS, Chen WQ, Hartman M, Lim WY, Chia KS, et al. Female breast cancer incidence among Asian and Western populations: more similar than expected. J Natl Cancer Inst. 2015;107(7):djv107. https://doi.org/10.1093/jnci/djv107.
4. Lei S, Zheng R, Zhang S, Wang S, Chen R, Sun K, et al. Global patterns of breast cancer incidence and mortality: a population-based cancer registry data analysis from 2000 to 2020. Cancer Commun (Lond). 2021;41(11):1183–94. https://doi.org/10.1002/cac2.12207.
5. National Cancer Center of Japan. Cancer incidence NCR (2016–2019). cancer_incidenceNCR (2016–9). https://view.officeapps.live.com/op/view.aspx?src=https%3A%2F%2Fganjoho.jp%2Freg_stat%2Fstatistics%2Fdata%2Fdl%2Fexcel%2Fpref_cancer_incidenceNCR(-9).xls&wdOrigin=BROWSELINK. Available from: https://ganjoho.jp/reg_stat/statistics/stat/summary.htm. Last accessed 31 May 2024. In Japanese.
6. Tavakoli B, Feizi A, Zamani-Alavijeh F, Shahnazi H. Factors influencing breast cancer screening practices among women worldwide: a systematic review of observational and qualitative studies. BMC Womens Health. 2024;24(1):268. https://doi.org/10.1186/s12905-024-03096-x.

7. Ohuchi N, Suzuki A, Sobue T, Kawai M, Yamamoto S, Zheng YF, et al. Sensitivity and specificity of mammography and adjunctive ultrasonography to screen for breast cancer in the Japan Strategic Anti-cancer Randomized Trial (J-START): a randomised controlled trial. Lancet. 2016;387(10016):341–8. https://doi.org/10.1016/S0140-6736(15)00774-6.
8. American Society of Clinical Oncology. Supportive Care and Treatment Related issues. Available from: https://old-prod.asco.org/practice-patients/guidelines/supportive-care-and-treatment-related-issues. Last assessed 19 Jan 2024.
9. Multinational Association for Supportive Care in Cancer. Every patient with cancer needs supportive care. Available from: https://mascc.org. Last accessed 19 Jan 2024.
10. European Society for Medical Oncology. ESMO Clinical Practice Guidelines: Supportive and Palliative Care. Available from: https://www.esmo.org/guidelines/guidelines-by-topic/esmo-clinical-practiceguidelines-supportive-and-palliative-care. Last accessed 19 Jan 2024.
11. Clark D. 'Total pain', disciplinary power and the body in the work of Cicely Saunders, 1958–1967. Soc Sci Med. 1999;49(6):727–36. https://doi.org/10.1016/s0277-9536(99)00098-2.
12. Saunders C. The treatment of intractable pain in terminal cancer. Proc R Soc Med. 1963;56(3):195–7.
13. Sohn KJ, Park SY, Kim S. A scoping review of return to work decision-making and experiences of breast cancer survivors in Korea. Support Care Cancer. 2021;29(4):1741–51. https://doi.org/10.1007/s00520-020-05817-y.
14. Sun Y, Shigaki CL, Armer JM. Return to work among breast cancer survivors: a literature review. Support Care Cancer. 2017;25(3):709–18. https://doi.org/10.1007/s00520-016-3446-1.
15. Akezaki Y, Nakata E, Kikuuchi M, Tominaga R, Kurokawa H, Hamada M, et al. Factors associated with return to work of breast cancer patients following axillary lymph node dissection. Work. 2021;70(1):271–7. https://doi.org/10.3233/WOR213571.
16. Saito N, Takahashi M, Sairenchi T, Muto T. The impact of breast cancer on employment among Japanese women. J Occup Health. 2014;56(1):49–55. https://doi.org/10.1539/joh.13-0140-oa.
17. Ministry of Health Labor and Welfare Japan. Guidelines for balancing treatment and work support in the workplace. March 2024 edition. Available from: https://www.mhlw.go.jp/content/11200000/001225327.pdf. Last accessed 31 May 2024. In Japanese.
18. Ministry of Health Labor and Welfare Japan. Treatment and work at the workplace – Guidelines for supporting work-life balance. Available from: https://chiryoutoshigoto.mhlw.go.jp/guideline/. Last accessed 31 May 2024. In Japanese.

Gastric Cancer

9

Mikiko Sakuraya and Naoki Hiki

Abstract

Loss of muscle mass after gastrectomy has a negative impact on the continuation of S-1 adjuvant chemotherapy and may also affect prognosis, but various oral nutritional supplements (ONS) have been administered to patients after gastrectomy to prevent muscle loss. However, there are problems with compliance, and the efficacy of ONS is poor. We will discuss the problems of amino acid administration after gastrectomy and examine methods for effectively administering amino acids after gastrectomy.

Keywords

Branched-chain amino acids · Gastric cancer · Muscle loss · Weight loss · Nutrition therapy · Surgery

9.1 Introduction

Gastric cancer remains one of the most prevalent malignancies in Asia, with particularly high incidence rates in Japan, South Korea, and China. According to GLOBOCAN data, gastric cancer ranks as the fifth most common cancer worldwide and the fourth leading cause of cancer-related death, with the majority of cases occurring in East Asia.

The primary risk factors for gastric cancer include *Helicobacter pylori* (*H. pylori*) infection, which is responsible for the majority of non-cardia gastric cancers. Additional risk factors include a high-salt diet, consumption of smoked or processed foods, low intake of fresh fruits and vegetables, smoking, and a family history of gastric cancer. Chronic atrophic gastritis and intestinal metaplasia are recognized as precancerous conditions. Notably, many of these risk factors are modifiable, underscoring the importance of workplace health promotion, dietary education, and screening programs—particularly in high-risk Asian populations.

Early detection through endoscopic screening, as widely practiced in Japan and South Korea, has significantly improved survival outcomes. Curative surgical resection (gastrectomy) remains the cornerstone of treatment for resectable gastric cancer, and understanding the nutritional consequences of gastrectomy is essential for supporting patients in maintaining their quality of life and work capacity after surgery.

Loss of muscle mass after gastrectomy has a negative impact on the continuation of S-1 adjuvant chemotherapy and may also affect prognosis, but various oral nutritional supplements (ONS) have been administered to the patients after gastrectomy to prevent muscle loss. However, there are problems with compliance, and the efficacy of ONS is poor. We will discuss the problems of amino acid administration after gastrectomy for gastric cancer.

9.2 Loss of Muscle Mass After Gastrectomy and Its Effects

After a gastrectomy, the function of storing, stirring, and digesting food decreases, and appetite decreases due to the loss of ghrelin. Therefore, even if oral intake is started from an early stage after gastrectomy, it is difficult to orally ingest a sufficient amount. In 2011, Abdiev et al. reported on changes in body weight and muscle mass after gastrectomy. They measured body composition using Bioelectrical Impedance Analysis (BIA) and reported that body weight decreased by 10–20% and muscle mass decreased by 10–15% by 3 months after surgery [1]. Loss of lean body mass after gastrectomy may affect the continuation of S-1 adjuvant chemotherapy, and in particular, it has been reported that a loss of 5% of lean body mass (LBM) within 1 month after gastrectomy poses a risk of it [2, 3]. On the other hand, it has been reported that among elderly patients with Stage I gastric cancer after curative gastrectomy, postoperative early

M. Sakuraya · N. Hiki (✉)
Department of Upper Gastrointestinal Surgery, Kitasato University School of Medicine, Sagamihara, Kanagawa, Japan
e-mail: sakuraya.mikiko@kitasato-u.ac.jp; nhiki@med.kitasato-u.ac.jp

© The Author(s), under exclusive license to Springer Nature Singapore Pte Ltd. 2026

M. Endo et al. (eds.), *Cancer and Work in Asia Volume 2*, https://doi.org/10.1007/978-981-95-6537-5_9

mortality was high, and deaths from other diseases were frequently observed [4]. Elderly people may experience a loss of muscle mass as a result of the aging process [5], and curative gastrectomy may result in further loss of muscle mass. Furthermore, it has been reported that sarcopenia with loss of muscle mass is a risk factor for death from other diseases in patients with gastrectomy for gastric cancer [6], and loss of muscle mass may be a contributing factor to death from other diseases. Therefore, sustaining muscle mass is an important goal in the perioperative management of patients who are undergoing gastrectomy.

9.3 Effectiveness of Amino Acid Administration

Nutrition is one of the interventions to sustain body weight and muscle mass after gastrectomy. Branched-chain amino acids (BCAAs) have been reported to be effective in increasing muscle mass and improving muscle strength in patients with primary sarcopenia [7], and were one of the candidates for improving muscle metabolism in postoperative patients [8, 9]. Marta et al. planned a prospective randomized controlled trial in which 5.2 g of BCAA was administered for 12 weeks to sarcopenia patients with liver cirrhosis and reported that muscle mass increased significantly in the intervention group [10]. In addition, during hospitalization after gastrectomy, amino acids were administered by combining forced feeding with Parenteral Peripheral Nutrition (PPN) and oral intake of enteral nutrition. It was reported that body weight loss on the seventh day and 1 month after gastrectomy, and muscle mass loss on the seventh day after gastrectomy were improved [11]. There are no reports of multicenter randomized controlled trials, and it is unclear whether amino acid administration is effective for weight loss and muscle mass loss after gastrectomy.

9.4 Amino Acid Content of Enteral Nutrition (Elental®) and Clinical Challenges

Imamura et al. planned a prospective randomized controlled trial in which 300 kcal of an enteral nutritional supplement (Elental®) was administered for 6–8 weeks after surgery for gastric cancer in addition to regular meals. It was reported that weight loss after 6–8 weeks was significantly suppressed (intervention group: 4.86 ± 3.72%, control group: 6.60 ± 4.90%, P = 0.047). In particular, the rate of weight loss was even lower in cases of total gastrectomy (intervention group: 5.03 ± 3.65%, control group: 9.13 ± 5.43%, P = 0.012) [12], and weight loss was significantly suppressed up to 1 year after surgery (intervention group: 9.66 ± 5.98%, control group: 15.11 ± 6.78%, P = 0.015, average value) [13]. One packet (80 g) of Elental® contains 14.1 g of amino acids (2.24 g of BCAA), and the intake rate was 81.2% (median), which is good compared to trials using other enteral nutritional supplements. In addition, the long administration period of 6–8 weeks after surgery may also have had an effect. The problem is that dietary calorie intake has not been examined, and it is unclear how the intake of enteral nutritional supplements affects the amount of oral intake.

9.5 Amino Acid Content of Enteral Nutrition (Prosure®) and Clinical Challenges

Ida et al. planned a prospective randomized controlled trial in which 600 kcal of an enteral nutritional supplement (Prosure®) was administered for 7 days before surgery and 21 days after surgery in addition to regular meals after total gastrectomy for gastric cancer. They reported that there was no significant difference in weight loss rate between 1 month and 3 months (1 month after surgery: intervention group: 8.5%, control group: 8.5%, P = 0.818; 3 months after surgery: intervention group: 13.5%, control group: 13%, P = 0.529) [15]. Similarly, no significant difference was observed in the rate of lean body mass loss at 1 month and 3 months postoperatively (1 month postoperatively: intervention group: 6.89%, control group: 6.74%, P = 0.794; 3 months postoperatively: intervention group: 7.77%, control group: 8.59%, P = 0.393) [16]. On the other hand, the rate of lean body mass loss of 5% or more was 76.8% in the intervention group and 91.1% in the control group (P = 0.070, median), which tended to be lower in the intervention group, but no significant difference was observed. Furthermore, no relationship was observed with the presence or absence of postoperative complications [16]. Prosure® (600 kcal/480 ml) contains 42.66 g of amino acids (8.7 g of BCAA), which has a higher amino acid content than other enteral nutritional supplements, but the intake rate is 100% before surgery/54% after surgery, and postoperative intake was particularly poor.

Due to the problems with compliance, enteral nutrition may not be administered sufficiently, and its effectiveness may not be fully evaluated.

9.6 Amino Acid Content of Enteral Nutrition (Racol®NF) and Clinical Challenges

Kobayashi et al. planned a prospective intervention trial in which 400 kcal of an enteral nutritional supplement (Racol®NF) was administered in addition to regular meals

Table 9.1 Nutrition therapy for gastric cancer after gastrectomy (modified from Ref. [14])

References	Imamura et al. [12]	Ida et al. [15]	Kobayashi et al. [17]
Date of publication	2016	2017	2017
Study design	RCT	RCT	Prospective, single arm
Sample size	106	123	82
Type of gastrectomy	TG and DG	TG	TG and DG
Formula administered	Elental®	Prosure®	Racol®NF
Calorie (kcal/day)	300	600	400
Amino acid (g/day)	14.1	42.66	8.76
BCAA (g/day)	2.24	8.7	1.73
Periods (days)			
Pre-	0	7	0
Post-	42–56	21	90
Compliance rate: mean (%)			
Pre-	N/A	92	N/A
Post-	68.7	61	52.7
Primary outcome:	Control: 6–8 W (mean ± SD)	Control: 1 M–3 M (median)	<200 ml: 1 M:3 M (mean ± SD)
Body weight loss rate (%)	6.60 ± 4.9	8.9:13.0	7.7 ± 2.6:10.4 ± 5.2
	Intervention: 6-8 W	Intervention: 1 M:3 M	≥200 ml:1 M:3 M
	4.86 ± 3.72[a]	8.8:12.9	6.3 ± 2.7[a]:6.1 ± 4.3[a]

Abbreviations: *DG* distal gastrectomy, *M* months, *N/A* not applicable, *RCT* randomized control trial, *SD* standard deviation, *TG* total gastrectomy, *W* weeks

[a]Statistical significance: $P < 0.05$

after gastrectomy, starting within 7 days after surgery and continuing for 3 months. It has been reported that patients who intake 200 ml or more of Racol®NF had significantly less weight loss 3 months after gastrectomy (<200 ml:3 M: 10.4 ± 5.2%, control group: 6.1 ± 4.3%, $P < 0.001$, average value above) [17]. Racol®NF (200 kcal/200 ml) contains 8.76 g of amino acids (1.73 g of BCAA), which is low in amino acid content compared to other enteral nutrition, but after long-term administration for 3 months, weight loss may have been suppressed (Table 9.1).

9.7 Future Prospects

BCAA may improve weight loss and muscle mass loss after gastrectomy, but due to problems with compliance of enteral nutrition, BCAA is not administered in sufficient amounts, and the clinical effects of BCAA on body weight and muscle mass are unknown. Although there are many enteral nutrition sources rich in BCAA, they are generally difficult to consume, and compliance is often poor. It is necessary to consider the taste and amount of enteral nutrition. In addition, forced feeding such as PPN, which does not affect compliance, may be used in combination, especially in the early postoperative period when oral intake is reduced. On the other hand, it has been reported that BCAA administration and exercise therapy prevent muscle loss in elderly patients with primary sarcopenia, and a combination of forced feeding and exercise therapy may be effective in reducing muscle mass in the early postoperative period.

References

1. Abdiev S, et al. Nutritional recovery after open and laparoscopic gastrectomy. Gastric Cancer. 2011;14:144–9.
2. Aoyama T, et al. Loss of lean body mass an independent risk factor for continuation of S-1 adjuvant chemotherapy for gastric cancer. Ann Surg Oncol. 2015;22:2560–6.
3. Aoyama T, et al. Risk factors for the loss of lean body mass after gastrectomy for gastric cancer. Ann Surg Oncol. 2016;23:1963–70.
4. Nunobe S, Oda I, Ishikawa T, Akazawa K, Katai H, Isobe Y, et al. Surgical outcomes of elderly patients with stage I gastric cancer from the nationwide registry of the Japanese Gastric Cancer Association. Gastric Cancer. 2020;23:328–38.
5. Cruz-Jentoft AJ, Sayer AA, et al. Sarcopenia. Lancet. 2019;393:2636–46.
6. Kuwada K, Kuroda S, Kikuchi S, Yoshida R, Nishizaki M, Kagawa S, Fujiwara T. Sarcopenia and comorbidity in gastric cancer surgery as a useful combined factor to predict eventual death from other causes. Ann Surg Oncol. 2018;25:1160.
7. Geng-Hao B, et al. Effects of branched-chain amino acid-rich supplementation on EWGSOP2 criteria for sarcopenia in older adults: a systematic review and meta-analysis. Eur J Nutr. 2022;61:637–51.
8. Freund H, Hoover HC Jr, Atamian S, Fischer JE. Infusion of the branched chain amino acids in postoperative patients. Anticatabolic properties. Ann Surg. 1979;190:18–23.
9. Johnson DJ, Jiang ZM, Colpoys M, Kapadia CR, Smith RJ, Wilmore DW. Branched chain amino acid uptake and muscle free amino acid concentrations predict postoperative muscle nitrogen balance. Ann Surg. 1986;204:513–23.

10. Hernández-Conde M, Llop E, Gómez-Pimpollo L, Fernández Carrillo C, Rodríguez L, Van Den Brule E, et al. Adding branched-chain amino acids to an enhanced standard-of-care treatment improves muscle mass of cirrhotic patients with sarcopenia: a placebo-controlled trial. Am J Gastroenterol. 2021;116:2241–9.
11. Kikuchi S, et al. Impact of amino acids nutrition following gastrectomy in gastric cancer patients. Anticancer Res. 2022;42:3637–43.
12. Imamura H, et al. Effects of an oral elemental nutritional supplement on post-gastrectomy body weight loss in gastric cancer patients: a randomized controlled clinical trial. Ann Surg Oncol. 2016;23:2928–35.
13. Kimura Y, Nishikawa K, Kishi K, Inoue K, Matsuyama J, Akamaru Y, et al. Long-term effects of an oral elemental nutritional supplement on post-gastrectomy body weight loss in gastric cancer patients (KSES002). Ann Gastroenterol Surg. 2019;3(6):648–56.
14. Ida S, Kumagai K, Nunobe S, et al. Current status of perioperative nutritional intervention and exercise in gastric cancer surgery: a review. Ann Gastroenterol Surg. 2021;6:197–203.
15. Ida S, Hiki N, Cho H, Sakamaki K, Ito S, Fujitani K, et al. Randomized clinical trial comparing standard diet with perioperative oral immunonutrition in total gastrectomy for gastric cancer. Br J Surg. 2017;104(4):377–83.
16. Aoyama T, Yoshikawa T, Ida S, et al. Effects of perioperative eicosapentaenoic acid-enriched Oral Nutritional Supplement On the long-term oncological outcomes after total gastrectomy for gastric cancer. Oncol Lett. 2022;23:151.
17. Kobayashi D, Ishigure K, Mochizuki Y, Nakayama H, Sakai M, Ito S, et al. Multi-institutional prospective feasibility study to explore tolerability and efficacy of oral nutritional supplements for patients with gastric cancer undergoing gastrectomy (CCOG1301). Gastric Cancer. 2017;20(4):718–27.

Colorectal Cancer

10

Toshiki Mimura

Abstract

The incidence of colorectal cancer (CRC) is 120 new cases per 100,000 population, being the first among all kinds of cancer in Japan. CRC is associated with so-called western lifestyle habits and diet as well as obesity and genetic factors. Symptoms of CRC include bloody stool, altered bowel habits, abdominal pain, anemia, and body weight loss. Colonoscopy is the best examination to find and diagnose CRC. Its treatment depends on local invasion depth, lymph node involvement, and presence of distant metastases. These factors are combined into an overall stage definition of UICC classification, which provides the basis for treatment decisions. The treatment of CRC includes endoscopy, surgery, chemotherapy, radiation therapy, and palliative care. The UICC classification provides valuable prognostic information, and the measured 5-year survival rates of CRC are 83% in Stage I, 76% in Stage II, 68% in Stage III, and 19% in Stage IV. Because more than 60% of patients with CRC survive more than 5 years, many CRC survivors are still living and working in the world. This section provides important information on how to live and work during and after treatment, with follow-up examinations, adjuvant chemotherapy, low anterior resection syndrome, permanent stoma, therapeutic chemotherapy, and palliative care.

Keywords

Colorectal cancer · Colonoscopy · UICC classification
Endoscopic treatment · Surgery · Chemotherapy
Radiation therapy · Palliative care · Low anterior resection syndrome · Permanent stoma

T. Mimura (✉)
Division of Gastroenterological, General and Transplant Surgery, Department of Surgery, Jichi Medical University, Tochigi, Japan
e-mail: mimurat@jichi.ac.jp

10.1 Introduction

Epidemiology Colorectal cancer (CRC) is the third most common cause of cancer mortality worldwide, with more than 1.85 million cases and 850,000 deaths annually. Its incidence is higher in men than women, strongly increases with age, and varies globally, being closely linked to elements of a so-called western lifestyle.

According to the national statistics of Japan in 2018, its incidence is 120 new cases per 100,000 population, being the first among all kinds of cancer in Japan [1]. It is in third place after prostatic and gastric cancer in men, while in second place after breast cancer in women. Its death rate is 42 patients per 100,000 population, being the second after lung cancer. It is in third place after lung and gastric cancer in men, while it is in first place followed by lung and pancreatic cancer in women.

Anatomy and Function The colon and rectum, also called the large bowel, are the last parts of the digestive tract, which starts from the cecum, followed by the ascending, transverse, descending, and sigmoid colon, and ends as the rectum connecting to the anal canal (Fig. 10.1) [2].

The rectum is classified into three parts: the upper rectum, so-called rectosigmoid (RS); the middle rectum, so-called rectum above peritoneal reflection (Ra); and the lower rectum, so-called rectum below peritoneal reflection (Rb).

The main functions of the large bowel include the formation and storage of stool by absorbing water from food debris as well as the fermentation of dietary fiber with the intestinal microbiome, including bacteria. The fermentation produces short-chain fatty acid, such as butyric, acetic, and propionic acid, which are important energy sources for colonic epithelium. The intestinal microbiome contributes to the intestinal immune system, protection from pathogen, and the production of various vitamins, dopamine, and serotonin. It is also recognized to play an important role in colorectal carcinogenesis as an environmental factor.

© The Author(s), under exclusive license to Springer Nature Singapore Pte Ltd. 2026
M. Endo et al. (eds.), *Cancer and Work in Asia Volume 2*, https://doi.org/10.1007/978-981-95-6537-5_10

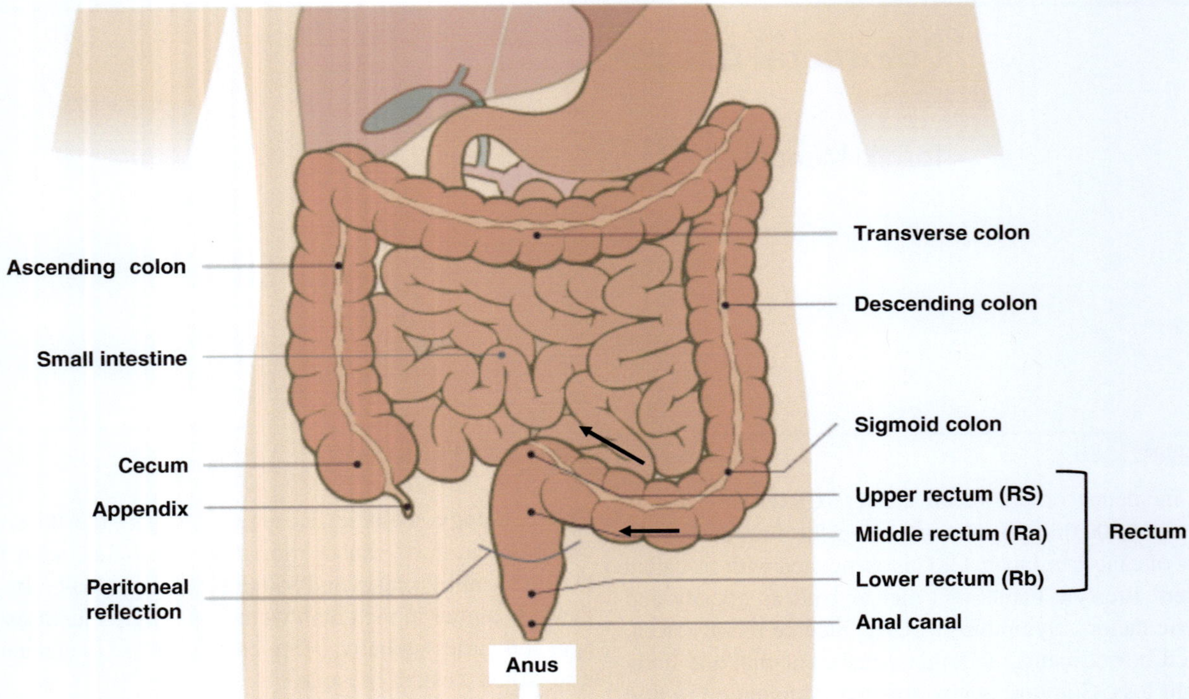

Fig. 10.1 Anatomy of colon and rectum. The colon and rectum, also called large bowel, are the last parts of the digestive tract, which starts from cecum, followed by ascending, transverse, descending and sigmoid colon, and ends as rectum connecting to anal canal. Rectum is classified into three parts: upper rectum, so called rectosigmoid (RS); middle rectum, so called rectum above peritoneal reflection (Ra); and lower rectum, so called rectum below peritoneal reflection (Rb)

Risk factors CRC is associated with lifestyle habits such as diet, alcohol intake, and smoking, as well as obesity and genetic factors of family history. The risk factors of diet include red meats, processed meats, preserved foods, saturated/animal fats, cholesterol, high-sugar foods, spicy foods, and refined carbohydrates. Inversely, a protective role against CRC risk is played by calcium/dairy foods, general vegetable/fruit/fiber consumption, soybean/soy products, alpha-carotene, beta-carotene, and folic acid, as well as vitamins C, D, E, and B12. Obesity is also one of the risk factors for CRC. Epidemiological data suggest that obesity is associated with a 30–70% increased risk of colon cancer in men, whereas the association is less consistent in women.

Most cases of CRC are sporadic, and family history is associated with less than 10% of CRC. Hereditary conditions such as familial adenomatous polyposis and Lynch syndrome confer an extremely high lifetime risk of CRC but account for a minority of all CRCs. A much larger proportion have moderately elevated risk of CRC due to a family history of CRC, likely due to a combination of shared polygenic and shared environmental risk.

Natural history Two different mechanisms are considered for the development of CRC: One is the adenoma-carcinoma sequence, in which an adenoma develops from a normal colorectal mucosa and slowly progresses into a carcinoma over several years, and the other is de novo CRC, in which a carcinoma directly develops from a normal colorectal mucosa.

A higher prevalence of adenomas in people with a family history of CRC is found in men, but adenoma progression is not accelerated in people with a family history. Small studies have suggested that adenoma growth may be accelerated in people with a family history of CRC.

10.2 Diagnosis

Symptoms Most patients with early and/or small CRC are asymptomatic, while symptoms occur as CRC progresses into an advanced and/or large tumor. They include bloody stool, thin stool, altered bowel habits such as constipation and diarrhea, abdominal pain and/or bloating, anemia, and body weight loss. When the tumor becomes large enough to obstruct the colon and rectum, it causes large bowel obstruction with symptoms of vomiting and severe abdominal pain. In a minority of patients with CRC, it is found with jaundice due to multiple liver metastases.

Images Colonoscopy is the best examination to find and diagnose CRC, particularly at an early stage. However, it requires an intake of a large amount of laxatives, usually with 2000 ml of polyethylene glycol, for colonic preparation. Such preparation is important to find small polyps and CRCs, but if the CRC is large enough to obstruct the colon and rectum, such intake of laxatives could induce large bowel obstruction, which might result in life-threatening perforation of the large bowel. Therefore, if nausea, vomiting, or severe abdominal pain occurs during the intake of the laxatives for colonoscopy, you should stop their intake and consult with your doctor in charge.

While colonoscopy can be used not only for examination but also for treatment, in which an early CRC can be endoscopically resected, computed tomography (CT) colonography can be used only for examination to detect CRCs with similar accuracy to colonoscopy. Although CT colonography is less invasive than colonoscopy, if some polyps or CRCs are suspected with CT colonography, they are to be confirmed with further colonoscopy.

Colonoscopic ultrasonography and magnifying chromoendoscopy are used to diagnose the invasion depth of CRC to decide whether it can be endoscopically resected. CRC also can be found by barium enema and CT, although their diagnostic accuracy is lower than colonoscopy and CT colonography.

CT and magnetic resonance imaging (MRI) are useful to detect and diagnose liver and lung metastasis as well as lymph node involvement. MRI is particularly useful to evaluate the invasion of rectal cancer into adjacent organs such as the prostate, vagina, uterus, and bladder. Positron emission tomography (PET) is sometimes used to evaluate systemic metastasis in patients with advanced CRC.

Pathology CRC is pathologically classified as adenocarcinoma, squamous cell carcinoma, and adenosquamous carcinoma. More than 95% of CRC is adenocarcinoma, which is further classified as papillary, well differentiated, moderately differentiated, poorly differentiated, and mucinous adenocarcinoma, as well as signet-ring cell and medullary carcinoma. Approximately 70% of adenocarcinomas are well differentiated with a good prognosis, and 17% are moderately differentiated with a poorer prognosis than well differentiated, while the prognosis of poorly differentiated adenocarcinoma and signet ring cell carcinoma is generally poor.

10.3 Treatment

The treatment algorithm of CRC is shown in Fig. 10.2 according to the 2019 guidelines for the treatment of colorectal cancer by the Japanese Society for Cancer of the Colon and Rectum [3, 4]. The treatment of CRC depends on local invasion depth (T stage) (Fig. 10.3) [3], lymph node involvement (N stage), and presence of distant metastases (M stage). These stages are combined into an overall stage definition of Union Internationale Contre le Cancer (UICC, Table 10.1) [5, 6], which provides the basis for treatment decisions. Although this UICC classification provides valuable prognostic information and guides therapeutic decisions, oncological and functional outcomes of individual patients' treatment cannot be certainly predicted. Therefore, a decision for an individual patient's treatment should be made depending on each patient's conditions and preference.

Endoscopic treatment Most of CRC at Stage 0 with tumors restricted to mucosa and some of CRC at Stage I with tumors infiltrating into the superficial part of submucosa (usually less than 1 mm beyond lamina muscularis mucosae) can be treated with endoscopic polypectomy, endoscopic mucosal resection (EMR), or endoscopic submucosal dissection (ESD). If the entire tumor cannot be resected endoscopically, or the histological findings of the resected specimen are unfavorable, such as deep invasion into submucosa or positive lymphatic and vascular infiltration, additional surgical resection of the colon or rectum with lymph node dissection should be discussed.

Surgery Most of CRC at Stage II or III and some of CRC at Stage I with tumors infiltrating into deep parts of the submucosa (usually 1 mm or over beyond the lamina muscularis mucosae) are treated with surgical resection of the colon or rectum with lymph node dissection. It can be performed with open, laparoscopic, or robotic surgery, depending on patients' conditions and preferences as well as surgeons' experience and preferences, while the proportion of laparoscopic surgery has been increasing. It is because laparoscopic surgery can now be performed more safely with less operating time compared with its early stage of development, thanks to the improvement of laparoscopic devices and surgeons' skills. Several meta-analyses have shown that laparoscopic resection of CRC achieves the same long-term results as open surgery and is associated with a reduced number of patients requiring blood transfusions, faster return of bowel function, and a shorter duration of hospital stay. Some evidence supports the use of robotic surgery for rectal cancer, but further data are needed.

Most colon cancer can be simply treated with colonic resection, while there are many surgical procedures to choose for rectal cancer, as is shown in Table 10.2 and Fig. 10.4, although the basic principle of total mesorectal excision is the same, that is, removal of the rectum together with the mesorectum containing involved lymph nodes and tumor deposits.

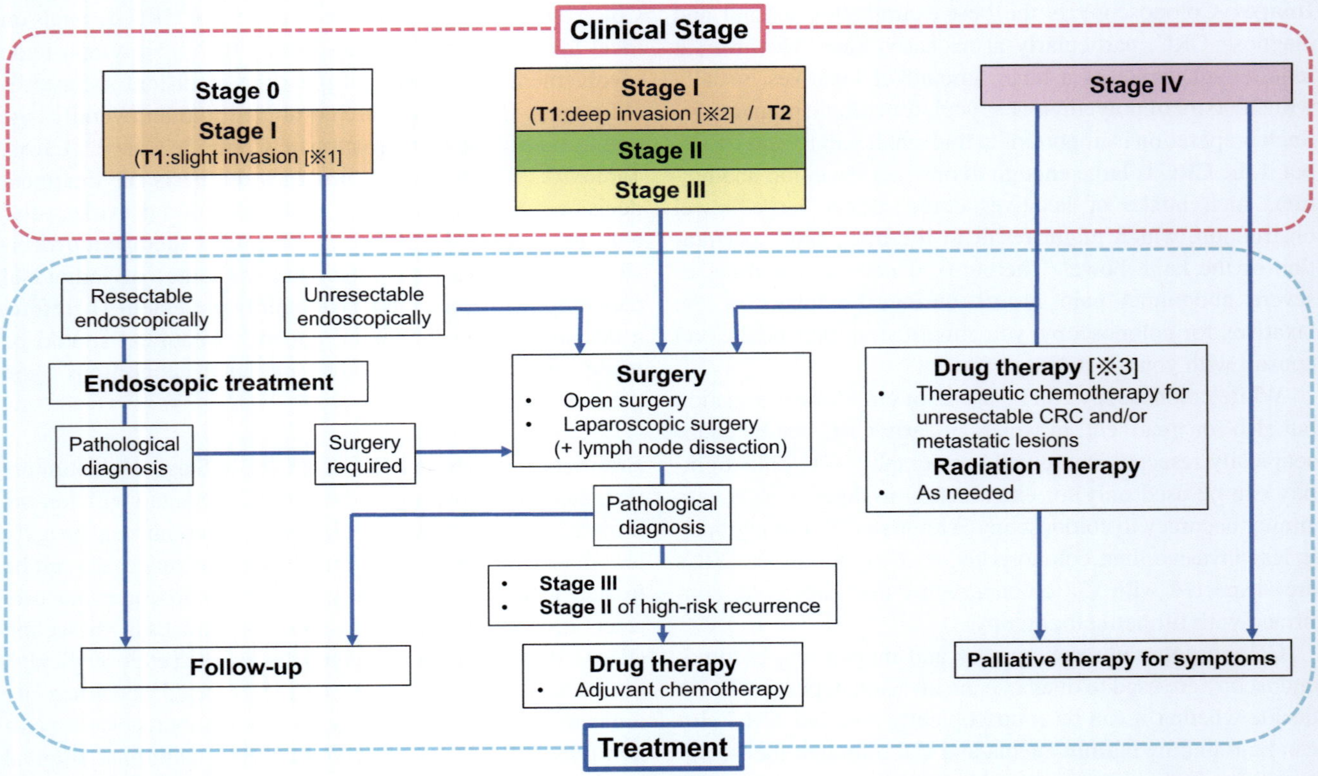

Fig. 10.2 Treatment algorithm of colorectal cancer. (1) slight invasion: infiltrating into submucosa less than 1mm beyond lamina muscularis mucosae; (2) deep invasion: infiltrating into submucosa less than 1mm or over beyond lamina muscularis mucosae; (3) Genomic profiling is conducted before chemotherapy to decide which agents to be used (Cited from Ref. [3] with translation from Japanese to English (https://ganjoho.jp/public/cancer/colon/treatment.html))

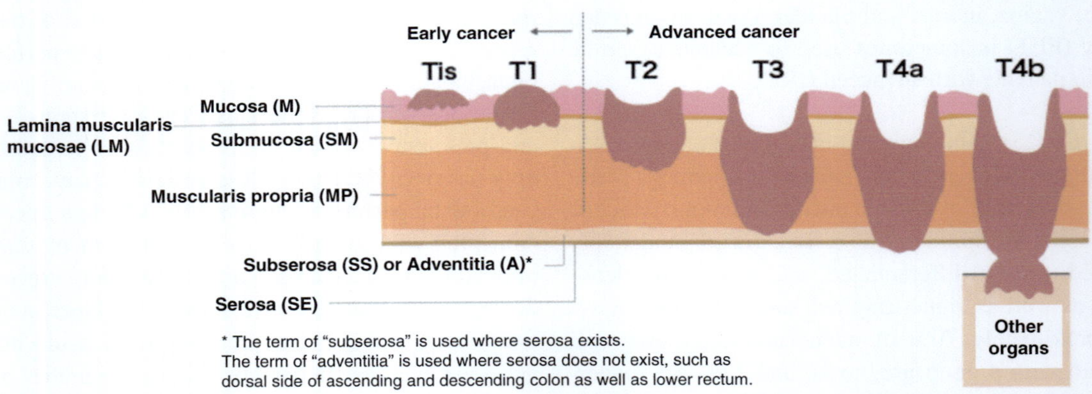

Tis	Tumor restricted to mucosa, no infiltration of lamina muscularis mucosae
T1	Infiltration through lamina muscularis mucosae into submucosa, no infiltration of muscularis propria
T2	Infiltration into, but not beyond, muscularis propria
T3	Infiltration into subserosa or adventitia, or both; no infiltration of serosa or neighboring organs
T4a	Infiltration into or beyond the serosa
T4b	Infiltration of neighboring tissues or other organs

Fig 10.3 T stage (classification of local invasion depth). (Cited from Ref. [3] with translation from Japanese to English (https://ganjoho.jp/public/cancer/colon/treatment.html))

Table 10.1 Stage classification of colorectal cancer by UICC

	T	N	M
Stage 0	Tis	N0	M0
Stage I	T1/T2	N0	M0
Stage II	T3/T4	N0	M0
IIA	T3	N0	M0
IIB	T4a	N0	M0
IIC	T4b	N0	M0
Stage III	Any	N+	M0
IIIA	T1-T2	N1	M0
	T1	N2a	M0
IIIB	T3-T4a	N1	M0
	T2-T3	N2a	M0
	T1-T2	N2b	M0
IIIC	T4a	N2a	M0
	T3-T4a	N2b	M0
	T4b	N1-N2	M0
Stage IV	Any	Any	M+
IVA	Any	Any	M1a
IVB	Any	Any	M1b

Created based on Ref. [5, 6]
UICC Union Internationale Contre le Cancer

Table 10.2 Surgical procedures for rectal cancer

Surgical procedures		Tumor location
1. High anterior resection (HAR)		RS (upper rectum)
2. Low anterior resection (LAR)		Ra (middle rectum)
3-1. Low anterior resection (LAR) with or without temporary stoma	Anus Preserving Operation (APO)	Rb (lower rectum)
3-2. Intersphincteric resection (ISR) with temporary stoma		Rb close to anus
3-3. Abdominoperineal resection (APR) with permanent stoma = Mile's operation		Rb close to anus
3-4. Transanal minimally invasive surgery (TAMIS)		Rb at Stage 0 and at Stage I with slight invasion into submucosa

1. High anterior resection (HAR) is performed for rectal cancer located in the upper rectum (Rs).
2. Low anterior resection (LAR) is performed for rectal cancer located in the middle rectum (Ra).
3. For cancer in the lower rectum (Rb), an appropriate surgical procedure is chosen among LAR, intersphincteric resection (ISR), abdominoperineal resection (APR) with permanent colostomy, and transanal resection, also called transanal minimally invasive surgery (TAMIS), depending on the location and stage of the tumor as well as the patients' preference.
   - 3-1. LAR is performed for Rb cancer, which is located far enough from the anus not to necessitate the resection of the internal anal sphincter (IAS).
   - 3-2. On the other hand, ISR is performed for Rb cancer, which is located very close to the anus, requiring resection of IAS partially or totally to have enough surgical margin at the anal side.

The LAR and ISR are also called anus-preserving operations (APO), in which your natural anus is preserved so that you can pass stool through it as is before the operation. In a case of very low anastomosis at APO, a temporary ileostomy or transverse colostomy is created to reduce the risk of anastomotic leakage. When the integrity of the anastomosis is confirmed radiologically or colonoscopically, usually 3–6 months after the original surgery, the temporary stoma is closed.

   - 3-3. In APR, also called Mile's operation, your anus is resected with the rectum, and peritoneal skin is closed so that you pass stool not through your natural anus but through your stoma created at your abdomen.
   - 3-4. TAMIS is performed as a local resection without lymph node dissection for Rb cancer at Stage 0 with the tumor restricted to the mucosa and some of Rb

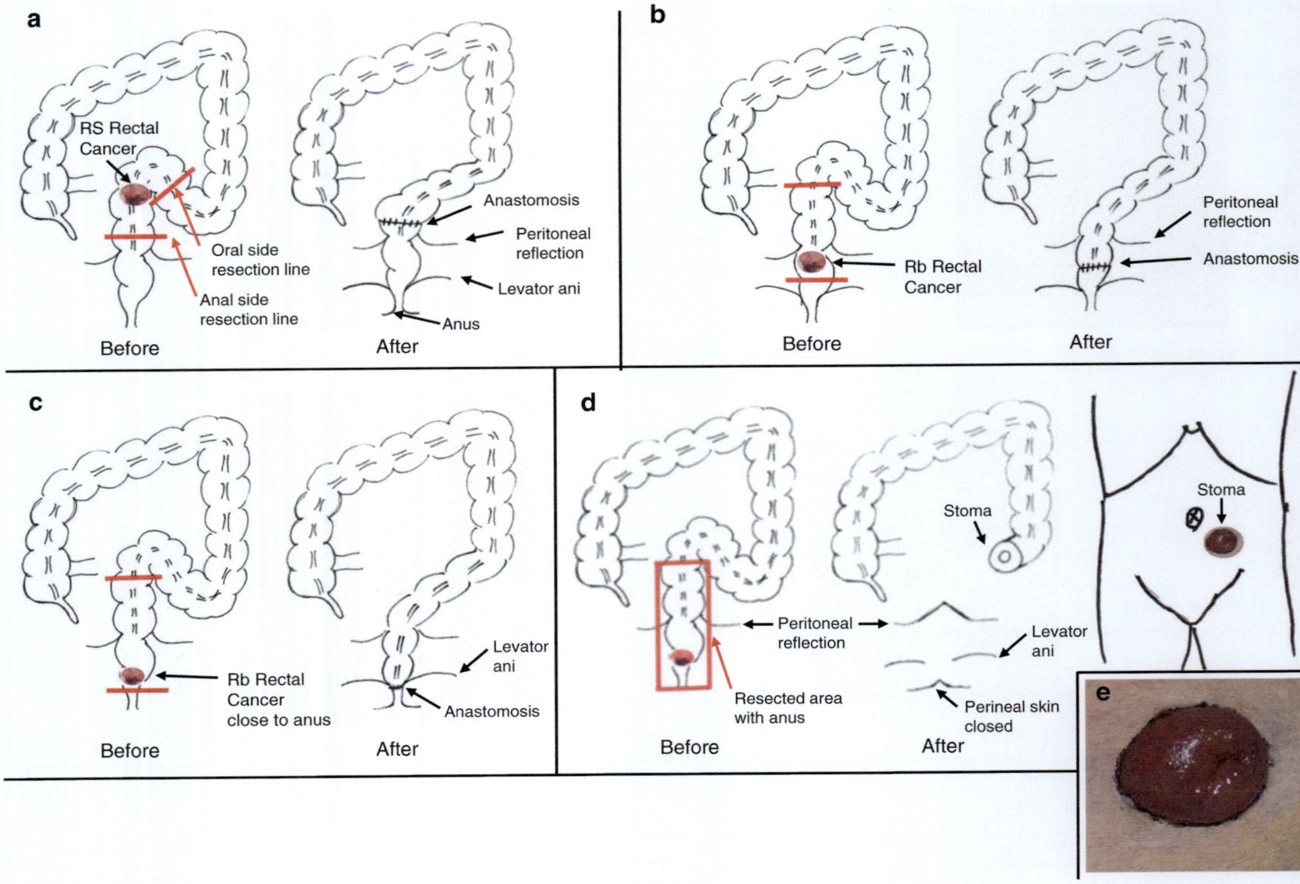

Fig. 10.4 Before and after each surgical procedure for rectal cancer. (**a**) High anterior resection, (**b**) Low anterior resection, (**c**) Intersphincteric resection, (**d**) Abdominoperineal resection, (**e**) Magnified view of stoma. RS: upper rectum (rectosigmoid); Rb: lower rectum (rectum below peritoneal reflection)

cancer at Stage I with the tumor infiltrating into the superficial part of the submucosa. In selected cases of frail patients who are not suitable for radical surgery of LAR, ISR, and APR and those who decline to undergo the radical surgery to avoid associated morbidities, TAMIS can be performed as a palliative surgery with or without radiotherapy for CRC at Stage I with a tumor infiltrating into the deep part of the submucosa and Stage II.

In patients with Rb cancer, the choice of APO or APR hugely affects their life and work. If you choose APO without a permanent stoma, you can keep your body image the same as others without a stoma and pass stool through your natural anus. However, you might be troubled with a constellation of defecatory symptoms, so-called low anterior resection syndrome (LARS), which includes frequent bowel movements, fecal urgency and incontinence, evacuation difficulty, feeling of incomplete defecation, and so on. LARS could disturb and interrupt your work as well as impair your quality of life (QOL). On the other hand, if you choose APR with permanent colostomy, you are not troubled with LARS without passing stool through your natural anus. However, you might be troubled with stoma-related complications, including stomal necrosis and retraction of the stoma in the short term, as well as peristomal dermatitis, parastomal hernia, stomal prolapse, and so on in the long term. These long-term stoma-related complications could disturb and interrupt your work as well as impair your QOL. The influence of LARS and permanent stoma over your daily life and work, as well as their management, will be discussed in the section "Cancer and Work."

Drug therapy Recent progress in chemotherapy has remarkably improved the prognosis of curatively resected CRC with adjuvant chemotherapy, which is given after curative resection of CRC to prevent its recurrence. It has been clearly demonstrated to be beneficial for node-positive CRC at Stage III and could be beneficial for CRC with high-risk recurrence at Stage II in the adjuvant setting. A number of trials in the adjuvant setting have analyzed the efficacy of multiple-agent combinations, including fluorouracil, levofolinate, irinotecan, oxaliplatin, capecitabine, bevacizumab, and cetuximab. Standard treatment options for adjuvant chemotherapy include fluorouracil or capecitabine with or without oxaliplatin, although oxaliplatin is associated with cumulative dose-dependent neurotoxicity, characterized by distal or perioral paresthesias or dysesthesias.

Of new colorectal cancer diagnoses, 20% of patients have metastatic lesions at presentation, and another 25% who present with localized disease will later develop metastases. Therapeutic chemotherapy has also remarkably improved the prognosis of unresectable, recurrent, and metastatic CRC. It is administered to treat unresectable CRC and/or metastatic lesions in the liver, lung, peritoneum, brain, bone, and so on, to reduce their size and number of metastatic lesions. When the unresectable CRC is brought into a respectable situation and/or the size and number of metastatic lesions are reduced after effective therapeutic chemotherapy, the CRC and/or metastatic lesions can be surgically resected. The other purposes of therapeutic chemotherapy are to prolong the rest of patients' lives with unresectable CRC and/or metastatic lesions and to alleviate uncomfortable symptoms due to them. For therapeutic chemotherapy, cytotoxic agents of fluorouracil, irinotecan, and oxaliplatin, as well as biologic therapies such as *molecularly targeted drugs,* antibodies to cellular growth factors, immunotherapy, and their combinations, are used. Genomic profiling of CRC to detect somatic variants is as important as tailoring treatment because it identifies the chemotherapy that is more likely to be effective. For the 50% of patients with metastatic CRC with KRAS/NRAS/BRAF wild-type tumors, cetuximab and panitumumab in combination with conventional chemotherapy can extend median survival by 2 to 4 months compared with the conventional chemotherapy alone. Other d*rugs for metastatic CRC include bevacizumab,* ramucirumab, *aflibercept, regorafenib, trifluridine, regorafenib, and pembrolizumab (an immune checkpoint inhibitor).*

These chemotherapies could cause unfavorable adverse events, including gastrointestinal symptoms (nausea, anorexia, *diarrhea, and stomatitis), bone marrow suppression,* neurotoxicity (distal, perioral paresthesias, or dysesthesias), hand and foot syndrome, skin pigmentation, alopecia and so on. In a limited number of patients, *bevacizumab,* ramucirumab, and *aflibercept are reported to cause serious adverse events, including intestinal perforation,* thromboembolism, and encephalopathy. Although cures remain uncommon in metastatic CRC, more patients can anticipate extended survival. Genomic profiling allows treatment selection so that more patients derive benefit and fewer are exposed to toxicity from ineffective therapies. *Therefore, you should discuss the benefits and disadvantages of chemotherapy with your doctor to decide whether or not you should receive it, and if you do, which chemotherapy you would opt for.*

Chemotherapy used to be administered by surgeons who performed the surgery, but because of its complexity with various combinations of many available agents, its role is now being transferred to specialized clinical oncologists.

Radiation therapy Radiation therapy is generally performed for rectal cancer with the following four purposes: One is preoperative radiation therapy to reduce local recurrence after curative resection of Rb rectal cancer. It is usually performed with neoadjuvant chemotherapy (chemoradiation therapy), and its indication is patients at Stage III, particularly those with T4 and advanced T3 tumors infiltrating mesorectal fascia. Second is preoperative chemoradiation therapy to reduce the size of Rb rectal cancer located very close to the anus. If such downstaging is effective, the tumor can be curatively resected with LAR or ISR, rather than APR, and a permanent stoma can be avoided, although LARS seems more severe after radiation therapy. The third is postoperative radiation therapy to reduce local recurrence after noncurative resection of Rb rectal cancer, particularly when the surgical margin of the resected specimen turns out positive after surgery. Last, but not least, is palliative radiation therapy to alleviate uncomfortable symptoms due to unresectable tumors and/or metastatic lesions. They include abdominal and pelvic pain, rectal bleeding and intestinal obstruction due to unresectable tumors, and pain due to bone metastasis, as well as nausea and vertigo due to brain metastasis.

Radiation therapy could cause adverse events not only during but also after the therapy. Early-stage side effects during the therapy include nausea, anorexia, dermatitis, and leukopenia. Late-stage complications after the therapy include bleeding from irradiated intestine, bladder, and vagina, as well as proctitis, cystitis, intestinal stricture, and fistula formation between irradiated organs. These late-stage complications could occur more than 10 years after the radiation therapy.

Palliative care For patients with unresectable CRC, recurrent and metastatic lesions who are not candidates for active therapies of surgery, chemotherapy, and radiotherapy, best supportive care (BSC) and therapies are provided physically and psychologically to alleviate their uncomfortable symptoms and maintain their QOL as best as possible. The BSC is essential to let these patients end their life peacefully in their own way with their family and friends.

10.4 Prognosis

The measured and relative 5-year survival rates of CRC are 63% and 73%, respectively [7]. The measured survival rate includes all deaths irrespective of their causes, and the relative survival rate includes only deaths due to CRC. The measured 5-year survival rates are more or less the same between

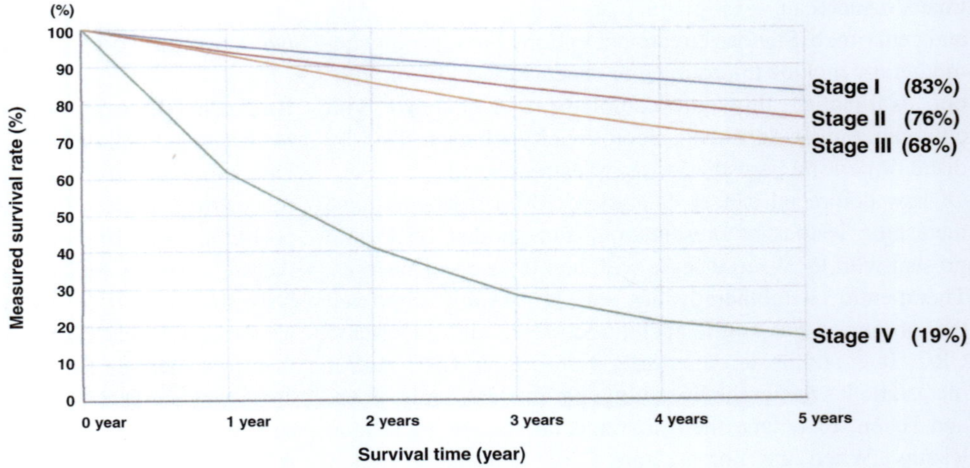

Fig. 10.5 Measured survival rates of colorectal cancer at each stage. The measured survival rate includes all death irrespective of its causes. The data are based on patients who were diagnosed as colorectal cancer between 2013 and 2014

colon and rectal cancer (63% vs. 65%). The UICC classification provides valuable prognostic information, as is shown in Fig. 10.5 [7]. The measured 5-year survival rates of CRC are 83% in Stage I, 76% in Stage II, 68% in Stage III, and 19% in Stage IV.

10.5 Cancer and Work (Table 10.3)

Because more than 60% of patients with CRC survive more than 5 years, many CRC survivors are still living and working in the world. Therefore, it is important for them to learn how to live and work during and after treatment of CRC.

Live and work with follow-up examinations:

1. If you are a patient with colorectal cancer at Stage 0, which was treated with endoscopic resection or TAMIS, no additional therapies are required. You can live and work in the same way as before your treatment without significant sequelae, unless some rare complications occurred. Follow-up colonoscopy is optional depending on the pathological diagnosis of the resected specimen.
2. If you are a patient with colon cancer or RS rectal cancer at Stage I or Stage II without adjuvant chemotherapy, which was resected by colectomy or HAR, respectively, no additional therapies are required. You can live and work in the same way as before your treatment without significant sequelae, unless some rare complications occurred. However, you have to undergo follow-up examinations for 5 years to detect recurrence, if any, at an early stage. They include laboratory tests such as tumor markers, chest XP, abdominal ultrasonography, chest and/or abdominal CT, and colonoscopy. Their interval is between 3 and 12 months depending on each examination and your conditions, and you must manage your work schedule to have the follow-up examinations without fail.

Live and work with adjuvant chemotherapy:

3. If you are a patient with colon cancer or RS rectal cancer at Stage II or Stage III with adjuvant chemotherapy, which was resected by colectomy or HAR, respectively, it is better for you to give priority to the adjuvant chemotherapy over your work. It is usually administered in an outpatient setting for 6 months. Therefore, you can work, if you wish, during the chemotherapy if you can manage its side effects. After the adjuvant chemotherapy is completed, you can live and work in the same way as before your treatment without significant sequelae, unless some rare complications occurred. However, you have to undergo follow-up examinations for 5 years to detect recurrence, if any, at an early stage.

Live and work with low anterior resection syndrome:

4. If you are a patient with rectal cancer at Stage I or Stage II without adjuvant chemotherapy, which was resected by anus-preserving operations (APOs), including LAR and ISR, you might be troubled with a constellation of defecatory symptoms, so-called low anterior resection syndrome (LARS), after the surgery. They include frequent bowel movements, fecal urgency and incontinence, evacuation difficulty, feeling of incomplete defecation, and so on. The etiologies of LARS include loose stool, anal sphincter dysfunction, impaired rectal sensation, reduced volume and compliance of the neorectum, and colonic dysfunction. LARS could occur in about 70% of

Table 10.3 Live and work with follow-up, therapy, and sequelae after treatment of colorectal cancer

Situations	Influence on and management of your daily life and work
Endoscopic resection or TAMIS for colorectal cancer at Stage 0	No additional therapies or sequela; Follow-up colonoscopy is optional
Surgy for colon cancer or HAR for rectal cancer at Stage I or Stage II without adjuvant chemotherapy	No additional therapies or sequela; Follow-up examinations for 5 years
Surgy for colon cancer or HAR for rectal cancer at Stage II or III with adjuvant chemotherapy	Live and work during adjuvant chemotherapy for 6 months, managing its side effects; Follow-up examinations for 5 years
LAR or ISR for rectal cancer at Stage I or Stage II without adjuvant chemotherapy	Follow-up examinations for 5 years; Live and work managing LARS for the rest of life
LAR or ISR for rectal cancer at Stage II or Stage III with adjuvant chemotherapy	Live and work during adjuvant chemotherapy for 6 months, managing its side effects; Follow-up examinations for 5 years Live and work managing LARS for the rest of life
APR for rectal cancer at Stage I or Stage II without adjuvant chemotherapy	Follow-up examinations for 5 years; Live and work managing stoma care and any stoma-related complications for the rest of your life
APR for rectal cancer at Stage II or Stage III with adjuvant chemotherapy	Live and work during adjuvant chemotherapy for 6 months, managing its side-effects; Follow-up examinations for 5 years Live and work managing stoma care and any stoma-related complications for the rest of your life
Unresectable colorectal cancer and/or metastatic lesions at Stage IV	Live and work with therapeutic chemotherapy managing its side effects and with palliative care for uncomfortable symptoms due to unresectable tumors and/or metastatic lesions

TAMIS transanal minimally invasive surgery; *HAR* high anterior resection; *LAR* low anterior resection; *ISR* intersphincteric resection; *LARS* low anterior resection syndrome; *APR* abdominoperineal resection

patients with Rb rectal cancer after LAR or ISR, while it happens only in about 15% of those with RS rectal cancer after HAR. LARS could disturb and interrupt your social and daily activities, including work, with unpredictable bowel function, toilet dependence, and preoccupation with bowel function. It also could impair your relationships and intimacy with your family, friends, and colleagues; the roles, commitments, and responsibilities in your community; as well as your mental and emotional well-being. Although their symptoms improve with time over 1 and 2 years after surgery or closure of a temporary stoma, they could last for the rest of your life. Therefore, you have to learn how to manage LARS with medication as well as modifications of your lifestyle and diet. Because they could be improved with biofeedback therapy, transanal irrigation, and sacral neuromodulation, you could consult about these treatments with your doctor if they disturb your daily life and work. Because a stoma can remarkably improve QOL in patients with refractory LARS, you also could discuss it with your doctor.

5. If you are a patient with rectal cancer at Stage II or Stage III with adjuvant chemotherapy, which was resected by APOs, you have to manage your work to undergo the adjuvant chemotherapy for 6 months as well as manage various symptoms of LARS. If you have a temporary stoma, it would be better to complete the adjuvant chemotherapy before its closure so that you can concentrate on the chemotherapy without worrying about various symptoms of LARS.

Live and work with a permanent stoma:

6. If you are a patient with rectal cancer at Stage I or Stage II without adjuvant chemotherapy, which was resected by abdominoperineal resection (APR) with permanent colostomy, you are not troubled with LARS without passing stool through your natural anus. However, you have to take care of your stoma (stoma care), and stool could leak from a stoma bag, although it is rare these days thanks to the progress of ostomy appliances and stoma care. Also, you might be troubled with stoma-related complications, including stomal necrosis and retraction of the stoma in the short term, as well as peristomal dermatitis, parastomal hernia, stomal prolapse, and so on in the long term. The stoma care and long-term stoma-related complications could disturb and interrupt your work as well as impair your QOL. The stoma can also affect your body image, which has now become different from others without stomas. However, life with a stoma is more predictable than life with LARS, and all you have to do is to dispose of stool from the stoma bag a couple of times a day at your convenient time and to change ostomy appli-

ances every 2 and 3 days if there are no serious stoma-related complications. Many studies have compared QOL between patients after APO and those after APR, and most of them concluded that there is no significant difference between them. Therefore, it is very important for you to decide whether you undergo APO or APR by fully discussing the advantages and disadvantages of each procedure with your surgeon, which is called shared decision making (SDM).

7. If you are a patient with rectal cancer at Stage II or Stage III with adjuvant chemotherapy, which was resected by APR with permanent colostomy, you have to manage your work to undergo the adjuvant chemotherapy for 6 months as well as manage stoma care and stoma-related complications. The importance of SDM is the same for adjuvant chemotherapy as for the choice of the surgical procedures.

Live and work with therapeutic chemotherapy or palliative care:

8. Even if you are a patient with unresectable colorectal cancer and/or metastatic lesions at Stage IV, the measured 5-year survival rate is not 0% but 19%, as is shown in Fig. 10.5. The data are based on patients who were diagnosed with colorectal cancer between 2013 and 2014. This means that there is a possibility, albeit small, that you might survive them by their down-staging with therapeutic chemotherapy ± radiation therapy, followed by their curative resection with surgery. Most therapeutic chemotherapies can be performed in an outpatient setting so that you can work during or in between each course of chemotherapy, although you have to manage its side effects. While you can keep a hope to survive them, you also have to accept the fact that 81% of patients with CRC at Stage IV decease within 5 years after its diagnosis. Therefore, it is better for you to prepare yourself to live, and possibly work if you wish, along with your tumors until the end of your life. Palliative care and therapy will support you all the way, alleviating your uncomfortable symptoms due to them. With these best supportive cares, you will be able to end your life peacefully in your own way with your family and friends.

References

1. National Cancer Center Japan: Statistics of colorectal cancer, Services for Cancer Information https://ganjoho.jp/reg_stat/statistics/stat/cancer/67_colorectal.html#anchor. Latest access 28 Feb 2022.
2. National Cancer Center Japan: About colon and rectum, Services for Cancer Information. https://ganjoho.jp/public/cancer/colon/about.html. Latest access 28 Feb 2022.
3. National Cancer Center Japan: Treatment of colorectal cancer, Services for Cancer Information. https://ganjoho.jp/public/cancer/colon/treatment.html. Latest access 28 Feb 2022.
4. Hashiguchi Y, Muro K, Saito Y, et al. Japanese Society for Cancer of the colon and Rectum (JSCCR) guidelines 2019 for the treatment of colorectal cancer. Int J Clin Oncol. 2020;25:1–42.
5. Brenner H, Kloor M, Pox CP. Colorectal cancer. Lancet. 2014;383:1490–502.
6. Sobin LH, Gospodarowicz M, Wittekind C. TNM classification of malignant tumours. 7th ed. New York: Wiley-Blackwell; 2009.
7. National Cancer Center Japan: Statistics of survival rate in colorectal cancer, Services for Cancer Information. https://hbcr-survival.ganjoho.jp/graph?year=2013-2014&elapsed=5&type=c02#h-title. Latest access 28 Feb 2022.

Evolution of Mode of Surgery for Lung Cancer: Historical Moment

11

Kenji Suzuki

Abstract

The mode of surgery for lung cancer has been changed in these 100 years. The first surgery for lung cancer was performed as a pneumonectomy in 1933. The standard pulmonary lobectomy was established in 1960, and then thoracic surgeons in the United States tried to minimize pulmonary parenchyma resected for lung cancer. The first randomized controlled trial was done comparing lobectomy and sublobar resection for lung cancer in 1995. The result was negative; that meant lobectomy was still the standard surgery for lung cancer. Due to the failure of the trial, the thoracic surgeon had to perform a lobectomy even for subcentimeter lung cancer. In the late 1990s, thin-section computed tomography was found to be useful for grading lung cancer preoperatively, and early peripheral lung cancer was defined by the results. As a result, investigations of sublobar resection were conducted in two ways: wedge for early lung cancer and segmentectomy for invasive lung cancer. After several clinical trials, such as JCOG0201, JCOG0802/WJOG4607L, and JCOG0804/WJOG4507L, the standard mode of surgery for lung cancer 2 cm or less in size was set to sublobar resection in 2023. Nowadays, sublobar resections are investigated for additional indications such as bigger tumors and lung cancer having nodal metastasis. Selection of mode of surgery for patients should be decided based on patients' tolerability for surgery as well as tumor characteristics. In this aspect, artificial intelligence would be used for the selection in the near future.

Keywords

Sublobar · Consolidation tumor ratio · Ground glass opacity · Lobectomy · Artificial intelligence

K. Suzuki (✉)
Department of General Thoracic Surgery, School of Medicine, Juntendo University, Bunkyo-ku, Tokyo, Japan
e-mail: kjsuzuki@juntendo.ac.jp

11.1 Introduction

Intrathoracic pressure is under zero. The thoracic cavity is the only place in the human body that is maintained at negative pressure. This notion did not prevail in the old days, and so lung resection was not successfully performed until the 1960s. Pneumonectomy, which is one of the most invasive procedures, was the only procedure for lung cancer. The change from pneumonectomy to lobectomy was not established based on clinical trials, but sublobar resection needed to be investigated compared to lobectomy for the standard mode of surgery. There were huge differences between the oriental and western ways of the investigations for establishing sublobar resection as a standard.

11.2 Historical "Ginsberg Study"

A lung cancer study group in the United States started to investigate sublobar resection for making a new standard for lung cancer surgery. The study was the first randomized trial comparing sublobar resection and lobectomy for clinical stage I non-small cell lung cancer (NSCLC). The study showed that lobectomy was superior to sublobar resection for cStage I NSCLC as to local control and prognosis [1]. Interestingly, survival curves were similar up to three years after operation, but in five years survival was better in the lobectomy group. As to local recurrence, 18% after wedge, 12% after segmentectomy, and 6% after lobectomy were the results; it was a multiple of 6! (Fig. 11.1) Ginsberg, who was the study's principal investigator as well as Rubenstein, said that as of the 3-year survival data, sublobar resection should become the new standard for clinical stage I NSCLC but ultimately stated that overall survival at 5 years was better in the lobectomy group. The results taught thoracic surgeons that small-sized lung cancers are more likely to recur later than more advanced lung cancers.

© The Author(s), under exclusive license to Springer Nature Singapore Pte Ltd. 2026
M. Endo et al. (eds.), *Cancer and Work in Asia Volume 2*, https://doi.org/10.1007/978-981-95-6537-5_11

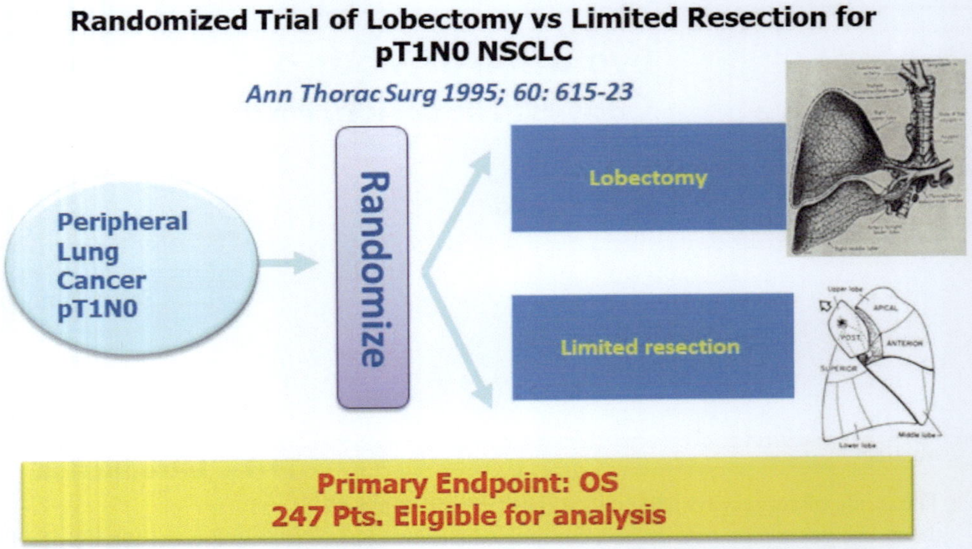

Fig. 11.1 "Ginsberg study" compared sublobar resection and lobectomy for lung cancer—the first randomized trial in the lung cancer surgical community

11.3 Scar Cancer

Carcinoma in situ of the lung had been defined in centrally located lung cancer, mostly squamous cell carcinoma, based on the findings of bronchoscopy [2, 3]. On the other hand, peripherally located cancer in situ, mostly adenocarcinoma, had not. Pathologists at the National Cancer Center Tokyo investigated the latter carcinoma in situ, i.e., adenocarcinoma in situ, and reported several important findings [4]. "Scar cancer" was the notion that prevailed among pathologists all over the world in the 1960s, which insisted that lung cancer developed from the preceding pulmonary scar formation. Shimosato et al. revised this notion to the upside down and proposed the adenoma-carcinoma sequence of the lung. One of the most striking reports was published by Noguchi et al. in 1995 [5]. This paper insisted on the first notion of peripheral, not central hilar, carcinoma in situ in lung cancer, i.e., peripheral in situ adenocarcinoma. The definition was established based on the revised notion of "scar cancer." After this report, adenocarcinoma, which is almost always developing peripheral lung parenchyma, could be graded in respect to prognosis. However, thoracic surgeons could not use this prognostic factor preoperatively, for no modalities were available to evaluate the factors until the development of thin-section computed tomography (TSCT). Radiologic ground glass opacity is related to pathological lepidic growth on TSCT, and therefore, radiological-pathological correlations were investigated. These correlation studies could be done based on the findings of the central scar formation reported by Shimosato et al. in 1980 [4]. The size of the central scar itself was shown to be prognostic, and then this was evaluated by the findings of TSCT [6] (Fig. 11.2). Japan Clinical Oncology Group (JCOG) conducted the first prospective multi-center prospective study for the correlation in 2002 and finally defined early peripheral lung cancer radiologically [7].

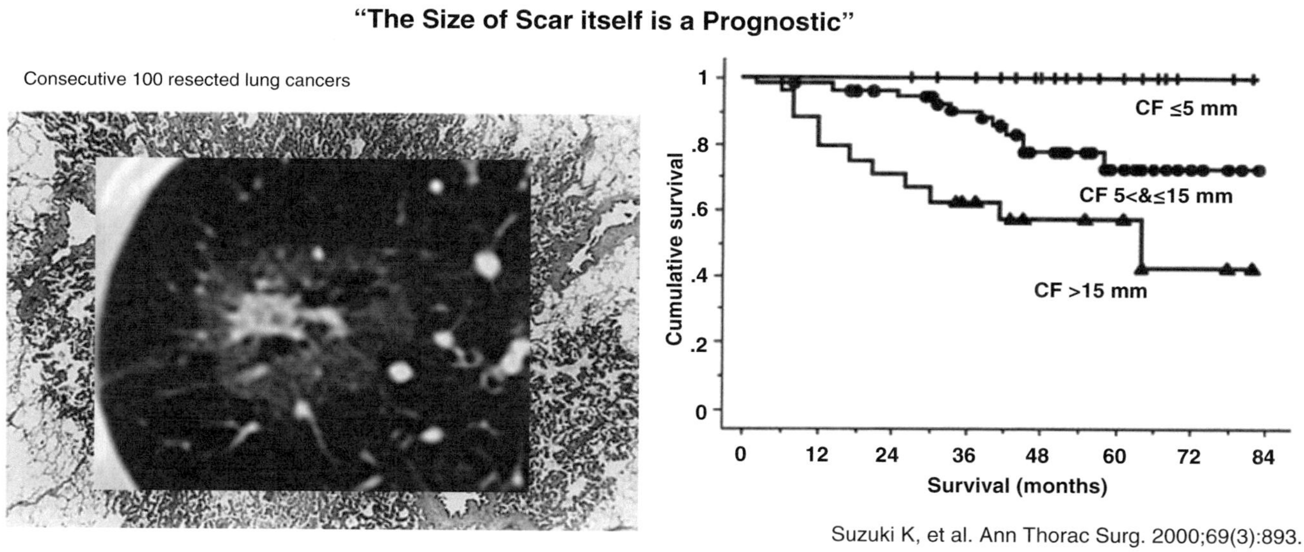

Fig. 11.2 Central scar formation in lung adenocarcinoma was evaluated with thin-section computed tomography

11.4 Radiological Early Lung Cancer

The prognosis of clinical stage I NSCLC is approximately 70% [8]. Stage I NSCLC can be broken down into six categories pathologically, which was reported in the Noguchi's classification [5]. Similar classification was reported based on radiological findings [9]. According to the classification, sublobar resection was indicated. However, the definition was not equally made by observers, and interobserver variation was not small. Thus, JCOG decided to perform a multi-institutional prospective study dealing with radiological-pathological correlation and define radiological early lung cancer, JCOG0201. Finally, early lung cancer was defined as peripherally located lung cancer 2 cm or less in size with a consolidation/tumor ratio (CTR) of 0.5 or less [7, 10, 11]. This definition was widely used in Japan, but in Western countries, it was not so accepted because they have no practice in which physicians evaluate thin-section CT routinely. For evaluation of GGO, TSCT is always necessary. Investigation of sublobar resection was divided into two parts in Japan and one way in the western country. Japanese trials were sublobar resection for radiological early lung cancer and invasive ones diagnosed with CTR, JCOG0804/WJOG4507L, and JCOG0802/WJOG4607L. The former trial adopted wide wedge resection, and the latter did segmentectomy for investigative sublobar resection. The Western trial was just one way of the investigation of sublobar resection, including both wide wedge and segmentectomy, CALGB140503.

11.5 JCOG0804/WJOG4507L Study

Peripheral GGO tends to be less invasive, and wide wedge resection was widely used all over the world. However, some authors warned about this strategy, and they reported a very high percentage of loco-regional recurrence after wedge resection [12, 13]. In this prospective study, they confirmed intraoperative pathological invasiveness in each lung cancer to select the mode of surgery, sublobar or lobectomy. During this study, I was one of the residents at the center and remember that it took approximately one hour to diagnose invasiveness based on frozen section diagnosis. This is because the pathologist confirmed the findings of the Elastica von Gieson stain as well as the hematoxylin and eosin stain. If the tumor has invasive natures, such as interruption of elastic fiber or activated fibroblast formation, lobectomy is performed [14]. Wide wedge resection was performed only for lung cancer having no invasion at all. However, they observed such a high local recurrence rate after wedge. One of the reasons for confirming wide wedge resection for GGO on a multi-institutional basis was the above. Wide wedge resection for GGO 2 cm or less in size having CTR less than 0.25 was investigated as a one-arm study, for the survival should be excellent, which meant it is not suitable to perform randomized trial [15]. Wide wedge for GGO should be very simple in practice, but the scheme was so complex when it was performed on a multi-institutional and prospective basis (Fig. 11.3). The 5-year relapse-

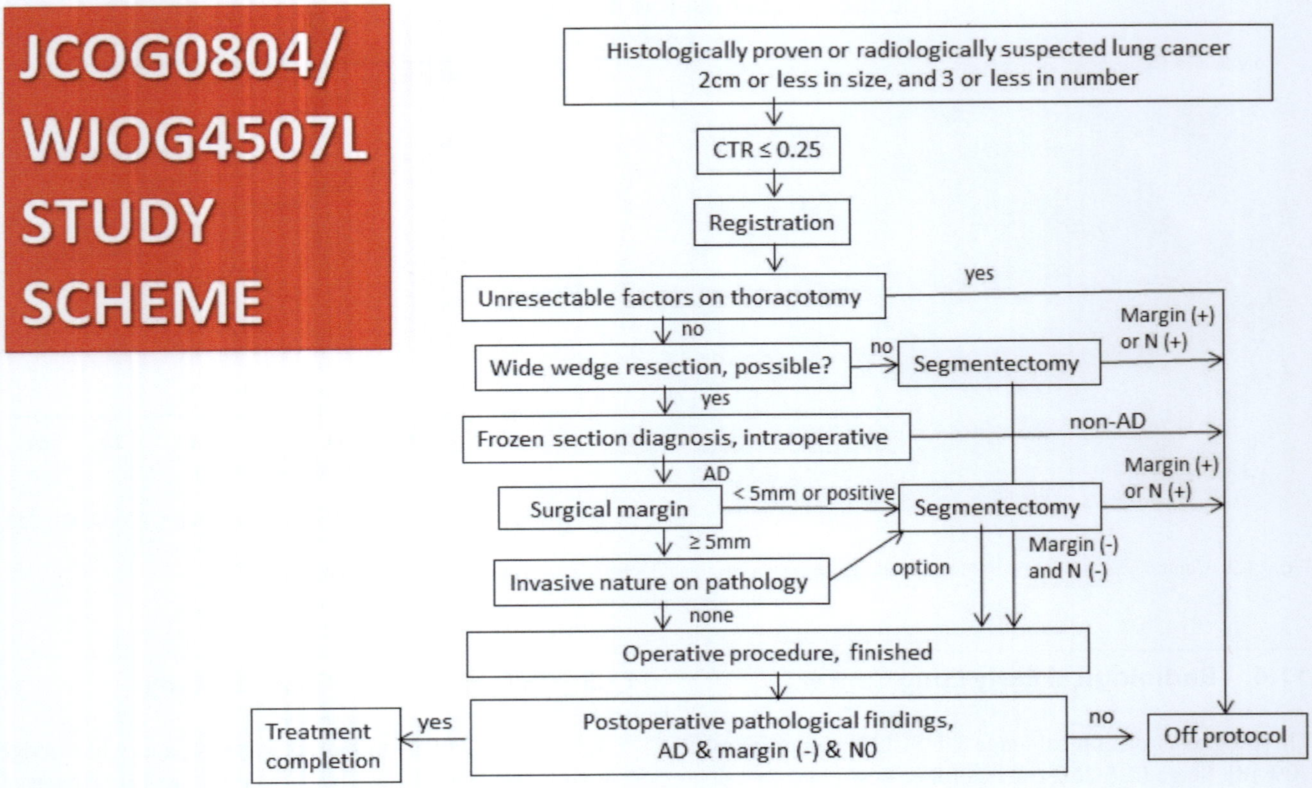

Fig. 11.3 JCOG0804/WJOG4507L study investigated sublobar resection for GGO-dominant lung cancer

free survival was 99.7% with a 95% confidence interval of 97.7 to 100.0, which met the primary endpoint. Thoracic surgeons should be careful to understand this study, and segmentectomy instead of wedge was performed in 58 cases, as well as lobectomy in 11 cases. Enough surgical margin is necessary for sublobar resection for GGO.

11.6 Another Fruit of the JCOG0804/WJOG4507L Study

One of the most popular questions on lung cancer is the probability of cancer when preoperative histological diagnosis was not possible. In practice, preoperative diagnosis of lung tumors is not always made, especially for small-sized tumors. Actually, in the prospective study of JCOG0804/WJOG4507L, preoperatively diagnosed lung cancer was just 1% of the patients, resulting in adenocarcinoma histology in 91% and atypical adenomatous hyperplasia (AAH) of the lung in 5% [16]. This meant the probability of a neoplastic lesion in persistent GGO is approximately 96% in total, because AAH has been shown to be neoplastic, verified by using clonal analysis [17, 18]. Based on the prospective study, we confirmed the accuracy of TSCT for diagnosing lung cancer.

11.7 JCOG0802/WJOG4607L Study

Adenocarcinoma peripherally located is classified into three: non-invasive, minimally invasive, and invasive. Non- and minimally invasive adenocarcinomas rarely metastasize to regional lymph nodes, and wedge resection with enough surgical margin is adequate for curative resection. On the other hand, the invasive nature of adenocarcinoma may result in nodal metastasis, and segmentectomy at least is necessary for complete resection. So, we selected segmentectomy for the investigative arm, and wedge was not permitted in the JCOG0802/WJOG4607L study (Fig. 11.4). This is the most striking difference between Japanese and US studies. The difference came from the lack of the definition of radiological early lung cancer in the US.

This historical randomized trial focused on lung cancer peripherally located 2 cm or less in size with a CTR of 0.5 or more on TSCT [19]. The first randomized "Ginsberg trial" performed in the US enrolled lung cancers 3 cm or less in size. JCOG reduced the maximum tumor size because of several positive studies for segmentectomy in lung cancer 2 cm or less in size [20–24]. The study was designed as a non-inferiority randomized trial, and the prognosis of sublobar resection was permitted to inferior up to 5% compared to lobectomy. The targeted number of patients was more than

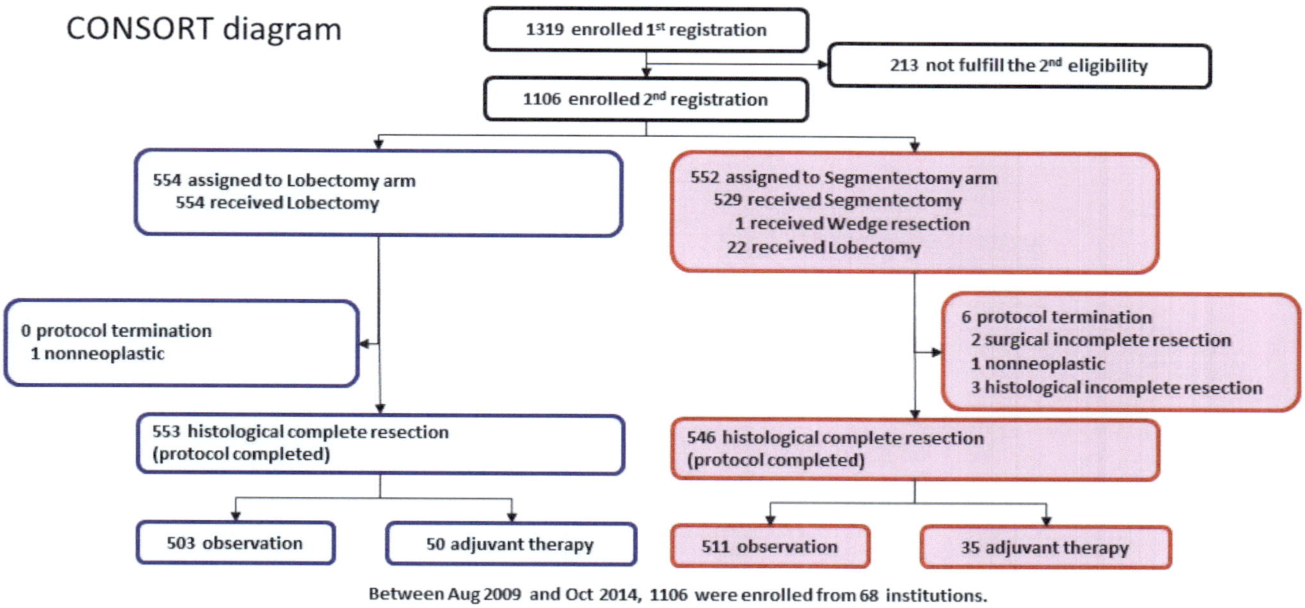

Fig. 11.4 JCOG0802/WJOG4507L study compared segmentectomy with lobectomy in a randomized setting

1000, having 500 for each arm. The primary endpoint of the study was overall survival, and the secondary endpoints were respiratory function, relapse-free survival, postoperative morbidity/mortality, operative time, local recurrence, and blood loss. Finally, the primary endpoint was met for the unexpected superiority of sublobar resection as to overall survival, and sublobar resection should be a standard mode of surgery for stage I NSCLC 2 cm or less in size. This is the historical study of deciding sublobar resection for invasive lung cancer for the first time.

11.8 Oncological Paradox "Less Is More"

Our practice in the thoracic surgical community has been widely changed due to the unexpected results of the JCOG 0802 study (Fig. 11.5). However, all secondary endpoints favored lobectomy. As to local control, local failure after sublobar resection was double compared to lobectomy. Some of the patients who had local failure after sublobar resection should have undergone completion lobectomy or pneumonectomy, and those operations are basically very invasive for patients [25]. That is why we continue to debate matters of controversy on the indication of sublobar resection. The "less is more" notion is one of the controversies in our field. Based on exploratory analysis, lobectomy was superior to sublobar resection as to relapse-free survival in selected lung cancer patients. For example, lobectomy would be indicated for lung cancer 2 cm or less in size in females 70 years old or less [26].

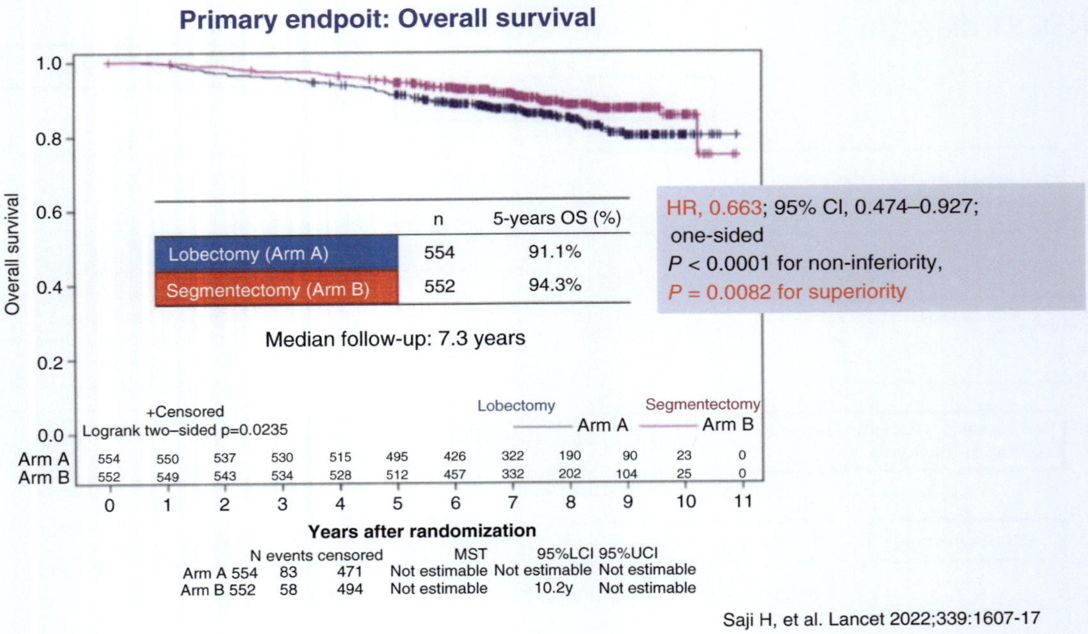

Fig. 11.5 Overall survival of sublobar resection was significantly superior to that of lobectomy

11.9 Next Clinical Questions

JCOG has made a sequence of clinical trials on the mode of surgery for lung cancer (Fig. 11.6). Most of the trials focused on lung cancer 2 cm or less in size except JCOG1211 [15, 19, 27]. JCOG1211 investigated the mode of surgery for lung cancer bigger than 2 cm, for which the standard was lobectomy [27]. The study dealt with CTR 0.5 or less, for those tumors rarely metastasize hilar nodes. The primary endpoint was met, and segmentectomy was set as the new standard for lung cancer 2–3 cm with CTR 0.5 or less. One of the next clinical questions should be sublobar resections for bigger tumor, which was investigated in the first "Ginsberg trial" in 1995. Nowadays, we have several technologies, such as computed tomography, magnetic resonance imaging, and/or positron emission tomography, which were not available in 1995. Therefore, the same design study would not show the same results. Neoadjuvant or adjuvant treatment has developed, which would make it possible for thoracic surgeons to select sublobar resection for lung cancer having N1 or N2 disease. Those questions were already investigated by the two randomized trials conducted by WJOG and JCOG.

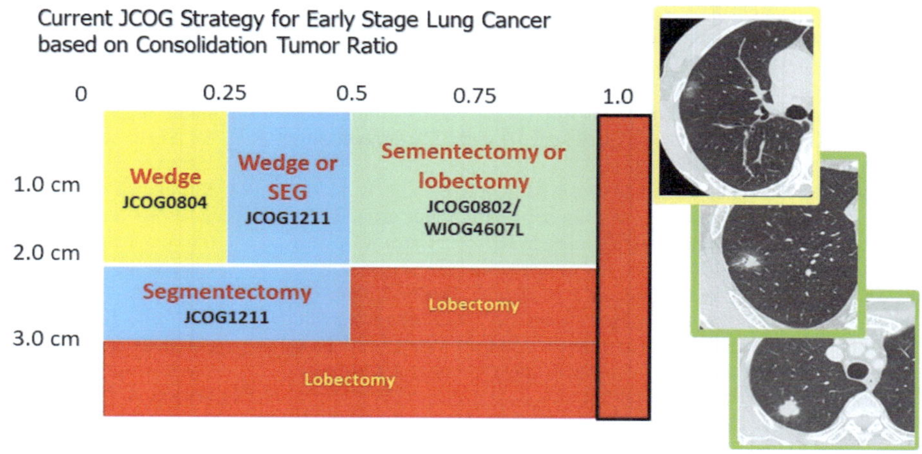

Fig. 11.6 JCOG trials

11.10 Recovery from Surgical Treatment of Lung Cancer

Thoracic surgery was performed with a big incision for a long time, for the procedure is quite complicated and has a risk of massive bleeding intraoperatively. In the 1990s, thoracotomy with cutting ribs was common, and the length of hospital stay was more than two weeks. Postoperative enhanced recovery after surgery (ERAS) was not considered at that time. Therefore, there were just one or two patients 80 years or older who were operated on. Nowadays there are many more patients 80 years or older in thoracic communities. ERAS is one of the most important factors in thoracic surgery [28].

11.11 Future Perspectives

The sequence of events in the evolution of the surgical mode for lung cancer has been described above. Selection of the surgical mode should be decided by the patient's tolerability for the planned surgery as well as tumor characteristics. However, this is one of the most difficult aspects for surgeons, and experiences are quite important for the selection. In this aspect, artificial intelligence (AI) should have a role in it in the near future. Our department is also planning to perform extensive investigations as to AI use for practical decision-making on the treatment of lung cancer [29].

References

1. Ginsberg RJ, Rubinstein LV. Randomized trial of lobectomy versus limited resection for T1 N0 non- small cell lung cancer. Lung Cancer Study Group [see comments]. Ann Thorac Surg. 1995;60(3):615–22; discussion 22–3.
2. Sobin LH. The World Health Organization's Histological Classification of Lung Tumors: a comparison of the first and second editions. Cancer Detect Prev. 1982;5(4):391–406.
3. Watanabe Y, Shimizu J, Oda M, Iwa T, Takashima T, Kamimura R, et al. Early hilar lung cancer: its clinical aspect. J Surg Oncol. 1991;48(2):75–80.
4. Shimosato Y, Suzuki A, Hashimoto T, Nishiwaki Y, Kodama T, Yoneyama T, Kameya T. Prognostic implications of fibrotic focus (scar) in small peripheral lung cancers. Am J Surg Pathol. 1980;4(4):365–73.
5. Noguchi M, Morikawa A, Kawasaki M, Matsuno Y, Yamada T, Hirohashi S, et al. Small adenocarcinoma of the lung. Histologic characteristics and prognosis. Cancer. 1995;75(12):2844–52.
6. Suzuki K, Yokose T, Yoshida J, Nishimura M, Takahashi K, Nagai K, Nishiwaki Y. Prognostic significance of the size of central fibrosis in peripheral adenocarcinoma of the lung. Ann Thorac Surg. 2000;69(3):893–7.
7. Suzuki K, Koike T, Asakawa T, Kusumoto M, Asamura H, Nagai K, et al. A prospective radiological study of thin-section computed tomography to predict pathological non-invasiveness in peripheral clinical IA lung cancer (JCOG0201). J Thorac Oncol. 2011;6:751–6.
8. Goya T, Asamura H, Yoshimura H, Kato H, Shimokata K, Tsuchiya R, et al. Prognosis of 6644 resected non-small cell lung cancers in Japan: a Japanese lung cancer registry study. Lung Cancer. 2005;50(2):227–34.
9. Suzuki K, Kusumoto M, Watanabe S, Tsuchiya R, Asamura H. Radiologic classification of small adenocarcinoma of the lung: radiologic-pathologic correlation and its prognostic impact. Ann Thorac Surg. 2006;81(2):413–9.
10. Asamura H, Hishida T, Suzuki K, Koike T, Nakamura K, Kusumoto M, et al. Radiographically determined noninvasive adenocarcinoma of the lung: survival outcomes of Japan Clinical Oncology Group 0201. J Thorac Cardiovasc Surg. 2013;146(1):24–30.
11. Ito H, Suzuki K, Mizutani T, Aokage K, Wakabayashi M, Fukuda H, Watanabe SI. Long-term survival outcome after lobectomy in patients with clinical T1 N0 lung cancer. J Thorac Cardiovasc Surg. 2020;161:281–90.
12. Nakao M, Yoshida J, Goto K, Ishii G, Kawase A, Aokage K, et al. Long-term outcomes of 50 cases of limited-resection trial for pulmonary ground-glass opacity nodules. J Thorac Oncol. 2012;7(10):1563–6.
13. Yoshida J, Ishii G, Yokose T, Aokage K, Hishida T, Nishimura M, et al. Possible delayed cut-end recurrence after limited resec-

tion for ground-glass opacity adenocarcinoma, intraoperatively diagnosed as Noguchi type B, in three patients. J Thorac Oncol. 2010;5(4):546–50.
14. Yoshida J, Nagai K, Yokose T, Nishimura M, Kakinuma R, Ohmatsu H, Nishiwaki Y. Limited resection trial for pulmonary ground-glass opacity nodules: fifty-case experience. J Thorac Cardiovasc Surg. 2005;129(5):991–6.
15. Suzuki K, Watanabe SI, Wakabayashi M, Saji H, Aokage K, Moriya Y, et al. A single-arm study of sublobar resection for ground-glass opacity dominant peripheral lung cancer. J Thorac Cardiovasc Surg. 2022;163(1):289–301.e2.
16. Suzuki K, Watanabe S, Mizusawa J, Moriya Y, Yoshino I, Tsuboi M, et al. Predictors of non-neoplastic lesions in lung tumours showing ground-glass opacity on thin-section computed tomography based on a multi-institutional prospective study†. Interact Cardiovasc Thorac Surg. 2015;21(2):218–23.
17. Niho S, Yokose T, Suzuki K, Kodama T, Nishiwaki Y, Mukai K. Monoclonality of atypical adenomatous hyperplasia of the lung [In Process Citation]. Am J Pathol. 1999;154(1):249–54.
18. Suzuki K, Ogura T, Yokose T, Nagai K, Mukai K, Kodama T, et al. Loss of heterozygosity in the tuberous sclerosis gene associated regions in adenocarcinoma of the lung accompanied by multiple atypical adenomatous hyperplasia. Int J Cancer. 1998;79(4):384–9.
19. Saji H, Okada M, Tsuboi M, Nakajima R, Suzuki K, Aokage K, et al. Segmentectomy versus lobectomy in small-sized peripheral non-small-cell lung cancer (JCOG0802/WJOG4607L): a multicentre, open-label, phase 3, randomised, controlled, non-inferiority trial. Lancet. 2022;399(10335):1607–17.
20. Okada M, Koike T, Higashiyama M, Yamato Y, Kodama K, Tsubota N. Radical sublobar resection for small-sized non-small cell lung cancer: a multicenter study. J Thorac Cardiovasc Surg. 2006;132(4):769–75.
21. Okada M, Nishio W, Sakamoto T, Uchino K, Yuki T, Nakagawa A, Tsubota N. Effect of tumor size on prognosis in patients with non-small cell lung cancer: the role of segmentectomy as a type of lesser resection. J Thorac Cardiovasc Surg. 2005;129(1):87–93.
22. Okada M, Yoshikawa K, Hatta T, Tsubota N. Is segmentectomy with lymph node assessment an alternative to lobectomy for non-small cell lung cancer of 2 cm or smaller? Ann Thorac Surg 2001;71(3):956–960; discussion 61.
23. Tsubota N, Ayabe K, Doi O, Mori T, Namikawa S, Taki T, Watanabe Y. Ongoing prospective study of segmentectomy for small lung tumors. Study Group of Extended Segmentectomy for Small Lung Tumor [In Process Citation]. Ann Thorac Surg. 1998;66(5):1787–90.
24. Yoshikawa K, Tsubota N, Kodama K, Ayabe H, Taki T, Mori T. Prospective study of extended segmentectomy for small lung tumors: the final report. Ann Thorac Surg. 2002;73(4):1055–8. discussion 8-9.
25. Hattori A, Matsunaga T, Watanabe Y, Fukui M, Takamochi K, Oh S, Suzuki K. Repeated anatomical pulmonary resection for metachronous ipsilateral second non-small cell lung cancer. J Thorac Cardiovasc Surg. 2021;162(5):1389–98.e2.
26. Hattori A, Suzuki K, Takamochi K, Wakabayashi M, Sekino Y, Tsutani Y, et al. Segmentectomy versus lobectomy in small-sized peripheral non-small-cell lung cancer with radiologically pure-solid appearance in Japan (JCOG0802/WJOG4607L): a post-hoc supplemental analysis of a multicentre, open-label, phase 3 trial. Lancet Respir Med. 2024;12(2):105–16.
27. Aokage K, Suzuki K, Saji H, Wakabayashi M, Kataoka T, Sekino Y, et al. Segmentectomy for ground-glass-dominant lung cancer with a tumour diameter of 3 cm or less including ground-glass opacity (JCOG1211): a multicentre, single-arm, confirmatory, phase 3 trial. Lancet Respir Med. 2023;11(6):540–9.
28. Batchelor TJP, Rasburn NJ, Abdelnour-Berchtold E, Brunelli A, Cerfolio RJ, Gonzalez M, et al. Guidelines for enhanced recovery after lung surgery: recommendations of the Enhanced Recovery After Surgery (ERAS®) society and the European Society of Thoracic Surgeons (ESTS). Eur J Cardio-thorac Surg. 2019;55(1):91–115.
29. Yan H, Niimi T, Matsunaga T, Fukui M, Hattori A, Takamochi K, Suzuki K. Preoperatively predicting survival outcome for clinical stage IA pure-solid non-small cell lung cancer by radiomics-based machine learning. J Thorac Cardiovasc Surg. 2024;169:254–66.

12 Brain Cancer

Akihide Kondo

Abstract

Symptoms and disabilities caused by brain tumors vary widely from person to person. Moreover, there is no well-established understanding in society because the incidence is low. As a result, the working environment has not been able to accept the return to work properly. Brain tumors include fatal tumors, in other words, malignant tumors, but there are also benign tumors that cause only temporary or reversible disability. Even if the expected prognosis of life expectancy is short due to a malignant tumor, work may still motivate a person to live as long as they remain in a healthy state of mind. In such cases, it is possible that depriving the patient of the right to work may, in fact, shorten the time they can live as a person. In addition, some central nervous system dysfunctions make it difficult to empathize or guess. For example, simultaneous executive dysfunction, estimation of distance, and half-blindness are challenging to understand without experiencing them, and even the assistance to be offered is difficult to guess. Therefore, to provide an appropriate working environment, it is necessary to understand what the individual is suffering from. With a bit of help in the work environment, the worker should be able to reach their full potential.

Keywords

Central nervous system · Brain tumors · Subsequent impairment · Higher cerebral dysfunction · Work environment · Sensory disturbance

A. Kondo (✉)
Department of Neurosurgery, School of Medicine, Juntendo University, Bunkyo-ku, Tokyo, Japan
e-mail: knd-aki@juntendo.ac.jp

12.1 Introduction

Whether malignant or benign, neoplasms of the central nervous system (CNS) cause a great deal of stress to the affected individuals. They often have some residual functional abnormalities and a common perception that this disease is fatal. This is true not just for the patient but also for family members and those involved with the patient at the workplace.

On the other hand, in modern medicine, some CNS tumors are not merely curable; they often have no permanent disability. We will discuss the impact of CNS tumors on affected individuals and the potential impact of the treatments they receive on their work lives.

12.2 Overview

The definition of the CNS in the human body includes the brain and spinal cord. The brain and spinal cord are protected by the skull and vertebrae (spinal canal) and exist in water called cerebrospinal fluid. The area where this cerebrospinal fluid exists is called the intrathecal space. From the brain and spinal cord, countless nerves are distributed from the base of the skull and intervertebral foramen to the limbs, trunk, and organs, but this group of nerves is strictly a peripheral nerve. Therefore, CNS tumors are brain tumors and spinal cord tumors, but they will be synonymous with brain tumors in this text. By convention, tumors in the intrathecal space are included in CNS tumors, even if they originate in peripheral nerves. Cancer and carcinoma are pathological terms for malignant tumors arising from epithelial cells, while sarcoma refers to malignant tumors of connective tissue origin. CNS malignant tumors are not epithelial cell-derived, and connective tissue-derived tumors are often benign, so these two names are not being used. However, the term "brain cancer" has been used to promote general understanding recently.

The CNS, the part of the brain responsible for essential functions such as the movement of limbs, sensation, higher-

© The Author(s), under exclusive license to Springer Nature Singapore Pte Ltd. 2026

M. Endo et al. (eds.), *Cancer and Work in Asia Volume 2*, https://doi.org/10.1007/978-981-95-6537-5_12

level judgment, memory, and the maintenance of one's own life, is located in a specific part of the brain. Therefore, symptoms and their severity vary greatly depending on the tumor's location. If the tumor occurs in the so-called eloquent areas, it is likely to result in a functional disability that can impair the quality of life. In other words, even though the classification of tumors is the same type, the potential disability varies based on the tumor's location.

Recent advances in molecular biological analysis techniques have revealed that a group of tumors thought to be the same type based on conventional histopathological findings may be composed of multiple tumors. It has also become clear that molecular biological characteristics can predict prognosis more accurately than histopathological characteristics, and then the conventional tumor types have been subdivided into more than 150 types.

Consequently, various degrees of life expectancy and disability arise depending on the site of tumor origin and tumor type.

In contrast to the common perception that brain tumors are fatal and disabling for all affected people, each patient has different symptoms and prognoses, requiring individualized treatments. This is one of the most important facts in understanding workers with brain tumors. It should also be understood that the patients themselves may be more bound by the aforementioned common understanding than by this fact.

It is also true that brain tumors include "fatal" diseases. Table 12.1 shows the 5-year survival rates for the CNS tumor. It shows that brain tumors collectively include a group of tumors with a poor prognosis and those that pose almost no risk to life [1].

Table 12.1 Brain tumor type and prognosis

Tumor type	Overall survival for 5 years (%)
Pilocytic astrocytoma	92.1
Diffuse astrocytoma	75.0
Oligodendroglioma	90.0
Anaplastic astrocytoma	41.1
Glioblastoma	10.1
Ependymoma	86.3
Ganglioglioma	98.1
Medulloblastoma	68.7
Germ cell tumor	97.1
Meningioma	97.9
Schwannoma	98.8
Hemangioblastoma	96.3
Primary CNS lymphoma	42.3
Craniopharyngioma	96.5

The 5-year survival rate for high-incidence brain tumors was shown according to Ref. [1]

12.3 Symptoms in Patients with Brain Tumors

The most critical aspect of evaluating a brain tumor in terms of workability is where the tumor originates. In clinical practice, we classify tumors as parenchymal or extraparenchymal.

Most parenchymal tumors, called gliomas, infiltrate the surrounding normal brain, and the boundary between the tumor and the normal brain is often unclear. This means they are difficult to remove entirely and require continuous post-treatment for residual tumors, such as radiation and chemotherapy. For this reason, if the tumor is malignant, the life expectancy is about 2 years. However, the patient should not be prevented from returning to work, as it is often possible to live with only minimal symptoms until recurrence. If the tumor is highly malignant, the patient may only be able to work for about a year.

Even if the grade is low for glioma, a cure is often impossible. It is necessary to keep searching for recurrence through regular visits to the medical institution. Recurrence may occur 7–8 years after the initial diagnosis, making it a disease that requires long-term treatment. The disability associated with the tumor varies greatly depending on the site of origin. In other words, if the tumor is located in the area responsible for language functions, aphasia will occur. If the tumor is located in the area responsible for motor functions, paralysis will remain. These cannot be expected to improve dramatically. Another characteristic of parenchymal tumors is that they may have higher functional impairment due to their treatments, including radiation therapy.

In contrast, extraparenchymal tumors arise from intracranial structures and peripheral nerves and are less likely to invade the central nervous system, which does not recover. Those tumors are often a meningioma or schwannoma, and a cure can be expected.

However, because schwannomas are tumors of the cranial nerves themselves, their neurological functions are often lost. The most common type of schwannoma is vestibular schwannoma, but dizziness and hearing impairment remain even if the tumor is cured. In particular, the hearing impairment is such that although the patient can hear, the directional perception of sound is impaired. The patient may not recognize when someone is speaking to them and may not be able to hear necessary conversations in noisy situations. This is a very characteristic disorder of this tumor.

Meningioma is a benign disease that is unlikely to affect life expectancy. It can be surgically removed and is a curable tumor. However, this is not the case when it occurs at the skull base. The base of the skull contains countless cranial nerves and peripheral nerves that transmit commands from the brain to the limbs and take in information about events in the limbs and trunk. Tumors in the vicinity of these nerves can prevent proper transmission of commands, impair movement, and make it difficult to take in sensory information. It is difficult to peel off the tumor from the nerves completely, and it is impossible to remove the entire tumor without damaging countless nerves, which may remain and continue to grow, worsening the symptoms. In this case, radiation therapy is used in combination. Nerve symptoms vary depending on the tumor's location, from visual to sensory disturbance and numbness. If the tumor is located in the spinal canal, it may cause difficulty walking and bladder and rectal problems such as incontinence. Large tumors not situated at the base of the skull may irreversibly damage the brain parenchyma due to pressure from the tumor. The resulting disability is very similar to that of a parenchymal brain tumor.

Brain tumors include metastatic brain tumors. Metastatic brain tumors result from the metastasis of malignant tumors in the neck, trunk, or extremities, most of which are intraparenchymal. It is not uncommon to have more than one tumor. Patients with metastatic brain tumors often suffer from the same disabilities as the parenchymal tumors described previously. In the past, metastatic brain tumors occurred when primary lesions could not be controlled, and the life expectancy was about 6 months, so there was no need to consider returning to work. However, with recent advances in anti-tumor drugs, the life expectancy has been extended to about 2.5 years. Therefore, the number of people with metastatic brain tumors who wish to return to work increases.

Patients with metastatic brain tumors require different considerations than patients with primary brain tumors because they need treatment for metastases while already receiving intensive treatment for primary cancer. With the recent advances in anti-tumor drugs, it is not uncommon for the primary lesion to be well controlled and the brain to remain the only lesion. This is because antitumor drugs may not reach brain lesions due to the brain-blood barrier in the brain. Therefore, radiation therapy is often used to treat metastatic brain tumors. There are two types of radiation therapy: whole brain radiation and stereotactic radiation. Either is selected depending on the medical concept and the nature of the primary cancer. After whole-brain irradiation, patients are likely to experience gradual impairment of cognition and memory over 1–2 years, so it is advisable to evaluate their ability to work continuously. The disability caused by CNS tumors may be caused by the tumor itself or treatment-related complications.

12.4 Work and Life Prognosis

The terminal stage of CNS tumors is rarely life-threatening due to multi-organ invasiveness by the tumor. The most direct causes of death are pneumonia and urinary tract infections. This is because aspiration during food intake is an immediate trigger as a result of impaired consciousness caused by the progression of the brain tumor. In other words, the brain tumor slowly deprives the patient of the ability to perform activities necessary to sustain life. This is thought to include the ability to persist in life. When parenchymal tumors are resected with a safety margin to achieve radical resection of the tumor, resulting in language impairment and paralysis, it is known that the group of patients with a residual tumor but no language or motor impairment has a better long-term prognosis. This means that maintaining human dignity can result in a long-term prognosis for this disease group.

There are many people for whom work is the primary reason for their identification. Depriving such people of working life may deprive them of their will to live, resulting in a short prognosis. Work-related support for patients with CNS tumors can provide the same value to patients as participation in treatment.

12.5 CNS Tumors and Depression

Although many of the disorders that occur by CNS tumors can be explained neuroanatomically, some conditions arise that are difficult to link to them. One such condition is depression. It is most likely due to neurophysiological changes associated with brain tumors. About 20% of affected patients have a depressive mood disorder [2]. To date, coexisting depression is known to have a worse prognosis than non-coexisting cases.

Higher rates of treatment-related complications and difficulties in establishing relationships, including with health care providers, are believed to be reasons for the poorer prognosis in comorbid cases [3].

Anxiety and depressive disorders may also develop due to brain tumor exposure. In response, psychosocial interventions have been reported to improve patients' quality of life [4].

A similar relationship-building problem occurs when a person has tumor-induced memory impairment. Tumors, especially in the temporal lobe and in areas associated with memory circuits, can cause seizure-induced memory loss. These are considered to be epileptic seizures and are called complex partial seizures. In complex partial seizures, consciousness is not attenuated, and general behavior is possible. However, because the affected part of the brain is not functioning, there is a significant loss of judgment and cognition, leading to accidents and misguided behavior. The biggest problem with memory impairment is the inability to understand events that occur when there is no memory, which may lead to the breakdown of relationships when errors are pointed out. The inability to hold people accountable when accidents happen because they cannot grasp the events. Furthermore, they may not be able to gain awareness of the seriousness of their illness, making it difficult for them to continue their social life. In many of these cases, the physician has already pointed out the dangers of the disease and given appropriate guidance. Hence, it is a disorder that should be shared by society.

12.6 Employers and Workers

There is a global trend of legislation requiring employers to provide an appropriate work environment for people with brain tumors. However, the extent and level of enforcement vary by government and region.

Under these laws, employers have specific responsibilities when accepting a person with a brain tumor into the workplace. Employers are obligated to protect the patient and the patient's family from discrimination and harassment due to the disability caused by the disease and are obligated to provide a working environment and assistance for the patient to remain on the job.

On the other hand, employees have the right not to have their personal information disclosed to anyone without their permission, the right to take leave for urgent medical treatment, and the right to take time off without sufficient notice.

Therefore, it is necessary to change the way work is done, to provide physical changes in the work facility environment, and, in some cases, to provide exceptional help and support. In other words, it is necessary to propose ways to deal with problems that may prevent employees from continuing to work or returning to work.

12.7 Symptoms and Management of Symptoms

Symptoms of a CNS tumor are difficult for anyone to predict. It is necessary to ask about symptoms and management at different times repeatedly. It is socially and therapeutically beneficial to utilize the patient's abilities effectively in the workplace. The focus should be on what they can do and their strengths, not on what they cannot do. Supportive coworkers who are responsible for helping in the workplace can be effective, and records such as occupational health plans can be helpful for similar cases. The following is a list of symptom-related disorders that have been reported to date and suggestions for workplace management of these disorders [5].

12.7.1 Fatigue

CNS tumors themselves, radiation therapy, and other factors can lead to mental and physical fatigue. Decreased immunity has also been implicated. The degree of fatigue is difficult for those around the patient to grasp because there is no objective indicator. Only the patient knows the degree of fatigue, and it fluctuates. Therefore, it is vital to understand the current situation through regular discussions. A step-by-step plan to return to work according to the individual's condition, adjustment of working hours, change to a part-time job, and reduction of work content are some of the actions that can be taken. Recently, teleworking is also a possible response, and in some cases, providing a temporary rest area and rest time at the workplace may dramatically improve work efficiency.

12.7.2 Movement Dysfunction

Hemiplegia or trunk ataxia is not always accompanied by decreased intelligence or impaired judgment. It is beneficial to consider appropriate aids such as transportation to work, handrails, and reduced periods of standing. Simply placing the person's work area on the entrance side of the building can improve mobility and help in an emergency evacuation. Proximity to restrooms is also a consideration. In some cases, only a sophisticated hand movement may be restricted, making it difficult to express oneself by type. In such cases, speech recognition software using recent computer technology can effectively assist expression.

12.7.3 Sensory Impairment

In addition to sensory impairment of the extremities, the five senses of sight, hearing, and taste are also affected. For vision, large letters and pictures, lighting adjustment in the work area, and voice reading software are effective. Photophobia is also common. It is known that environments with significant changes in light levels can lead to headaches and epileptic seizures. Workplaces should be provided far away from windows, and appropriate sunglasses should be allowed to be worn at work if necessary. Regarding hearing, it is recommended to offer individualized headphones and wear hearing impairment stickers or badges with the individual's consent. Hearing impairment may include hypersensitivity to hearing, and quiet workplaces may be provided. Taste disorders have been linked to decreased appetite and motivation and gastrointestinal symptoms such as diarrhea and constipation. Workplace eating alternatives need to be suggested.

Unfortunately, it is difficult to manage headaches completely when one has a CNS tumor. Headaches are more likely to be caused by prolonged periods of sitting and/or standing in the same position, indoor environments, and interpersonal relationships, so try to identify and eliminate triggers. The background should be conducive to taking oral medication at the appropriate time.

Repetition of the same task for a long time may aggravate neuropathic pain. Consider appropriate rest and alternative work assignments.

12.7.4 Epileptic Seizures

Focal or generalized damage to the brain results in seizures. This is often treated with antiepileptic drugs, but it is difficult to eliminate the seizures completely. In the workplace, train your staff to deal with attacks. There is no need for special training, such as measuring seizure duration or protecting oneself from trauma during a large seizure, which doctors are concerned about; knowledge of seizures is necessary. In the case of complex partial seizures, as described above, the patient often has no memory of the seizure, and the information is not conveyed to the physician in charge. Keeping these records will play a major role in the treatment progress. In seizure management, it is believed that a short rest at the aura of a seizure prevents a major seizure. Antiepileptic drugs can cause drowsiness and dizziness, so appropriate attention is desirable.

12.7.5 Higher Functional Impairment

Higher cerebral dysfunction associated with tumor incidence and related treatments is a significant issue in labor. Since the patient may not necessarily have an awareness of the symptoms, careful handling is required. A variety of intelligence testing methods have been established, and it is possible to compare the affected person with the same age group using a conversion table. One of the most useful intelligence tests is the Wechsler Adult Intelligence Scale-Revised (WAIS-R), which can identify weaknesses in 12 areas such as movement and language and suggest appropriate actions. However, because of the time and expense required for assessment, it is often not used in cases where the disease is in its progressive stage. Therefore, it is advisable to understand what can occur due to the disease as knowledge in the workplace and to manage the entire work environment without overreacting, with the appropriate intervention of medical personnel.

12.8 Communication

Decreased memory and attention lead to learning disabilities and difficulties in systematic behavior. It is not uncommon for personality changes to occur due to anxiety caused by these decreased abilities. Differences in behavior before and after the illness may result in communication disorders. Therefore, more time is needed to establish cooperation than before. It is also necessary to limit and record work assignments and job descriptions. Short, concise directions and sufficient response time are helpful, and providing a place and time for calm is part of the solution. However, if the continuation of the work that requires adjustment causes delays or affects the overall quality of the work, a change in duties should be proactively proposed.

12.9 Memory Impairment

In addition to epileptic seizures, short-term memory loss may be unstable due to impaired memory circuits caused by the tumor itself. In particular, the patient may ignore what has just happened and may ask the same questions repeatedly. Repetition and documentation of instructions are important, but an environment that allows for repetition can also prevent the disorder from deteriorating. Since memory impairment triggers communication disorders, obtaining the patient's consent and encouraging the cooperation of those around them will lead to the improvement of the workplace environment.

12.10 Labor Processing

It is known that CNS diseases in general cause concurrent executive dysfunction after the disease, which is difficult to recover from. Work support should be a single step. Instructions given in meetings are often incomprehensible, so documenting them will help understanding. It is important to simplify the directives because it is often the lack of understanding of the directives that takes time to respond. They may not be good at planning and processing labor, so color-coding the priority of tasks and indicating the time required will often help them respond appropriately.

12.11 Cognition

Concentration and attention are often more attenuated than before the disease. On the other hand, there may be no decline in processing ability, so limiting the scope of manageable or subdivided tasks may be beneficial. Moving the work area to a quieter location may help maintain concentration. If there is a decline in practical ability, indicate it and suggest realistic goals.

12.12 Endocrine Disorders

Some neoplastic diseases can cause hormonal abnormalities. Hormones are chemical messengers in the body that are necessary to maintain homeostasis. Insufficient or excessive levels of hormones can cause disorders. In general, they manage appetite, libido, and other physiological needs and regulate body temperature and urine output. Therefore, weight gain, appetite changes, short stature, and metabolic disorders such as lipid metabolism and diabetes may occur in addition to tumor burden. Concerning temperature dysregulation, easing the dress code, adjusting the room temperature, and providing a shower in more complicated cases are often effective.

12.13 Appearance

The cranium is an area that is not entirely covered by clothing. It can be subject to a wide range of cosmetic changes, including facial paralysis and other limitations in facial expression, hair loss due to radiation and chemotherapy, skin tissue deposition, and surgical scarring due to surgical intervention. More recently, tumor-treating field therapy has been used to control malignant brain tumors. This treatment involves shaving the patient's head and attaching large electrodes to a device that generates an electric field for an extended period. In such cases, private rooms may be necessary. In some cases, it is desirable to avoid contact with non-employees, but in other cases, a positive connection with others after counseling may help to eliminate excessive anxiety.

12.14 Social Conditions

Affected individuals are often subject to a variety of social restrictions. They often lose their driver's license due to brain dysfunction, and if they have epileptic seizures, they are often socially isolated. To avoid such a situation, it is necessary to discuss how and to what extent the information will be shared with those around the workplace after the patient has given consent. It is also essential to consider how much knowledge and experience the workplace should have about the disease. The proposed mental health environment does not have to be more excessive than in the traditional workplace. Instead, by suggesting support programs for the surrounding workers as well, we can find cooperation in the workplace and avoid overburdening the supporters.

12.15 Conclusion

We have presented the disabilities that can occur when a person is affected by a CNS tumor, and we have presented our current approach to returning to and maintaining work.

Difficulties in returning to work after a CNS tumor are not only caused by depressive symptoms and cognitive decline due to the tumor or by the poor prognosis of the tumor itself. It is due to the lack of an organization that can accept and deal with these difficulties in social life. In particular, work is essential in social life, and the existence of a work environment that can accommodate this has a tremendous impact on patients' lives. We as a society need to provide appropriate occupational rehabilitation programs for those who wish to return to work.

There is no need to always have large, high-cost programs in the works. Simply establishing a method of contacting people who are absent from work to manage their physical condition will reduce the burden on the patient. As staff, colleagues, and supervisors in the workplace, all we need to do is listen to what the patient wants, talk to them about the tumor if they're going to, and ask how it affects them. Having a work environment that listens to what they want and never assumes what they can or cannot do will best encourage them to return to work.

References

1. Brain tumor registry of Japan. Neurol Med Chir. 2014;57.
2. Monika J, et al. Quality of life among patients with a brain tumor and their carers. J Psychosom Res. 2007;63
3. Litofsky NS, et al. The relationships between depression and brain tumors. J Neuro-Oncol. 2009;94
4. Silvaggi F, et al. Employment and work ability of persons with brain tumors: a systematic review. Front Hum Neurosci. 2020;14
5. The brain tumour Charity; 2022. https://www.thebraintumourcharity.org.

13 Hepatic and Pancreatic Cancer

Yoshihiro Mise

Abstract

Hepatic (liver) and pancreatic cancers are considered refractory diseases. However, advances in treatment strategies have led to the prognosis of both cancers becoming more and more promising. This chapter provides a general outline of the two diseases and describes how medical treatment is given. It also discusses the impact the disease and its treatment have on the daily life of a patient with liver or pancreatic cancer.

Keywords

Return to work · Liver cancer · Pancreatic cancer · Multidisciplinary treatment · Cancer survivorship

13.1 Introduction

13.1.1 Liver Cancer

What Does the Liver Do?

The liver is a large organ located in the upper part of the abdomen (Fig. 13.1). It is protected by the lower ribs on the right side of your body. Two blood vessels, the hepatic artery and the portal vein, supply your liver with blood that comes through the gut. The blood reaching the liver contains nutrients, such as carbohydrates, proteins, fats, and vitamins. The liver stores nutrients, makes substances essential to your body, like bile and proteins, and breaks down harmful substances, such as drugs and alcohol.

What Is Liver Cancer?

Liver cancer is categorized into two types according to where it starts: primary and secondary liver cancer. A primary liver cancer starts growing in the liver, while a secondary liver cancer starts growing somewhere other than the liver. Secondary liver cancer occurs when cancer cells break away from this other primary site, such as the colon, travel to the liver, and start to grow a new cancer.

In this chapter, we will focus on primary hepatocellular carcinoma (HCC), a type of cancer that starts growing in the liver and is common in Asian countries. Asia has the highest occurrence of HCC in the world, with 80% of all cases globally occurring on the Asian continent and 55% in China and Hong Kong alone. HCC is the most common form of cancer in Laos, Mongolia, Taiwan, and Thailand.

Risk Factors of Liver Cancer

Some common risk factors for liver cancer, which are also risk factors for other cancers, are male gender, aging, obesity, and smoking. A risk factor specific to liver cancer is baseline liver cirrhosis, which can be caused by a hepatitis virus infection, long-term alcohol drinking, or a fatty liver (where the liver has an excessive amount of fat).

13.1.2 Pancreatic Cancer

What Does the Pancreas Do?

The pancreas is a small leaf-shaped organ located behind the stomach (Fig. 13.1). The main role of the pancreas is to promote food digestion and regulate blood sugar levels throughout the body. The pancreas has two parts: the exocrine pancreas produces digestive juices, while the endocrine pancreas produces hormones, such as insulin. Digestive juices produced by the exocrine pancreas flow down a tube (pancreatic duct) into the bowel.

What Is Pancreatic Cancer?

There are two types of pancreatic cancer: exocrine cancer and endocrine cancer. About 93% of all pancreatic cancers are exocrine cancers, and adenocarcinoma is the most common kind of exocrine pancreatic cancer. In this chapter, we will focus on pancreatic ductal adenocarcinoma, as this is

Y. Mise (✉)
Department of Hepatobiliary-Pancreatic Surgery, School of Medicine, Juntendo University, Bunkyo-ku, Tokyo, Japan
e-mail: y.mise.xb@juntendo.ac.jp

© The Author(s), under exclusive license to Springer Nature Singapore Pte Ltd. 2026

M. Endo et al. (eds.), *Cancer and Work in Asia Volume 2*, https://doi.org/10.1007/978-981-95-6537-5_13

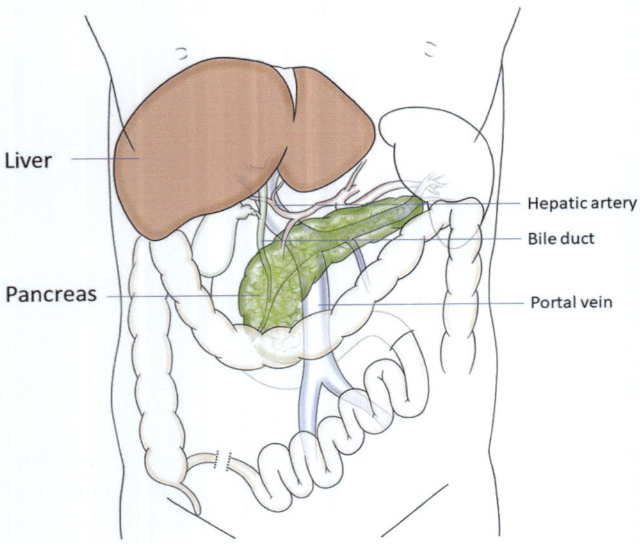

Fig. 13.1 Location of the liver, pancreas, and surrounding vessels within the abdomen

what people are usually referring to with pancreatic cancer. In 2018, over 200,000 cases of pancreatic cancers (including endocrine tumors) were reported in Asia. The crude incidence rate in Japan is 33.9 cases per 100,000 people, while in China the rate is 8.2 cases per 100,000 people [1].

Risk Factors for Pancreatic Cancer

Pancreatic cancer is more common in older people. Almost half of all new cases are diagnosed in people aged 75 years and over. Male gender, smoking, and obesity are also risk factors for pancreatic cancer.

Genetic factors have also been associated with pancreatic cancer, where between 5% and 10% of patients diagnosed with pancreatic cancer have a family history of the disease. The risk of developing pancreatic cancer increases if you have a first-degree relative with pancreatic cancer.

13.2 Diagnosis

13.2.1 Liver Cancer

Symptoms

Early-stage primary liver cancer does not show any symptoms. As such, it is frequently detected during screening for an underlying liver disease, such as viral hepatitis or alcoholic cirrhosis. Liver disease does have symptoms, which include

- Weight loss
- Swollen stomach (due to the growing cancer in the liver or liver cirrhosis producing ascites [fluid in the abdomen] that swells the abdomen)
- Jaundice (yellowing of the skin and whites of the eyes)
- Itching
- Nausea or vomiting.

Tests for Liver Cancer

Blood tests can check your liver function. Additionally, alpha-fetoprotein (AFP) is a useful tumor marker when diagnosing liver cancer. A steadily rising AFP level in the blood is indicative of liver cancer. If you have underlying liver disease, your AFP level will be checked every 3–4 months.

Imaging can identify tumors on your liver. Various imaging methods (described below) can create a detailed image of the abdominal area:

- Ultrasound scan: a very safe and simple procedure because it does not involve radiation. If you are at high risk of liver cancer, ultrasound screening may be done every 6 months to scan for any tumors.
- Computed tomography (CT): a powerful X-ray test that creates detailed pictures of the inside of your body. This test may be done after liver cancer is found by ultrasound to obtain more detailed images of the cancer, or when cancer is not detected by ultrasound despite blood tests indicating cancer may be present.
- Magnetic resonance imaging (MRI): creates pictures using magnetic waves. It is very safe and does not use radiation.

A liver biopsy means removing a sample of cells from a suspicious mass in your liver. It is not an essential test and is only performed when a definite diagnosis cannot be obtained with imaging. In a liver biopsy, a special needle is inserted through the skin into the liver under local anesthesia.

13.2.2 Pancreatic Cancer

Symptoms

Most people with pancreatic cancer do not show any symptoms in the early stages of the disease. As the cancer grows, it can start causing symptoms such as

- Upper abdominal pain that may spread to the back
- Jaundice (yellowing of the skin and whites of the eyes)
- Weight loss
- Light-colored feces
- Dark-colored urine
- Itching
- New or worsening diabetes.

Tests for Pancreatic Cancer

It is difficult to detect pancreatic cancer when the disease is in the early stages. If your doctor suspects pancreatic cancer, a blood test, ultrasound, and CT scan may be performed, as described earlier in the liver cancer section. Some pancreatic cancers produce proteins in the blood called CEA and CA19–9, which are used as tumor markers of pancreatic cancer. However, other conditions can also increase these proteins, so they cannot be used to make a definite diagnosis.

An endoscopic ultrasound (EUS) is a specific test for pancreatic cancer. An EUS uses a thin tube (endoscope) with a camera at the tip that is passed through the mouth and into the stomach. The ultrasound probe at the end of the endoscope allows imaging of the pancreas through the stomach wall. For a definite diagnosis of pancreatic cancer, a biopsy is performed during the EUS by passing a special needle into the pancreatic tumor through the endoscope.

Using information from imaging tests, your doctor assigns your pancreatic cancer a stage. The stages help determine what treatments are most likely to benefit you.

- Stage 0: characterized by abnormal cells in the lining of the pancreas.
- Stage I: cancer is only in the pancreas.
- Stage II: cancer is in the pancreas and has either spread to nearby tissues or lymph nodes.
- Stage III: cancer has spread to the major vessels near the pancreas and may have spread to nearby lymph nodes.
- Stage IV: cancer has spread to distant organs, such as the liver, lungs, or abdominal cavity.

13.3 Treatment

13.3.1 Liver Cancer

Several treatment options are effective for liver cancer. A team of doctors from different specialties, called a multidisciplinary team, will discuss the best treatment and care for you, based on the following conditions:

- The location and the size of your cancer
- The stage (where the cancer has spread)
- How well your liver is functioning
- Your general health and comorbidities (other diseases or conditions that you may have).

Surgery

Surgery gives the best chance of curing liver cancer. However, your cancer needs to be early stage, that is, localized within the liver. There are two different types of surgical treatment: liver resection and liver transplant.

Liver resection is an option if your liver cancer is localized and the rest of your liver is healthy. The amount of the liver that can be removed depends on how well your liver is working; up to 70% of the liver can be removed if your liver is healthy.

A liver transplant is an operation that removes your whole liver and replaces it with a healthy liver from a donor. Thorough reviews of your condition by liver transplant specialists are necessary beforehand, and it requires a donor liver that matches yours. Liver transplantations are categorized into two types depending on the source of the donor liver: a deceased donor liver transplantation and a living donor liver transplantation, where the donor liver is from a family member, relative, or close friend.

Ablation Therapy

Ablation therapy destroys tumor cells without removing them by inserting a special probe from the skin through to your liver. Unlike surgery, which is done under general anesthesia, ablation therapy is performed under local anesthesia. This treatment works best on small cancers, usually those smaller than 3 cm in size. Several clinical trials have demonstrated surgery and ablation therapy have equivalent therapeutic effects for smaller-sized liver cancer.

Intra-arterial Therapy

Liver cancer gets its blood supply from the hepatic artery. In intra-arterial therapy, anti-cancer drugs and particles that can block the blood supply are injected through the artery by interventional radiologists. This therapy is called trans-arterial chemoembolization (TACE) and is performed under local anesthesia. In some cases, patients that do not initially qualify for surgery can become eligible after TACE shrinks the liver cancer.

Drug Therapy

Drug therapy is used for advanced liver cancer that cannot be treated by the therapies described above. Recently, a drug therapy called a targeted cancer therapy has made revolutionary advances. Targeted cancer drugs work by 'targeting' the cancer cells, which are different from normal cells, and have reduced side effects compared with conventional chemotherapy drugs. Several targeted cancer drugs are available for treatment of liver cancer, such as sorafenib (Nexavar), envatinib (Lenvima) and regorafenib (Stivarga).

These drugs are taken as tablets or capsules, and treatment is continued as long as they control cancer growth and the side effects are not severe. Once a drug therapy has controlled the cancer, other treatments, such as surgery, can be an option.

Side effects depend on the type of drug, with the most common ones including:

- Diarrhea
- Hand-foot syndrome (soreness and redness of the palms and soles)
- Rash
- Fatigue
- Hypertension (high blood pressure)
- Increased risk of bleeding.

13.3.2 Pancreatic Cancer

Treatment for pancreatic cancer depends on the stage and location of the cancer. The primary goal of treatment is to eliminate the cancer, if possible by surgery. However, only 20% of patients with pancreatic cancer qualify for surgery. When surgery is not an option, the focus may be on improving quality of life and preventing the cancer from growing further.

Surgery

Surgery can be performed as a potentially curative treatment if the pancreatic cancer is localized within the pancreas and has not yet metastasized, that is, spread to another site. Research has shown that the safety of pancreatic surgery significantly depends on the experience of the hospital, with fewer complications occurring when pancreatic surgery is performed at hospitals that do lots of pancreatic surgery. For this reason, it would be better to have surgery at institutions performing at least 15–20 pancreatic surgeries a year.

Two different types of procedures are performed based on the location of the tumor:

- Pancreatoduodenectomy (Whipple procedure) (Fig. 13.2). This procedure is done if the cancer is located in the head of the pancreas (right side of the body). This operation is technically demanding because the surgeon needs to remove several organs, including the head of the pancreas, the duodenum, the gallbladder, and the bile duct. Part of the stomach may also be removed. After removal of the organs, a procedure called reconstruction is performed that reconnects the rest of the pancreas, the bile duct, the stomach, and the intestines.
- Distal pancreatectomy (Fig. 13.3). This surgery removes the body and tail of the pancreas (left side of the body). The spleen is also removed in this operation.

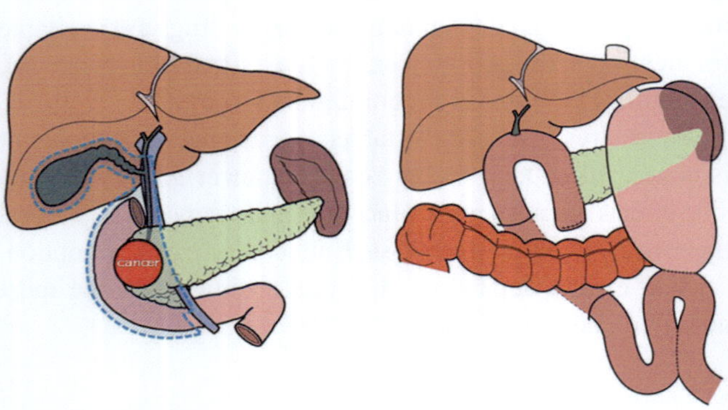

Fig. 13.2 Operation for the pancreatic tumor located at the head of the pancreas (pancreatoduodenectomy). In this operation, the head of the pancreas, duodenum, and bile duct are removed (resection). Reconstruction of the resected organs is performed following resection

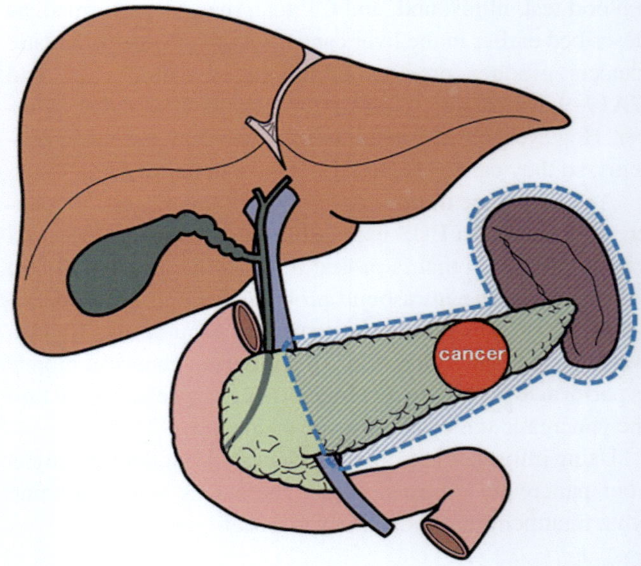

Fig. 13.3 Operation for the pancreatic tumor located at the body or tail of the pancreas (distal pancreatectomy). The left side of the pancreas (almost two-thirds of the whole volume) and the spleen are removed in this operation

Chemotherapy

There are two reasons to use chemotherapy for patients with pancreatic cancer. One is to control the disease before and after surgical treatment. Preoperative chemotherapy is called neoadjuvant chemotherapy, while postoperative chemotherapy is called adjuvant chemotherapy. Neoadjuvant chemotherapy is usually administered to patients with borderline resectable cancer, which means the cancer is located right next to a main vessel and needs to shrink before surgery. Clinical research has shown that adjuvant chemotherapy, which usually lasts for 6 months, significantly improves survival compared with that of patients having surgery alone.

Another reason to use chemotherapy is to reduce symptoms and improve the quality of life of patients with advanced cancer for which surgical treatment is not an option. Unfortunately, chemotherapy alone cannot cure advanced pancreatic cancer. However, in rare cases, patients with advanced disease may qualify for surgery if chemotherapy has dramatically shrunk the cancer.

Chemotherapy can also be combined with radiation therapy (chemoradiation) to help shrink the cancer.

Supportive Care

Supportive care, also called palliative care, is treatment that focuses on providing relief from pain and other symptoms of the disease. Supportive care may include:

- Pain management
- Jaundice treatment: a stent tube is inserted to expand the bile duct occupied by cancer

- Reducing intestinal blockage, a stent tube insertion or bypass surgery may be performed
- Emotional support and supportive care to help patients process their emotions.

Specialists work with you, your family, and your other doctors to provide an extra layer of support. It is often used while undergoing aggressive treatments, such as surgery or chemotherapy.

13.4 Impact on Daily Life

Owing to the evolution of treatment options, the prognosis of liver and pancreatic cancers is improving. Treatment strategies are becoming more and more complex and require a multidisciplinary approach involving surgeons, oncologists, endoscopists, radiologists, and other medical experts. The aim is to provide optimal treatment based on the cancer stage of each patient.

When you have a diagnosis of liver or pancreatic cancer, it is better to go to a high-volume hospital that has experienced a lot of cancer patients. Extensive research has shown that experienced hospitals offer better long-term as well as short-term outcomes after cancer treatment.

This section discusses the impact of cancer treatment on daily life in patients with liver and pancreatic cancers.

13.4.1 Liver Cancer

If you have localized liver cancer, radical treatment, such as surgery or ablation therapy, can remove the cancer. However, an unfortunate fact is that liver cancer often returns, as it never goes away completely. A recent clinical trial from Japan demonstrated that about 50% of patients who underwent surgery or ablation therapy for liver cancer, where they had less than three tumors, with each measuring 3 cm or less, had cancer recurrence within 3 years [2].

Although it is common for liver cancer to recur, repetitive treatment improves prognosis even after having liver cancer recurrence. In some patients, three or more repeat liver resections reportedly led to favorable survival [3]. Hence, even if you have completed treatment, your doctors will still want to monitor you regularly to detect any recurrence while still in an early stage. Blood tests that check liver function and tumor markers and imaging studies, such as ultrasound or CT scans, should be performed every 3–6 months.

How Does Liver Cancer Treatment Affect Your Quality of Life?

There has been much research assessing the impact of liver cancer on health-related quality of life (HRQoL) in patients with liver cancer. A diagnosis of liver cancer negatively affects the mental component of HRQoL, and it worsens as the disease advances [4]. However, optimal treatment can reportedly improve both physical and mental HRQoL in patients with liver cancer.

Pain and the consequential impairment of physical activity after surgery may be a concern. However, even after open liver surgery, physical status has been shown to recover within 6 months of surgery [5]. Furthermore, the mental component of HRQoL scores improves beyond preoperative scores, indicating surgical treatment improves mental health. Removal of the tumors may not only improve physical well-being but also enhance social and emotional health status. When there is a single and small (less than 3 cm) liver cancer, ablation therapy may be a better option in terms of maintaining HRQoL. A study found that compared with surgical resection, ablation therapy offered better HRQoL scores at 3, 6, 12, 24, and 36 months, without compromising prognosis [6].

As mentioned above, you may need repetitive surgery or ablation to treat cancer recurrence. Research has demonstrated that repetitive treatment for liver cancer does not adversely affect HRQoL. Following a second or third surgery, mental HRQoL scores were not impaired and were similar to those from the general population, suggesting previous operations may prepare you for repeated surgical treatment [5]. A survey of patients undergoing multiple therapies, such as surgery, chemotherapy, TACE, and ablation therapy, found ablation therapy was the least stressful, with 81% of patients having little or no fear undergoing repeat ablation [7].

For advanced liver cancer that does not qualify for radical treatment, drug therapy can prolong the lifetime. However, side effects may deteriorate your HRQoL [8]. As such, when choosing a treatment option, you need to discuss this balance between the benefit and harm of certain treatments with your doctors.

A recent report investigated the return-to-work rate in liver cancer patients in Taiwan [9] . The return-to-work rate after liver cancer diagnosis was assessed in 2451 patients with liver cancer in relation to cancer stage, income status, and industrial classification. Two and five years after treatment, patients who underwent surgery were more likely to return to work compared with those who had ablation therapy or chemotherapy. There were no differences in return-to-work rates in relation to industrial classification (such as agriculture, manufacturing, or food service), but patients that worked for a large company returned to work more frequently than those who worked for a small company. This suggests a large company may offer a better work environment and health care for its employees than a small enterprise, providing not only financial support but also occupational counseling and a supportive environment for cancer survivors.

13.4.2 Pancreatic Cancer

Pancreatic cancer is the most aggressive cancer among all solid tumors. Hence, a multidisciplinary approach including drug therapy or supportive care is essential. Supportive care is not hospice or end-of-life care. It is often used for patients undergoing aggressive treatment (such as surgery), and early administration of supportive care, including soon after diagnosis, can reportedly improve survival as well as quality of life.

Even with a localized cancer amenable to surgery, drug therapy is still used after surgery (adjuvant chemotherapy) to improve the prognosis. Evidence shows that adjuvant chemotherapy doubles life span compared with surgery alone. Recently, research from a Japanese group demonstrated that chemotherapy before surgery (neoadjuvant chemotherapy) improves survival even in patients with resectable pancreatic cancer. For this reason, your doctor may recommend drug therapy before surgery.

Unfortunately, 80% of patients diagnosed with pancreatic cancer do not qualify for surgery due to an advanced cancer stage. However, appropriate drug therapy can prolong life span and improve HRQoL. Recent data reveal that appropriate chemotherapy can offer a median survival of 24 months in patients with advanced pancreatic cancer [10]. Thus, your best treatment options will be based on your general status and cancer stage.

How Does Pancreatic Cancer Treatment Affect Your Quality of Life?

As described in the previous section, pancreatic surgery is invasive and removes several organs from your body. As expected, research has shown that HRQoL scores are impaired immediately after surgery. However, within 3–6 months after surgery, physical and mental HRQoL scores improve beyond before-surgery scores, implying surgical removal of cancer also alleviates patient anxiety [11–13].

You may worry that drug therapy before surgery (neoadjuvant chemotherapy) worsens your general condition due to the side effects of chemotherapy. However, research has shown that neoadjuvant chemotherapy does not compromise your HRQoL. To further investigate the feasibility of neoadjuvant chemotherapy, an observational survey of patient experiences using a smartphone app was recently launched [14].

In patients with advanced pancreatic cancer who do not qualify for surgical treatment, optimal drug therapy can improve prognosis as well as HRQoL by relieving cancer-related symptoms, such as pain or bowel obstruction. Although more than half of patients experience chemotherapy-related toxicity, including nausea, vomiting, diarrhea, or fatigue, the global health status of patients who have undergone at least four cycles of intensive chemotherapy is better than that of the general population [15].

Even when advanced pancreatic cancer is not amenable to cancer treatment, research on HRQoL highlights the importance of supportive care. In patients with advanced pancreatic cancer but not undergoing aggressive cancer treatment, all HRQoL scores that were lower than the average at diagnosis had improved at follow-up 3 months later [16].

Unfortunately, there has not yet been any comprehensive survey on return-to-work rates in pancreatic cancer patients. A Japanese study of 98 workers with pancreatic or liver cancer found the median time to return to work was 194 days after the initial day of sick leave [17]. However, larger, more comprehensive studies are required.

Treatment strategies for pancreatic cancer have become more complex as technology has advanced. As such, development of a large-scale program might be inevitable. A study to assess whether a nationwide implementation of cancer care may improve survival in pancreatic cancer patients is currently being conducted in the Netherlands, with the survey ending in 2025. A positive result in this study may further accelerate a comprehensive approach to pancreatic cancer that considers the medical aspect as well as the socio-economic viewpoint.

Conflicts of Interest and Source of Funding The author declares no conflicts of interest.

References

1. Ranganath R, Chu Q. Global trends in pancreas cancer among Asia-Pacific population. J Gastrointest Oncol. 2021;12(Suppl 2):S374–s86.
2. Izumi N, Hasegawa K, Nishioka Y, Takayama T, Yamanaka N, Kudo M, et al. A multicenter randomized controlled trial to evaluate the efficacy of surgery vs. radiofrequency ablation for small hepatocellular carcinoma (SURF trial). J Clin Oncol. 2019;37(15_suppl):4002.
3. Mise Y, Hasegawa K, Shindoh J, Ishizawa T, Aoki T, Sakamoto Y, et al. The feasibility of third or more repeat hepatectomy for recurrent hepatocellular carcinoma. Ann Surg. 2014;
4. Verma M, Paik JM, Younossi I, Tan D, Abdelaal H, Younossi ZM. The impact of hepatocellular carcinoma diagnosis on patients' health-related quality of life. Cancer Med. 2021;10(18):6273–81.
5. Mise Y, Satou S, Ishizawa T, Kaneko J, Aoki T, Hasegawa K, et al. Impact of surgery on quality of life in patients with hepatocellular carcinoma. World J Surg. 2013;38:958.
6. Huang G, Chen X, Lau WY, Shen F, Wang R-Y, Yuan S-X, et al. Quality of life after surgical resection compared with radiofrequency ablation for small hepatocellular carcinomas. Br J Surg. 2014;101(8):1006–15.
7. Schullian P, Gertl A, Laimer G, Putzer D, Siebert U, Levy E, et al. Quality of life analysis after stereotactic radiofrequency ablation of liver tumors. Sci Rep. 2020;10(1):12809.
8. Kudo M, Finn RS, Qin S, Han K-H, Ikeda K, Piscaglia F, et al. Lenvatinib versus sorafenib in first-line treatment of patients with unresectable hepatocellular carcinoma: a randomised phase 3 non-inferiority trial. Lancet. 2018;391(10126):1163–73.
9. Yang SW, Chen WL, Wu WT, Wang CC. Investigation on returning to work in liver cancer survivors in Taiwan: a 5-year follow-up study. BMC Public Health. 2021;21(1):1846.

10. Suker M, Beumer BR, Sadot E, Marthey L, Faris JE, Mellon EA, et al. FOLFIRINOX for locally advanced pancreatic cancer: a systematic review and patient-level meta-analysis. Lancet Oncol. 2016;17(6):801–10.
11. Chan C, Franssen B, Domínguez I, Ramírez-Del Val A, Uscanga LF, Campuzano M. Impact on quality of life after pancreatoduodenectomy: a prospective study comparing preoperative and postoperative scores. J Gastrointest Surg. 2012;16(7):1341–6.
12. Eaton AA, Gonen M, Karanicolas P, Jarnagin WR, D'Angelica MI, DeMatteo R, et al. Health-related quality of life after pancreatectomy: results from a randomized controlled trial. Ann Surg Oncol. 2016;23(7):2137–45.
13. Crippa S, Domínguez I, Rodríguez JR, Razo O, Thayer SP, Ryan DP, et al. Quality of life in pancreatic cancer: analysis by stage and treatment. J Gastrointest Surg. 2008;12(5):783–93; discussion 93–4
14. Cloyd JM, Hyman S, Huwig T, Monsour C, Santry H, Wills C, et al. Patient experience and quality of life during neoadjuvant therapy for pancreatic cancer: a systematic review and study protocol. Support Care Cancer. 2021;29(6):3009–16.
15. van der Sijde F, Schafthuizen L, van 't Land FR, Moskie M, van Laarhoven HWM, van Dijk M, et al. Quality of life of locally advanced pancreatic cancer patients after FOLFIRINOX treatment. Support Care Cancer. 2021;
16. Mackay TM, Dijksterhuis WPM, Latenstein AEJ, van der Geest LG, Sprangers MAG, van Eijck CHJ, et al. The impact of cancer treatment on quality of life in patients with pancreatic and periampullary cancer: a propensity score matched analysis. HPB (Oxford). 2021;
17. Endo M, Haruyama Y, Takahashi M, Nishiura C, Kojimahara N, Yamaguchi N. Returning to work after sick leave due to cancer: a 365-day cohort study of Japanese cancer survivors. J Cancer Surviv. 2016;10(2):320–9.

Hematological Cancer

14

Shintaro Kinoshita, Hajime Yasuda, Yoshiki Furukawa, Yoko Azusawa, Jun Ando, and Miki Ando

Abstract

Hematological malignancies are extremely diverse, and treatment can range from very mild to extremely intense depending on the type of malignancy. Thus, during treatment, some patients may enjoy nearly unchanged daily life and work, while others may require long-term hospitalization and a temporary leave from work. The treatment strategy would be decided depending on factors such as the type of hematological malignancy, disease stage, and patient status, and the patient would be requested to have different lifestyles and working formats depending on the treatment strategy. Treatment modalities for hematologic malignancies include observation, surgery, radiotherapy, chemotherapy, autologous and allogeneic stem cell transplantation, and chimeric antigen receptor T (CAR-T) cell therapy, and we describe how these modalities are incorporated into the treatment of individual hematological malignancies along with a discussion of how work is affected and what kind of precautions are to be taken by the patient. Hematological malignancies discussed here include diffuse large B-cell lymphoma, follicular lymphoma, classic Hodgkin's lymphoma, multiple myeloma, acute myeloid leukemia, acute lymphoblastic leukemia, and chronic myeloid leukemia. Although obstacles and restrictions accommodate, working while being treated can be possible for many hematological malignancies if treatment-related adverse events are mild and certain safety measures are taken.

Keywords

DLBCL · FL · AML · CML · ALL · MM · HSCT · Infections · Precautions · Working styles

14.1 General Facts

Hematological malignancies arise from both mature and a wide variety of immature blood cells. All blood cells are derived from a common hematopoietic stem cell, but the differentiation and maturation process is extremely complex (Fig. 14.1). Different cells of origin, including cells of different maturation stages, lead to distinct malignancies, and therefore the types of hematological malignancies are extremely diverse. Frequently used terms like "leukemia" and "lymphoma" mean very little by themselves, because even these categories engulf so many types of malignancies that are extremely diverse in nature, with some malignancies requiring immediate attention and treatment due to accommodating life-threatening events, while others may be observed without treatment for years due to their indolent clinical course. Thus, accurate diagnosis of the exact type of hematological malignancy is indispensable for building treatment strategies for the attending physician, and the patient would be requested to have different lifestyles and working formats depending on the treatment strategy.

Treatment modalities for hematologic malignancies include observation, surgery, radiotherapy, and chemotherapy, and adoption depends on the type of malignancy and patient characteristics (age, general condition, stage of malignancy, etc.). However, because hematological malignancies are usually systemic, chemotherapy is often the treatment of choice.

S. Kinoshita (✉) · H. Yasuda · Y. Furukawa · M. Ando
Department of Hematology, School of Medicine, Juntendo University, Bunkyo-ku, Tokyo, Japan
e-mail: s-kinoshita@juntendo.ac.jp; hyasuda@juntendo.ac.jp; y-furukawa@juntendo.ac.jp; m-ando@juntendo.ac.jp

Y. Azusawa
Division of Cell Therapy & Blood Transfusion Medicine, Juntendo University School of Medicine, Tokyo, Japan
e-mail: y.azusawa.ce@juntendo.ac.jp

J. Ando
Department of Hematology, School of Medicine, Juntendo University, Bunkyo-ku, Tokyo, Japan

Division of Cell Therapy & Blood Transfusion Medicine, Juntendo University School of Medicine, Tokyo, Japan
e-mail: j-ando@juntendo.ac.jp

© The Author(s), under exclusive license to Springer Nature Singapore Pte Ltd. 2026

M. Endo et al. (eds.), *Cancer and Work in Asia Volume 2*, https://doi.org/10.1007/978-981-95-6537-5_14

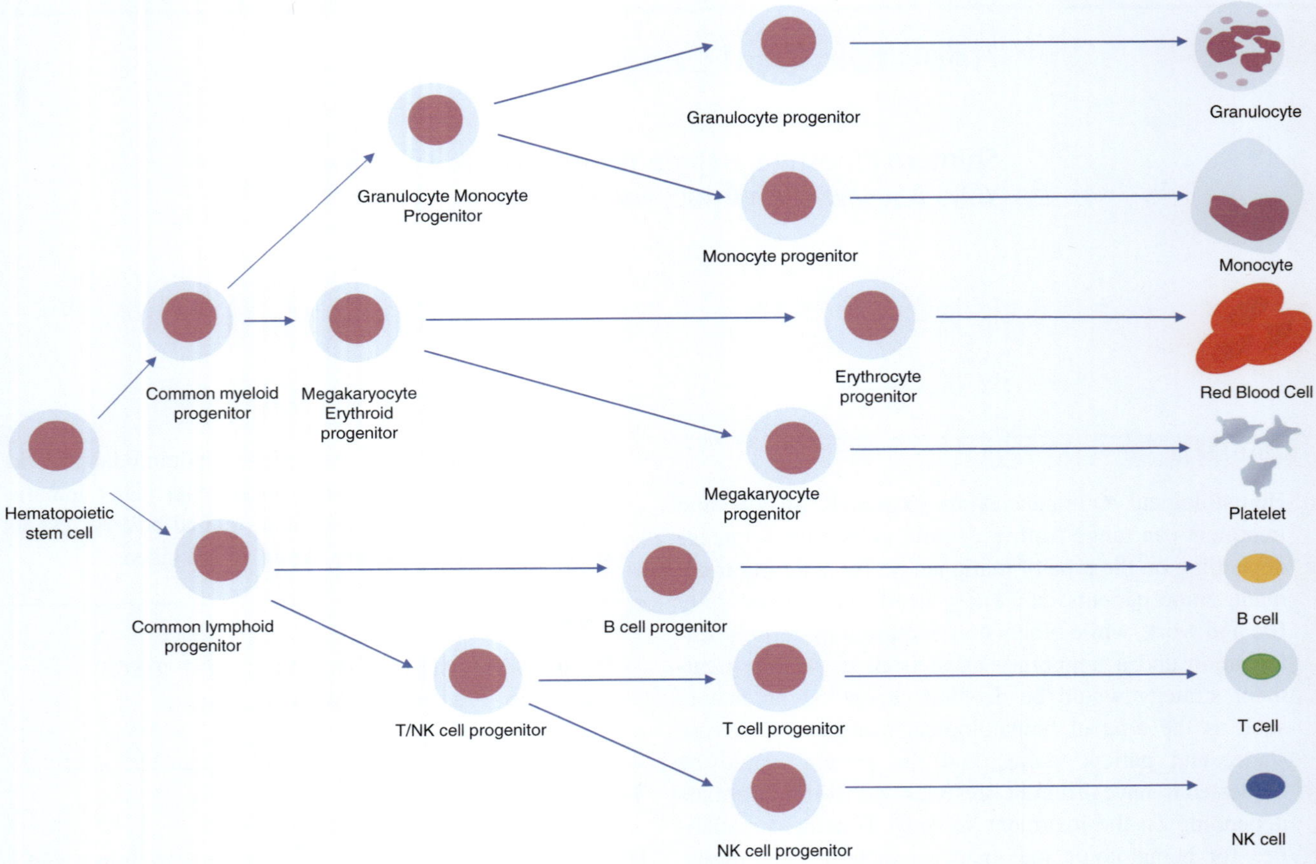

Fig. 14.1 Flowchart of normal hematopoiesis. Hematopoietic stem cells reside in the bone marrow and possess the ability to differentiate into diverse blood cell types

14.2 Chemotherapy

Chemotherapy can range from oral or intravenous administration with minimal outpatient visits to high-intensity multiple-agent therapy requiring months of in-hospital stay. Therefore, depending on the type of chemotherapy, some patients may enjoy near unchanged daily life, while others may be required to temporarily take a leave from work. Current-day intravenous chemotherapy administration at the outpatient clinic is efficiently carried out in a room specialized for chemotherapy patients and safely managed by nurses with expertise in the field (Fig. 14.2).

General precautions for the patient with hematological malignancies undergoing chemotherapy do not differ largely from patients with other malignancies, but one distinct trait is that patients with hematological malignancies are especially prone to infections. One reason for this is because the normal counterparts of most hematological malignancies are constituents of the immune system, and thus the malignancy itself contributes to immunodeficiency. Another reason is that the intensity of chemotherapy for hematological malignancies is in general high compared to that of other malignancies, and this leads to stronger immunosuppression. Therefore, when symptoms of infections such as fever appear during chemotherapy, the patient should consult his/her doctor as soon as possible. The patient should be educated that acquiring infectious diseases in normal states and during chemotherapy is a completely different scenario, and the latter may even be life-threatening within short periods of time. Opportunistic infections, including fungal infections, may also occur. The patient should also avoid meeting people with contagious diseases (including the common cold), which may be an obstacle for working without restrictions, but again, the intensity of chemotherapy for hematological malignancies ranges from very mild to extremely intense, and the attending physician should advise the patient concerning these restrictions depending on the type of hematological malignancy and chemotherapy administered. Feeling sick and vomiting are also frequently encountered adverse events of chemotherapy and often one of the biggest issues of concern for the patient. However, progress in supportive care has led to very potent antiemetics, and most patients fare well concerning this subject. Other frequent adverse events of chemotherapy include malaise, alopecia (usually

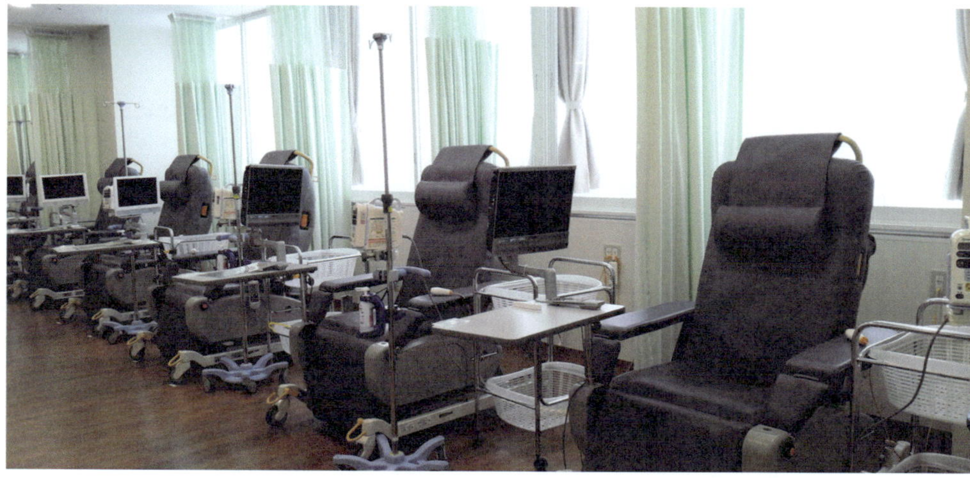

Fig. 14.2 Outpatient chemotherapy room. The outpatient chemotherapy room is a purpose-built treatment room for cancer patients. The room is managed by specialized nurses, and patients can receive chemotherapy safely and comfortably at the outpatient

reversible), myelosuppression (results in decreased white blood cells, hemoglobin, and platelets), allergic reactions, skin and respiratory disorders, renal and liver dysfunction, peripheral neuropathy, infertility, and secondary cancers. Some patients may be faced with multiple and heavy adverse events, while others may experience none. However, most of the adverse events are predictable, and the patient should be informed beforehand what to expect depending on the chemotherapeutics scheduled.

14.3 Therapeutic Methods Beyond Chemotherapy

Although systemic chemotherapy is the mainstay of treatment for most hematological malignancies, in certain diseases, chemotherapy alone may not be sufficient for disease cure or for treating patients with relapsed/refractory disease. In this section, we cover the major treatment methods utilized for hematological malignancies that go beyond systemic chemotherapy and discuss restrictions they impose on the patient, with a focus on work. These treatment methods often require use of the clean room (Fig. 14.3) due to severe immunosuppression.

14.3.1 Autologous Stem Cell Transplantation (Auto-HSCT)

Auto-HSCT is often utilized for treatment of hematological malignancies, including diffuse large B-cell lymphoma, classic Hodgkin's lymphoma, and multiple myeloma. In auto-HSCT, the patient's own stem cells are used for the source of transplantation. The stem cells are harvested from the patient in advance and cryopreserved. The stem cells are returned to the patient following administration of extreme-intensity chemotherapy (often referred to as "conditioning therapy"). The aim of auto-HSCT is restoration of the ability to produce normal blood cells following conditioning therapy, which may permanently deplete bone marrow cells. The self-derived transplanted hematopoietic stem cells become engrafted around 2–3 weeks post-transplant, and the bone marrow regains the ability of hematopoiesis. Blood transfusions will be required for a period of time until engraftment. The typical in-hospital stay for patients undergoing auto-HSCT is around 3–4 weeks.

14.3.2 Allogeneic Stem Cell Transplantation (Allo-HSCT)

Allo-HSCT is frequently used for treatment of disorders such as acute lymphoblastic leukemia/lymphoma and acute myeloid leukemia. Allo-HSCT is quite different from auto-HSCT in that the stem cells used for transplantation are derived from another individual (donor). The stem cell source may be from an HLA-matched related donor or a non-related donor, or from cord blood. Infusions of stem cells are carried out following extreme-intensity chemotherapy and/or radiation therapy (conditioning therapy). The conditioning therapy is often myeloablative, but the infused stem cells eventually become engrafted, and thus the bone marrow is restored. Blood transfusions are necessary for patients undergoing allo-HSCT until bone marrow restoration. The conditioning therapy not only helps exterminate the neoplastic cells but also aids the infused stem cells by acting as a powerful immunosuppressor so that the stem cells are not rejected by patient-derived immune cells. A major complication of allo-HSCT is graft-versus-host disease (GVHD), in which donor-derived immune cells attack the healthy cells of the patient's body. Organs commonly affected by GVHD are the skin, gastrointestinal tract, liver, mouth, eyes, joints, fascia, lungs, and genital tract. GVHD significantly contributes to mortality among patients undergoing allo-HSCT, and

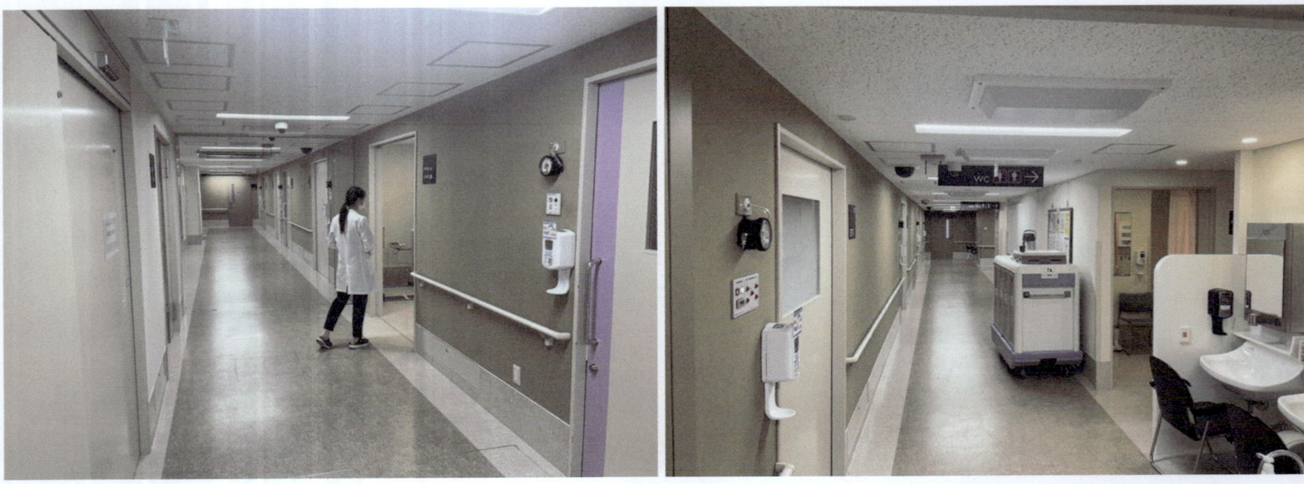

Fig. 14.3 Clean rooms. A clean room is a room in which clean air with minimal floating particles is circulated using high performance filters. Clean rooms are not necessary for all patients with hematological malignancies, but patients undergoing intensive treatment such as autologous and allogeneic stem cell transplantation are good candidates for the clean room because such patients are exposed to long periods of leukopenia and therefore are at higher risk of infections

even when not life-taking, the patient's quality of life is often drastically impaired by GVHD [1]. The mainstay of GVHD treatment is administration of immunosuppressants. Allo-HSCT typically requires around 3 months of in-hospital stay, and relatively frequent outpatient visits are usually necessary after discharge.

14.3.3 Chimeric Antigen Receptor T (CAR-T) Cell Therapy

CAR-T therapy was developed to augment the function of effector T-cells in the tumor microenvironment. CAR-T cells are genetically engineered T-cells expressing CARs consisting of a single-chain variable fragment (scFv) as an antigen recognition module, a cytoplasmic activation domain such as the co-stimulation domain, and the T-cell receptor (TCR) CD3-z chain. CAR-expressing T-cells recognize tumor antigens by the scFV region and subsequently transmit the signal into T-cells through the CD3ζ chain, which induces apoptosis in tumor cells by secreting cytotoxic granules such as perforin and granzyme B.

In order to provide CAR-T therapy, to begin with, T-cells are collected from patients via apheresis and cryopreserved at the cell processing center (Fig. 14.4). Subsequently, CARs are transduced into these T-cells and expanded ex vivo. Prior to infusion of the CAR-T cells, patients receive lymphodepleting chemotherapy to prevent rejection of CAR-T cells by the patient's immune system. After CAR-T cell infusion, special attention must be paid toward the development of

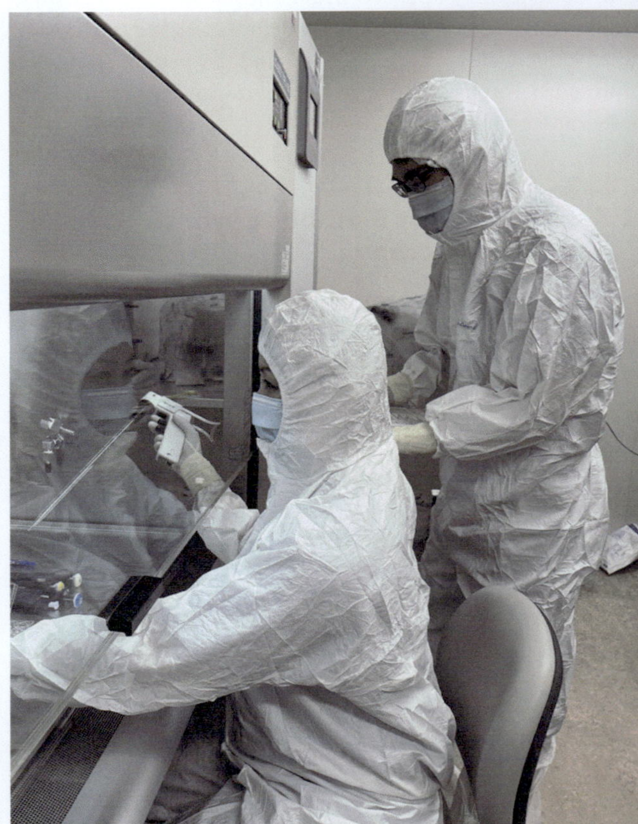

Fig. 14.4 Cell processing center. The cell processing center is managed and operated in accordance with laws and regulations of Good Manufacturing Practice standards to ensure the safety of cell therapy and regenerative medicine

cytokine release syndrome (CRS), which is a systemic inflammatory response that can be triggered by activated CAR-T cells. Common symptoms of CRS are hypotension, dyspnea, and high fever. Severe CRS can be life-threatening, and prompt recognition and treatment are indispensable. The typical in-hospital stay required for CAR-T therapy is roughly about a month, and patients can return to work within a relatively short period of time [2].

14.4 Common Hematological Malignancies

Although the types of hematological malignancies are extremely diverse, the number is only a handful when restricted to common disease types. In this section, we cover the major types of hematological malignancies and discuss treatment options in order to give readers a general idea of how work and lifestyle should be modified during treatment.

14.4.1 Diffuse Large B-Cell Lymphoma (DLBCL)

As the name indicates, DLBCL is a B-cell lymphoid malignancy showing diffuse infiltration of large neoplastic cells. DLBCL is one of the most common types of lymphoma found. DLBCL can arise from both nodal and extranodal sites, and as many as 40% of cases are initially confined to extranodal sites. DLBCL is an aggressive lymphoma, and disease progression is generally rapid [3]. Prognosis of DLBCL differs greatly depending on multiple factors, including disease site, immunophenotype, genetic mutations, and international prognostic index (IPI) category. However, as a whole, DLBCL is a potentially curable type of lymphoma, and thus treatment usually begins as soon as a diagnosis is made. R-CHOP (rituximab, cyclophosphamide, doxorubicin, vincristine, and prednisolone) is the most widely used treatment for DLBCL. Rituximab is a chimeric anti-CD20 monoclonal antibody, and infusion reactions are the characteristic side effects of this drug. Representative symptoms of infusion reactions are fever, mucocutaneous symptoms, hypotension, respiratory distress, and abdominal symptoms. Infusion reactions occur acutely and have been reported to occur in 77% of patients receiving their first administration of rituximab, and the percentage decreases in subsequent courses [4]. Doxorubicin is categorized as an anthracycline, which is a group of drugs known for cardiotoxicity, and thus risk of heart failure may become an issue for some patients. Vincristine is a vinca alkaloid of which the characteristic adverse events are peripheral neuropathy and intestinal obstruction. One course of R-CHOP is a 21-day cycle schedule, and R-CHOP is typically administered for 6–8 courses. R-CHOP can be administered at the outpatient, and the need for hospitalization is minimal. Immunosuppression is usually moderate, and although some patients work while they receive R-CHOP, patients should definitely avoid high-risk situations of contracting infectious diseases. In refractory and relapsed DLBCL, salvage chemotherapy followed by auto-HSCT is usually the treatment of choice in eligible patients. Some salvage chemotherapy regimens for DLBCL can be administered at the outpatient clinic, while others require long-term hospitalization. In younger and fit patients, auto-HSCT is applied to those responding to salvage chemotherapy. Auto-HSCT usually requires about a month of hospitalization, and thus patients are often required to ask for a temporary leave from work in this scenario. Newer drugs and treatment methods for DLBCL include polatuzumab vedotin and CAR-T therapy. Polatuzumab vedotin is an antibody-drug conjugate with an anti-CD79b antibody bonded to the anticancer drug monomethyl auristatin E (MMAE), and peripheral neuropathy is the characteristic adverse event. CAR-T therapy is discussed in Sect. 3.3.

14.4.2 Follicular Lymphoma (FL)

FL is the most common type of indolent B-cell lymphoma and accounts for approximately 20% of all lymphomas. FL predominantly involves the lymph nodes, and unlike DLBCL, cases with pure extranodal lesions are rare. The majority of patients present with widespread disease. Disease progression of FL is usually slow, typically taking months to years. However, approximately 25–35% of FL patients eventually experience transformation to DLBCL, and disease progression can suddenly accelerate in such situations. FL is basically an incurable disease by conventional treatment methods. One exception is a minority of patients with limited-stage disease who may be potentially cured by local radiotherapy. Because a cure cannot be expected in the majority of cases, the goal of therapy is disease control, and thus diagnosis of FL does not necessarily mean immediate therapy. Groupe d'Etude des Lymphomes Folliculaires (GELF) and British National Lymphoma Investigation (BNLI) have proposed criteria for treatment initiation and may be of guidance, but actual decision-making should be based on clinical significance and not on a strict adherence to the aforementioned criteria [5]. When the necessity of upfront treatment is denied, patients are followed up with observation only with outpatient visits until the need for treatment (watch and wait strategy), and patients can enjoy normal daily life and work. When treatment for FL is indicated, there are currently multiple chemotherapy regimens from which the attending physician can choose. R-CVP (rituximab, cyclophosphamide, vincristine, and prednisolone), R-CHOP (discussed in Sect. 7.1), and BR (bendamustine, rituximab) are some of the frequently used regimens, and rituximab may be substituted with obinutuzumab. R-CVP and R-CHOP are 21-day cycle regimens, and BR is a 28-day cycle regimen. When treating FL, R-CVP is typically administered for 8 courses, R-CHOP for 6–8 courses, and BR for 6 courses [6]. R-CVP, R-CHOP, and BR all require minimal hospitalization, and working while on chemotherapy is possible if safety measures are taken, such as avoiding high-risk infectious situations. Newer treatment strategies include rituximab-lenalidomide combination therapy and the EZH2 inhibitor tazemetostat. Upon relapse, patients are most often treated with chemotherapy regimens for FL not previously used in the patient, and auto-HSCT may be considered in selected cases.

14.4.3 Classic Hodgkin Lymphoma (cHL)

cHL is a lymphoid malignancy with a bimodal age distribution with peaks in the young (20 s) and in later life (60 s). cHL presents most often with lymphadenopathy, but the disease can also involve extranodal tissues such as the spleen, lungs, liver, and bone marrow. The so-called B symptoms (fever, night sweats, and weight loss) are seen in approximately one-third of cHL patients. cHL is a disease known for high cure rates compared to other lymphomas [7]. Treatment consists of combination chemotherapy with or without radiotherapy. The most widely used chemotherapy combination is ABVD, which consists of doxorubicin, bleomycin, vinblastine, and dacarbazine. One course of ABVD is constituted by a 28-day schedule, and chemotherapy is administered on days 1 and 15. ABVD is typically administered for 2–6 courses, and the number of courses depends on multiple factors, including disease stage. ABVD can for the most part be administered at the outpatient, and the need for hospitalization is usually minimal. Therefore, some patients may continue work if certain restrictions, such as not having to meet potentially sick people with infectious diseases, are considered. Dacarbazine is known to frequently cause nausea, and thus the risk of feeling sick during ABVD therapy is relatively higher compared to other regimens. However, as mentioned earlier, current-day antiemetics are usually capable of controlling these symptoms. Another major concern of ABVD therapy is bleomycin-induced lung toxicity because it can be fatal, and thus the patient should look out for the emergence of respiratory symptoms such as abnormal shortness of breath [8]. Newer drugs for cHL include brentuximab vedotin, nivolumab, and pembrolizumab. Brentuximab vedotin is an antibody-drug conjugate with an anti-CD30 antibody bonded to the anticancer drug (MMAE). Peripheral neuropathy is one of the characteristic adverse events of brentuximab vedotin. Nivolumab and pembrolizumab are both antibodies targeted towards PD-1, and because these drugs act as immune checkpoint inhibitors, various immune-related adverse events, including skin disorders, endocrinopathies, pneumonia, colitis, and hepatitis, are seen. In relapsed or refractory cHL, salvage chemotherapy followed by auto-HSCT is currently the standard of care in eligible patients. Salvage chemotherapy is chosen from a wide variety of regimens, of which many require hospitalization, and auto-HSCT also usually requires about a month of hospitalization.

14.4.4 Multiple Myeloma (MM)

MM is a plasma cell dyscrasia. The bone marrow is the primary site of disease, although a minority of patients present with extramedullary lesions. The major presentations of MM are often referred to by the acronym CRAB (hyper<u>c</u>alcemia, <u>r</u>enal dysfunction, <u>a</u>nemia, <u>b</u>one disease). Hypercalcemia can cause excessive thirst, nausea, appetite loss, constipation, and confusion. Renal dysfunction causes low urine output and edema. Anemia leads to shortness of breath, malaise, and palpitation. Bone disease can lead to bone pain and pathological fractures. MM is basically an incurable disease by conventional treatment methods, and thus the goal of therapy is disease control. Therefore, even when a diagnosis of MM is rendered, the asymptomatic patient may be observed with minimal outpatient visits, and the patient's working format may not need to be altered during this period. Chemotherapy is the mainstay of MM treatment when it is required. In recent years, extraordinary progress has been seen in the treatment of MM, and new chemotherapeutics and different chemotherapy combinations are constantly being introduced. The drugs most frequently used are bortezomib, lenalidomide, steroids, carfilzomib, ixazomib, daratumumab, isatuximab, melphalan, pomalidomide, and thalidomide. Treatment is usually carried out using various combinations of these drugs, and auto-HSCT is considered for eligible patients. Aside from auto-HSCT, most of the treatment of MM takes place at the outpatient, although one drawback is that treatment periods are often long and many regimens require relatively frequent hospital visits. Many patients work while they receive chemotherapy, but because MM is by nature a disease with excessively impaired humoral immunity, measures to avoid high-risk infectious situations should be taken.

14.4.5 Acute Lymphoblastic Leukemia/Lymphoma (ALL/LBL)

ALL is an extremely aggressive hematologic malignancy requiring immediate attention and treatment. ALL is a neoplasm of precursor lymphoid cells, presenting with expansion of neoplastic blasts in the bone marrow and often the peripheral blood, and may be accompanied by extramedullary lesions, which may be nodal or extranodal. LBL is basically considered the same disease as ALL, and the only difference is that extramedullary lesions are the primary site of disease and peripheral blood and bone marrow involvement are minimal in LBL [3]. Patients with ALL show signs and consequences of bone marrow failure, and bone pain and arthralgias are frequently seen symptoms. ALL is potentially curable, but prognosis differs depending on multiple factors, including the types of genetic mutations involved. Treatment consists of sequential courses of high-intensity multiagent chemotherapy followed by consideration for allo-HSCT in eligible patients. Chemotherapy usually requires months of hospitalization, and because treatment with allo-HSCT follows after chemotherapy for many, patients need to take a long-term leave from work, sometimes exceeding 1 year. Types of adverse events depend on what kind of chemotherapeutics are used, but a common issue of concern is infectious complications due to the extreme immunosuppression of ALL-oriented chemotherapy and allo-HSCT. Newer treatment methods for ALL include the bispecific T-cell engager blinatumomab, the antibody-drug conjugate inotuzumab ozogamicin, and CAR-T therapy (discussed in Sect. 3.3).

14.4.6 Acute Myeloid Leukemia (AML)

AML is a highly aggressive disease presenting with neoplastic blasts arising from precursor myeloid cells proliferating in the bone marrow and often the peripheral blood. Extramedullary disease involvement is seen only in a minority of patients. General symptoms of AML are similar to that of ALL. AML is a potentially curable disease, but the prognosis of AML is highly variable, and the type of genetic mutation involved is a major factor for deciding the prognosis. Treatment should be initiated as soon as possible, and sequential courses of high-intensity chemotherapy are the mainstay of treatment. In eligible patients, whether allo-HSCT subsequent to chemotherapy should be carried out is decided by weighing multiple factors, of which the risk category of genetic mutations involved plays a major role. As is the case with ALL, chemotherapy for young and fit AML patients is also extremely immunosuppressive and requires months of hospitalization, and patients cannot physically go to work during this period.

14.4.7 Chronic Myeloid Leukemia (CML)

CML is a hematological neoplasm with prominent proliferation of cells of various maturation stages of the myeloid lineage. Most patients with CML are asymptomatic, and thus the disease is frequently found incidentally on routine health checks. Although disease progression of CML is relatively slow, the disease evolves to life-threatening acute leukemia usually within years after onset if left untreated. However, timely treatment under current-day practice has led CML to become a disease with an extremely bright outlook. The vast majority of CML patients show excellent disease control with oral administration of tyrosine kinase inhibitors (TKIs), minimal hospital visits, and most patients enjoy basically unchanged daily life and working formats. There are currently many types of TKIs available, and some are more potent than others, while at the same time some are known for more serious adverse events.

14.5 Real-Life Experiences of a Hematological Malignancy Survivor

Although we have provided a general overview of hematological malignancies and given readers an idea of how long individual disorders and treatment methods take until work can be resumed, the optimal timing of returning to work (or continuing work) actually depends on a diverse number of personal factors, including disease status, type of work, financial situation, family support, and patient mentality. Therefore, listening to real-life experiences and how patients actually managed their disease and work by balancing the strengths and weaknesses of their diverse personal factors would be of precious reference for patients who are expecting treatment in the near future. The following letter is from a cHL patient who experienced disease relapse and underwent auto-HSCT, and he tells his story and how he resourcefully coped with the many obstacles of working while being treated for a hematological malignancy.

A letter from a hematological malignancy survivor:

I was 30 years old. After earning an MBA in the United States (US), I was working for a US-based investment bank in Tokyo. My career outlook was bright, I had never experienced major health issues, and I was feeling invincible. Then things took an unexpected turn.

In 2003, when my journey began, I started to experience symptoms that were similar to those of a common flu, such as low-grade fever and cough. I didn't find them to be concerning. However, over a couple of short months, the fatigue, night sweats, fever, and weight loss continued to worsen to the point where I knew there was something severely wrong with my health. On August 8, 2003, after 2 months of diagnostic testing at Juntendo Hospital in Tokyo, the results came back. I was diagnosed with Stage 4 Hodgkin lymphoma, a type of blood cancer.

A few days later, I was admitted to the hospital and started a chemotherapy regimen consisting of doxorubicin hydrochloride (Adriamycin), bleomycin, vinblastine, and dacarbazine (ABVD). It was the most common regimen, and it required six to eight cycles of chemotherapy. Each cycle of treatment was typically 4 weeks in duration, and chemotherapy was administered at the beginning of the first and third weeks. On August 18, 2003, my first cycle started, and the drugs were administered inpatient in case there were adverse reactions. Then the rest of the treatments were outpatient. Given that my diagnosis was a Stage 4, it required me to endure eight cycles of chemotherapy until I was in complete remission in March of 2004.

Receiving the news that I was in complete remission, however, did not immediately end this misery. Including a couple of months of rehabilitation following the chemotherapy, this ordeal consumed a year of my life. I returned to my former position with the firm after 12 months of medical leave, but I was able to reduce my hours and shift my schedule to avoid crowded trains for the first few months. I also dedicated time for rehabilitation to regain physical strength. It took yet another year for me to gradually acclimate back to my previous routine and energy level, which was about the same amount of time I spent in treatment.

After completing my treatment, I continued periodic checkups at Juntendo to ensure my complete remission status. Initially, the checkup was monthly. Then, it was reduced to every couple of months and finally down to every 6 months after my three-year anniversary of being in complete remission. Every milestone gave me additional confidence that cancer was behind me.

At the end of the three-year anniversary in 2006, I made a personal and professional decision to transfer to the headquarters office of the investment bank in New York City. Even after 3 years, continuing a periodic checkup was essential for me to maintain peace of mind. Through a serendipitous way of introduction, a prominent oncologist at New York-Presbyterian/Weill Cornell Medicine agreed to take me as a new patient. I was under his watch during my 3 years in New York when I surpassed my five-year milestone of being in complete remission.

Soon after, I returned to Tokyo. Almost a decade had passed since my initial diagnosis, I was now approaching the age of 40, and everything in my life was on track. I was happily married, my career was promising, and I was feeling strong physically. Without any hesitation, I went to my annual checkup at Juntendo, as I had done countless times in the past. This time, however, a tumor was identified on the superior vena cava. Cancer had relapsed. I had no subjective symptoms, so the finding was completely surprising and devastating.

On October 25, 2011, a median sternotomy was performed to surgically remove the tumor in my chest. Pathological analysis determined that it was a relapse from the previous Hodgkin lymphoma. The entire tumor was removed. However, the big question was, what to do next? Follow up with rigorous adjuvant therapy, which could develop secondary cancer, or wait and see? After thorough discussions with the Juntendo medical team and consultations with other doctors, including my previous oncologist in New York, we decided to take a wait-and-see approach. Following the surgery, I was cancer–free, and it may never come back.

I continued my monthly checkups, feeling as if I had a ticking time bomb in my chest. On January 28, 2013, a little over a year after the surgery, a PET scan detected a tumor in my chest once again. The bomb had exploded. In April of 2013, I underwent a laparoscopic surgery to pathologically confirm the type of lymphoma in order to determine appropriate adjuvant therapy. Again, after exhaustive discussions with my primary doctor, along with other oncologists in Tokyo and New York, the gemcitabine, dexamethasone, and cisplatin regimen (GDP) combined with autologous stem cell transplant was determined to be the most effective adjuvant therapy.

Overall, this time was a much more aggressive treatment than before. Unlike the first time, all of the treatment was administered inpatient given the stronger toxicity. Halfway through the treatment, I had completely lost my hair, and I was suffering from various side effects much more severely than the first time. During the last phase of the treatment for autologous stem cell transplant, I spent 6 weeks in a clean room due to immunosuppression. Adjuvant therapy lasted over six intense months.

In a case where curative surgery is an option, the maximum pain level of the treatment is typically immediately after the surgery. With each day or week thereafter, the pain subsides. In contrast, with chemotherapy treatment, the subsequent cycle is more painful than the prior cycle. With each round, damage accumulates in the body and the pain worsens. Physically, it felt like being punched round after round in a boxing match. Mentally, however, I had to focus on the big picture, which was to beat cancer.

Like the previous decade, I ended up taking another year of medical leave from the firm. I planned a similar approach as before in acclimating back to the work routine. In order to regain physical strength, I started Pilates to build core strength and improve flexibility and posture, and to regain my mental sharpness, I studied for a professional certification. Starting with reduced hours in the office, I eased back into the professional world. The amount of time to fully recover, again, took about the same amount of time I spent in treatment.

Looking back on the two events that disrupted not only my health but also my life, there were commonalities as well as differences. The major difference was my emotional reaction to hearing the word "cancer." The first time, I was already suffering from symptoms, and I knew something was severely wrong. So, when I was diagnosed with lymphoma, instead of feeling fear, I was actually relieved to finally find an answer. It meant that, at last, doctors knew what was causing those symptoms, and we were able to take a step toward treatment. The second time, however, cancer was found in a routine checkup after nearly 10 years of complete remission. Emotionally, it was much harder to accept given the surprise factor.

As for common factors, I had incredible support around me both times—a dedicated and knowledgeable medical team, an employer with generous employee benefit programs, and, of course, caring family and friends. Luckily for me, I believe these common factors I had for both times were the key factors in the successful outcome. Cancer is not something one can fight alone.

The key to receiving good medical care is to be resourceful and to have an open and trusting relationship with the doctors. As a patient, it was critical for me to understand the disease and treatment options in order to assess the situation and make the right decisions. I did not hesitate to maximize my effort to determine the best treatment. Fortunately for me, I had doctors that I could trust. Dr. J.A. was my treating doctor both times, and I had a renowned specialist in New York City to seek expert opinion outside of Japan. Once a patient is diagnosed with cancer, he or she needs to deal with it for a lifetime, so having a trusting doctor to partner with for years is critical.

Securing a supportive employer was also immensely important. The treatments required me to take two separate year-long medical leaves from the firm. I was fortunate to have incredibly understanding managers and to have worked for one of the premier investment banks in the world. Not only did the firm have one of the best healthcare benefits, providing extremely supportive programs, but I was also granted medical leaves with full salary and benefits both times to concentrate on my health. I underwent the treatment and had the luxury of not having to worry about work and finances.

Lastly, I could not have gone through this without the support of my family and friends. There were days when I felt extreme fatigue and pain, yet I had to stay positive and believe that I was headed in the right direction. In between cycles when I would partially recover from the treatment, I always made an effort to meet with friends who were the foundation of enormous emotional support and a source of energy to stay positive. The only downside was that I would only see them on "good" days, so many people assumed that I was not suffering too much from the treatment; however, there were certainly "bad" days when I could not even get out of bed or feel like talking to anyone. I now apologize to my family members who had to deal with me on those "bad" days. In general, my personal stance in regard to my illness was to be completely open, providing a full disclosure to those around me. From the beginning, I did not disguise my diagnosis and prognosis of the illness. I think this stance made it easier for everyone to communicate with me and stay in touch without any awkwardness.

December 2021 marked the eight-year anniversary of the second complete remission. I continue to be excited for life and what opportunities it holds for me in the future, but I realize cancer will always coexist with me. I just need to stay one step ahead of it so I can seize every opportunity and not allow cancer to hold me back. In Japan, the phrase "100-year life," has become prevalent recently. During a span of 100 years, hardships are both expected and unavoidable. My conviction is that a good life is not the absence of misfortunes but rather defined by how they are managed. I have had two misfortunes already before turning 50, yet I don't feel as if I am unlucky. In fact, I had the fortune of having amazing support around me to manage and overcome those difficult events. These experiences gave me a chance to realize what is truly important. For that, I am forever grateful.

To those fighting cancer, stay strong. Live the dream.

14.6 Concluding Remarks

Although obstacles and restrictions accommodate, working while being treated can be possible for many hematological malignancies if treatment-related adverse events are mild and certain safety measures are taken. Conversely, some hematological malignancies and situations may not allow for work during the most intense period of treatment, and patients would be required to ask for a leave from work. Planning working formats beforehand with the attending physician is indispensable, and if work is to be continued during therapy, a cautious self-monitoring of physical state would be required by the patient.

References

1. Wenzel F, Pralong A, Holtick U, Scheid C, Herling M, Simon ST. Burden and needs of patients with severe GvHD from the supportive and palliative care perspective-a literature review. Cancers (Basel). 2021;13(11)
2. Huguet M, Raimond V, Kaltenbach E, Augusto V, Perrier L. How much does the hospital stay for infusion of anti-CD19 CAR-T cells cost to the French National Health Insurance? Bull Cancer. 2021;108(12):1170–80.
3. Hasserjian RP, Gattermann N, Bennett JM, Brunning RD, Malcovati L, Thiele J. Myelodysplastic syndrome with ring sideroblasts. In: Swerdlow SH, Campo E, Harris NL, et al., editors. WHO classification of tumours of haematopoietic and lymphoid tissues. 4th ed. Lyon: IARC Press; 2017. p. 109–11.
4. Rosello S, Blasco I, Garcia Fabregat L, Cervantes A, Jordan K, Committee EG. Management of infusion reactions to systemic anti-

cancer therapy: ESMO Clinical Practice Guidelines. Ann Oncol. 2017;28(suppl_4):iv100–iv18.

5. Cartron G, Trotman J. Time for an individualized approach to first-line management of follicular lymphoma. Haematologica. 2022;107(1):7–18.
6. Federico M, Luminari S, Dondi A, et al. R-CVP versus R-CHOP versus R-FM for the initial treatment of patients with advanced-stage follicular lymphoma: results of the FOLL05 trial conducted by the Fondazione Italiana Linfomi. J Clin Oncol. 2013;31(12):1506–13.
7. Ansell SM. Hodgkin lymphoma: 2018 update on diagnosis, risk-stratification, and management. Am J Hematol. 2018;93(5):704–15.
8. Martin WG, Ristow KM, Habermann TM, Colgan JP, Witzig TE, Ansell SM. Bleomycin pulmonary toxicity has a negative impact on the outcome of patients with Hodgkin's lymphoma. J Clin Oncol. 2005;23(30):7614–20.

Urogenital Cancer

15

Koichiro Akakura

Abstract

In patients with localized kidney cancer, activities of daily living are usually maintained. But if renal function is disturbed, dietary restriction or hemodialysis may be necessary. In metastatic kidney cancer, systemic therapy is continued, and careful attention is needed for employment. Urinary bladder cancer is known as environmental and industrial cancer. In superficial bladder cancer, no serious restriction is demanded after endoscopic surgery. In muscle-invasive bladder cancer, urinary diversion is necessary upon resection of the urinary bladder, and stoma/ostomy bag care is crucial for working. In metastatic bladder cancer, chemotherapy and/or immunotherapy are performed, and management of side effects and disturbance of activities are important for employment. In localized prostate cancer, complications vary between surgery (erectile dysfunction and urinary incontinence) and radiotherapy (hematuria and rectal bleeding). In metastatic prostate cancer, hormone therapy is generally utilized. Although hormone therapy is less toxic, side effects consist of sexual dysfunction, hot flushes, osteoporosis, fatigue, cognitive impairment, and cardiovascular diseases. Because patients with testicular cancer are young, physical and psychological care are important for management of work. In advanced-stage testicular cancer, extensive and long-term chemotherapy must be applied to cure the disease, and working during and after therapy should be managed and supported appropriately.

Keywords

Urological cancers · Asia · Kidney cancer · Bladder cancer · Prostate cancer · Testicular cancer · Clinical features · Treatment · Work

K. Akakura (✉)
Department of Urology, Japan Community Health-care Organization (JCHO) Mishima General Hospital, Mishima, Japan
e-mail: akakurak@ae.auone-net.jp

15.1 Kidney Cancer

15.1.1 Clinical Features (Table 15.1)

In Japan, the National Cancer Center Japan reported that the diagnosis (2018) and death (2019) of kidney and ureter cancer were 29,763 and 9375 cases, respectively [1]. Kidney cancer is prevalent in male. The male-to-female ratio of kidney cancer is estimated at approximately 2:1. Pathologically, a majority of kidney cancer is renal cell carcinoma. Cancer of the renal pelvis is generally urothelial carcinoma and has distinct etiology and features. The three major classical symptoms of kidney cancer were macroscopic hematuria, abdominal mass, and back pain. In recent years, however, incidental cancer without symptoms is common, which is found by chance during imaging tests such as ultrasonography or CT scans. Further examinations, generally contrast-enhanced CT scan, are used to confirm the diagnosis of kidney cancer. Because imaging examinations are reliable for diagnosis, biopsy is not always performed before surgery for kidney cancer. Kidney cancer is frequently developed among patients in hemodialysis or with a certain hereditary disease such as von Hippel-Lindau disease. NCCN (National Comprehensive Cancer Network) Guidelines for Patients: Kidney Cancer is useful to understand kidney cancer in detail [2].

15.1.2 Treatment

Radiotherapy or conventional chemotherapy is less effective for kidney cancer. Surgery is a main or primary treatment for kidney cancer. Unless metastasis is found, kidney cancer is treated with surgery, which is total or partial resection of the kidney. Recently surgery for kidney cancer is performed mostly through endoscopic procedure. Even for metastatic disease, surgical resection of the kidney and metastatic site may be considered. For metastatic or unresectable kidney cancer, recently established molecular targeting drugs and

© The Author(s), under exclusive license to Springer Nature Singapore Pte Ltd. 2026

M. Endo et al. (eds.), *Cancer and Work in Asia Volume 2*, https://doi.org/10.1007/978-981-95-6537-5_15

Table 15.1 Clinical features of kidney cancer (renal cell carcinoma)

1. Prevalent in male (gender ratio: approximately 2:1)
2. Recently incidental cancer without symptom is common
3. Frequently diagnosed among patients in hemodialysis or with a certain hereditary disease
4. Localized cancer is treated with surgery (total or partial resection of kidney) mostly through endoscopic procedure
5. Even for metastatic disease, surgical resection may be considered
6. Radiotherapy or conventional chemotherapy is less effective
7. Molecular targeting drugs are effective
8. Immunotherapy (immune check point inhibitors) is effective

immune checkpoint inhibitors are effective and utilized to prolong progression and survival [3].

15.1.3 Cancer and Work

In patients with localized kidney cancer, kidney function is partially disturbed after curative resection of cancer. In most cases, because the contralateral kidney and possibly the residual part of the affected kidney (partial resection) are preserved, activities of daily living will be maintained. In some cases, however, for those who have chronic kidney disease as a comorbidity, restriction of diet or therapeutic intervention may be required. In patients with end-stage renal failure, hemodialysis for 2–3 h may be necessary 3 times per week at a clinic to replace kidney function, and limitation of fluid intake and dietary restriction are instructed, which result in significant deterioration of work [4].

In patients with metastatic or unresectable kidney cancer, systemic therapy by means of intravenous and/or oral administration of molecular targeting drugs and/or immune checkpoint inhibitors will be continued at the outpatient clinic for a long-term period. Therefore, careful attention is needed for scheduling employment and care of side effects.

15.2 Bladder Cancer

15.2.1 Clinical Features (Table 15.2)

In Japan, the National Cancer Center Japan reported that the diagnosis (2018) and death (2019) of bladder cancer were 23,230 and 8911 cases, respectively [1]. Urinary bladder cancer is prevalent in male. The male-to-female ratio of bladder cancer is estimated at approximately 3–4:1. Pathologically, most bladder cancer is urothelial carcinoma and frequently develops in multiple sites of the mucosa of the urinary bladder, ureter, and renal pelvis. Smoking and occupation in certain chemical and dye factories are risks of developing bladder cancer. Macroscopic hematuria without other symptoms is the typical symptom and may be a trigger of diagnosis. Bladder cancer is first diagnosed by endoscopy of the urinary bladder, and several imaging examinations, including MRI and CT scans are done to evaluate the stage of the disease. NCCN Guidelines for Patients: Bladder Cancer is useful to understand bladder cancer in detail [5].

Table 15.2 Clinical features of urinary bladder cancer

1. Prevalent in male (gender ratio: approximately 3–4:1)
2. Urothelial cancer is frequently multiple in urinary bladder, ureter, and renal pelvis
3. Smoking and certain occupations are risk of developing disease
4. Macroscopic hematuria without other symptoms is most frequent symptom
5. Endoscopic surgery (transurethral resection) is performed and the clinical stage is evaluated
6. For superficial disease, infusion therapy of BCG, etc., into bladder may be used to prevent recurrence
7. For muscle invasive disease, total resection of bladder with urinary diversion is a standard therapy
8. For metastatic or progressive disease, systemic chemotherapy and immunotherapy are effective

15.2.2 Treatment

Endoscopic surgery (TUR-BT: transurethral resection of bladder tumor) is performed and utilized for evaluation of disease grade and stage. For superficial disease (non-muscle invasive bladder cancer), infusion therapy of BCG or a chemotherapeutic agent into the bladder may be used to prevent recurrence after surgical resection. For muscle-invasive bladder cancer, total resection of the urinary bladder (total cystectomy) along with urinary diversion is a standard therapy. There are two types of urinary diversion: continent urinary diversion (neobladder) and non-continent urinary diversion (ileal conduit, uretero-cutaneostomy) (Fig. 15.1). For continent urinary diversion, a pouch is made inside the body from part of the intestines to hold urine. The urine is discharged through the urethra or by self-catheterization. Non-continent urinary diversion often involves linking the ureters to a piece of intestine that is brought out of the belly. The urine then drains continuously into an ostomy bag. Radiation therapy with or without chemotherapy is an alternative option for the treatment of muscle-invasive bladder cancer. For metastatic or progressive disease, systemic chemotherapy (platinum-based combination chemotherapy) and immunotherapy (immune checkpoint inhibitors) are effective and used to prolong progression and survival [6].

15.2.3 Cancer and Work

Urinary bladder cancer is well known as an environmental and industrial cancer. Aromatic amines secreted into urine

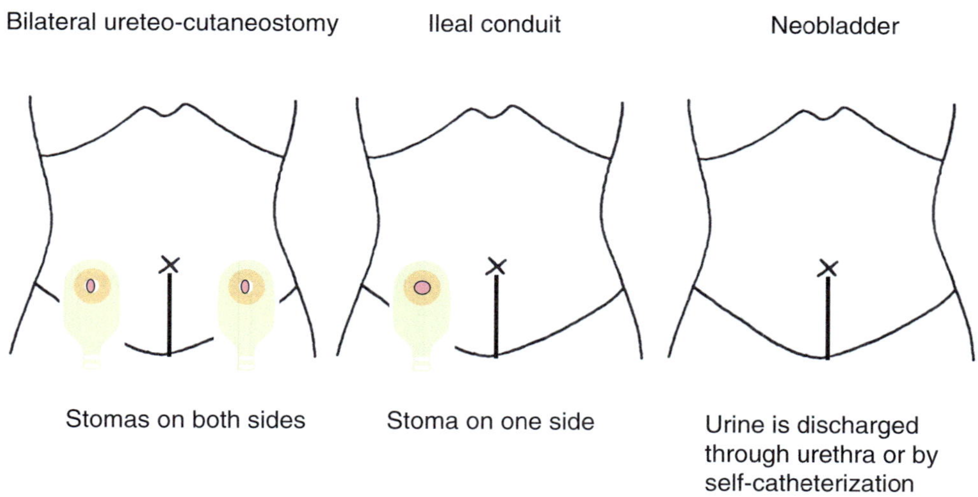

Fig. 15.1 Appearance after urinary diversion surgery for bladder cancer

are exposed to the urinary bladder and might develop cancer. Workers dealing with aromatic amines in chemical and dye factories have an increased risk of bladder cancer [7]. In addition, smoking is a risk factor for bladder cancer. Therefore, patient with bladder cancer is strongly recommended to avoid contacting aromatic amines and to quit smoking to decrease the risk of recurrence.

In patients with superficial bladder cancer, after curative resection of cancer by endoscopic surgery, no serious restriction is demanded except for visiting the clinic for monitoring and treatment against recurrence.

In patients with muscle-invasive bladder cancer, urinary diversion is necessary upon surgical resection of the urinary bladder. The patient will still be able to take part in strenuous physical activity, as well as daily routines. Therefore, self-catheterization or stoma/ostomy bag care will be a crucial issue for the patient to get and continue work.

In patients with metastatic or progressive bladder cancer, systemic therapy by chemotherapy and/or immunotherapy is usually performed. Management of the side effects of systemic therapy and disturbance of activities of daily living are important issues for employment.

15.3 Prostate Cancer

15.3.1 Clinical Features (Table 15.3)

Prostate cancer is one of the most common male malignancies in the Western countries [8]. Although the incidences of prostate cancer in Asian countries were considered to be low, recently they have been dramatically increasing, probably due to rapid aging of the population, change to the Western lifestyle, and spread of serum prostate-specific antigen (PSA) as a screening tool. In addition, the proportion of early-stage localized prostate cancer would be increasing in

Table 15.3 Clinical features of prostate cancer

1. Low incidence in Asian countries, but recently increasing
2. Prevalent in elderly men
3. No typical symptom in early stage
4. Serum tumor marker (PSA) is useful for screening and monitoring
5. Often metastasize to bone, and bone management is important
6. For early stage, several selections of curative treatment, such as surgery and radiotherapy
7. Hormone therapy is effective and utilized for advanced disease
8. Novel agents have been introduced for castration-resistant prostate cancer
9. Generally progresses slowly, and demonstrates favorable survival outcomes except in metastatic disease

Asian countries. In Japan, the National Cancer Center Japan reported that the diagnosis (2018) and death (2019) of prostate cancer were 92,021 (the most common in male) and 12,544 cases (the sixthy place in male), respectively [1]. Prostate cancer is frequently diagnosed among elderly males, and the most prevalent age of prostate cancer is 75–79 years. No typical symptom is evident in early-stage prostate cancer. Serum PSA is the most widely utilized biomarker among solid cancers. During the management of prostate cancer patients, measurement of serum PSA is useful for screening, diagnosis, risk classification, assessment of treatment effect, prediction of outcomes, and detection of recurrence or progression [9]. Pathological diagnosis and histological evaluation of prostate cancer are done by prostate needle biopsy. MRI, CT, and bone scans are used to examine the extent of disease spread. The most frequent site of metastasis from prostate cancer is bone, followed by lymph node. Generally prostate cancer is progressing slowly, and prognosis is expected to be relatively good except for the metastatic stage. NCCN Guidelines for Patients: Prostate Cancer is useful to understand prostate cancer in detail [10, 11].

15.3.2 Treatment

For decision-making on the therapeutic strategy for localized prostate cancer, risk classification is widely used based on T (tumor) stage, Gleason score (pathological classification), and serum PSA level [12]. Definitive therapy such as surgery (radical prostatectomy) or radiotherapy (external beam radiation therapy, interstitial irradiation) is conducted with curative intent. With the recent prevalence of robot-assisted surgery, minimally invasive therapy has been achieved. Hormone therapy may be combined according to risk classification. Active surveillance without therapeutic intervention, in which the patient is followed up with serial serum PSA measurements and periodical prostate biopsy, is one of the choices for small and slow-growing (low-risk) prostate cancer [13].

For advanced or metastatic prostate cancer, hormone therapy by means of androgen (male sex hormone) deprivation therapy (ADT) using LHRH agonists/antagonists or surgical castration is a standard treatment. Recently a new hormonal agent (ARTA: androgen receptor targeted agent) or docetaxel may be combined, especially for high-risk/volume disease. It was known that the prognosis of Asian prostate cancer patients who had been treated with hormone therapy was better than that of the Western countries [14], and that serious complications such as cardiovascular disease from hormone therapy are less common in Asian men. Based on these findings, the NCCN Asia Consensus Statement on Prostate Cancer was published and recommended more hormone therapy for Asian prostate cancer patients [15]. For castration-resistant prostate cancer (CRPC), which progressed after ADT, novel therapies including ARTA, chemotherapy (docetaxel, cabazitaxel), radionuclide therapy (Ra-223), and molecular targeted therapy (olaparib) are utilized to prolong survival and improve the quality of life of the patient.During the clinical course of advanced prostate cancer, the risk of fall and fracture will increase owing to a number of factors, including osteoporosis, muscular weakness and anemia due to ADT, bone metastasis, radiotherapy, and nocturia due to prostate enlargement and overactive bladder (Fig. 15.2). To overcome this risk, evaluation of bone mineral density, intake of enough calcium, appropriate exercise, and administration of bone-modifying agents (bisphosphonate, anti-RANKL antibody) are recommended [16].

15.3.3 Cancer and Work

Since prostate cancer is frequently diagnosed among aged men, it might be difficult to find a new job if the patient quits his job because of prostate cancer.

In patients with localized prostate cancer after curative treatment, complications vary between surgery and radiotherapy: erectile dysfunction and urinary incontinence after surgery, and hematuria and rectal bleeding after radiation. Urinary incontinence after radical prostatectomy is usually stress incontinence, in which urine is leaked upon increased pressure on the urinary bladder, such as coughing, laughing, sneezing, running, or heavy lifting. Radiation cystitis and radiation proctitis may occur owing to radiation therapy for prostate cancer, sometimes after a long-term period. Bleeding and irritative symptoms of the urinary bladder and rectum are causes of deterioration of activities of daily living. These symptoms due to complications may be disturbing problems at work.

In patients with metastatic or advanced prostate cancer, hormone therapy is generally utilized to prolong survival and improve the quality of life of the patient. Although hormone therapy is thought to be less toxic than chemotherapy, hormone therapy will be continued long-term, usually for life long, and thus the side effects of hormone therapy are an important issue for employment. Side effects of hormone therapy consist of a variety of symptoms: sexual dysfunction (decreased libido, erectile dysfunction), menopause (hot flush, sweating), osteoporosis, muscle weakness, depression, fatigue, cognitive impairment, metabolic disor-

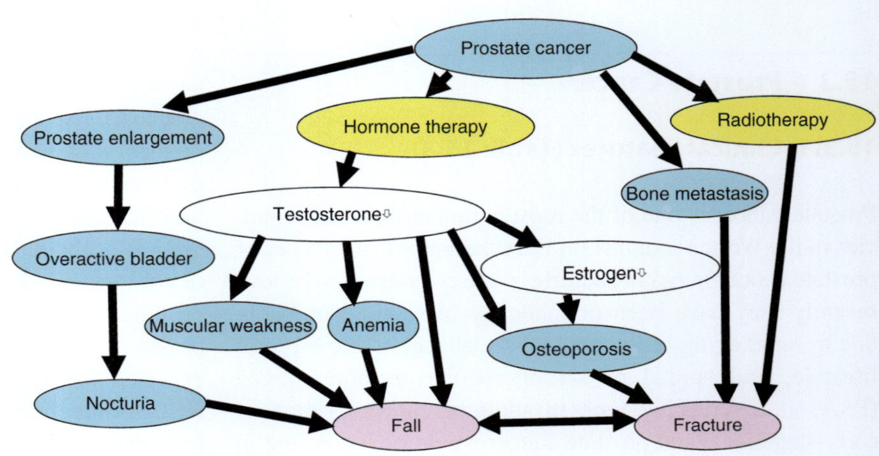

Fig. 15.2 Risk of fall and fracture in prostate cancer

Table 15.4 Side effects of hormone therapy for prostate cancer

Category of side effects	Symptoms
Deficiency of androgen	
Sexual function	Decreased libido, erectile dysfunction
Menopause	Hot flush, sweating
Bone and muscle	Osteoporosis, muscle weakness
Psychological function	Depression, fatigue, cognitive impairment
Metabolic disorders	Diabetes mellitus, hyperlipidemia, obesity
Cardiovascular diseases	Thrombosis, ischemic heart disease
Anemia	
Liver dysfunction	
Gynecomastia	Breast swelling and pain

ders (diabetes mellitus, hyperlipidemia, obesity), cardiovascular diseases (thrombosis, ischemic heart disease), anemia, liver dysfunction, and gynecomastia (Table 15.4). In patients with progressed prostate cancer, patients' preferences of goal of treatment, which are different from physicians' priority [17], were reported to be risk of fatigue, followed by risk of bone pain, and overall survival [18]. Also, unmet needs of prostate cancer patients varied between Asian countries [19]. Especially a study on patients' journeys revealed that symptoms of bone metastasis were variable and important for the management of prostate cancer patients with bone metastasis [20].

Since clinical features of prostate cancer are relatively specific, patient advocacy groups on prostate cancer have been acting to support physical, mental, and social issues, including working in several Asian countries.

15.4 Testicular Cancer

15.4.1 Clinical Features (Table 15.5)

Malignant tumor of the testis is prevalent in young-aged men. In men of 20–40 years old, testicular cancer is the most frequently diagnosed cancer among solid cancers. Enlargement of the testis without pain is a typical symptom. Serum tumor markers (alpha-fetoprotein, hCG, LDH) are useful for staging and monitoring. Radiotherapy is effective for testicular cancer and may be used to prevent or treat possible metastasis of lymph nodes. Chemotherapy is remarkably effective for testicular cancer, and therefore even in metastatic or advanced disease, a cure is expected by extensive chemotherapy. NCCN Guidelines for Testicular Cancer may be utilized to understand testicular cancer [21].

Table 15.5 Clinical features of testicular cancer

1. Prevalent in young-aged male
2. Enlargement of testis without pain is typical symptom
3. Diagnosed by prompt surgery (resection of testis, epididymis, and spermatic cord)
4. Serum tumor markers (alfa fetoprotein, hCG, LDH) are useful for diagnosis and monitoring
5. Decide therapeutic option based on pathology (seminoma or non-seminoma), serum markers, and stage
6. Chemotherapy is remarkably effective
7. Even in metastatic or advanced disease, cure is expected by chemotherapy

hCG human chorionic gonadotropin, *LDH* lactase dehydrogenase

15.4.2 Treatment

For the patient presenting enlargement of the testis and suspicion of testicular cancer by imaging (ultrasonography, MRI), high orchiectomy, in which all of the testis, epididymis, and spermatic cord are resected from the inguinal incision, is the first step of standard management. Based on pathological diagnosis (seminoma or non-seminoma) using resected specimen, results of serum tumor marker (alpha-fetoprotein, hCG, LDH), and evaluation of metastasis by imaging (CT), the therapeutic option, whether active surveillance, chemotherapy, or radiotherapy, will be decided. Platinum-based combination chemotherapy is significantly effective for testicular cancer.

15.4.3 Cancer and Work

In patients with early-stage testicular cancer, active surveillance without therapeutic intervention, prophylactic radiotherapy, or chemotherapy is performed. Because patients with testicular cancer are young, not only physical but also psychological care are important for the management of work.

In patients with advanced-stage testicular cancer, extensive and long-term chemotherapy, possibly longer than 1 year, must be applied to cure the disease. Therefore, working during as well as after cancer therapy should be managed and supported appropriately. Since extensive chemotherapy will cause spermatogenic dysfunction, preservation of frozen semen may be considered before the start of chemotherapy. In addition, secondary malignancy might arise after a long-term interval and should be checked carefully.

References

1. https://ganjoho.jp/reg_stat/statistics/stat/cancer/index.html
2. https://www.nccn.org/patients/guidelines/content/PDF/kidney-patient.pdf
3. Fujioka T, Obara W. Evidence-based clinical practice guidelines for renal cell carcinoma (Summary--JUA 2007 Edition). Int J Urol. 2009;16:339–53.
4. Nitta K, Masakane I, Tomo T, et al. Policy for developing clinical practice guidelines of Japanese Society for Dialysis Therapy. Renal Replace Ther. 2017;3:34.
5. https://www.nccn.org/patients/guidelines/content/PDF/bladder-patient.pdf
6. Matsumoto H, Shiraishi K, Azuma H, et al. Clinical practice guidelines for bladder cancer 2019 update by the Japanese Urological Association: summary of the revision. Int J Urol. 2020;27:702–9.
7. Heuper WC. Environmental and industrial cancer of the urinary bladder in USA. Acta Unio. 1962;18:585–96.
8. Torre LA, Bray F, Siegel RL, et al. Global cancer statistics, 2012. CA Cancer J Clin. 2015;65:87–108.
9. Gretzer MB, Partin AW. PSA markers in prostate cancer detection. Urol Clin North Am. 2003;30:677–86.
10. https://www.nccn.org/patients/guidelines/content/PDF/prostate-early-patient.pdf
11. https://www.nccn.org/patients/guidelines/content/PDF/prostate-advanced-patient.pdf
12. D'Amico AV, Whittington R, Malkowicz SB, et al. Biochemical outcome after radical prostatectomy, external beam radiation therapy, or interstitial radiation therapy for clinically localized prostate cancer. JAMA. 1998;280:969–74.
13. Bul M, Zhu X, Valdagni R, et al. Active surveillance for low-risk prostate cancer worldwide: the PRIAS study. Eur Urol. 2013;63:597–603.
14. Cooperberg MR, Hinotsu S, Namiki M, et al. Trans-Pacific variation in outcomes for men treated with primary androgen-deprivation therapy (ADT) for prostate cancer. BJU Int. 2016;117:102–9.
15. Hinotsu S, Namiki M, Ozono S, et al. NCCN Asia consensus statement prostate cancer. Jpn J Clin Oncol. 2018;48:964–5.
16. Kakehi Y, Sugimoto M, Taoka R, et al. Evidenced-based clinical practice guideline for prostate cancer (summary: Japanese Urological Association, 2016 edition). Int J Urol. 2017;24:648–66.
17. Suzuki K, Grillo V, Chen Y, et al. Understanding treatment strategies and preferences in nonmetastatic castration-resistant prostate cancer from the Japanese physician perspective. JCO Glob Oncol. 2021;7:302–10.
18. Uemura H, Matsubara N, Kimura G, et al. Patient preferences for treatment of castration-resistant prostate cancer in Japan: a discrete-choice experiment. BMC Urol. 2016;16:63.
19. Akakura K, Bolton D, Grillo V, et al. Not all prostate cancer is the same - patient perceptions: an Asia-Pacific region study. BJU Int. 2020;126(Suppl 1):38–45.
20. Akakura K, Uemura H, Miyazaki K, et al. A qualitative research study in Japan investigating patients' experience with metastatic castration-resistant prostate cancer: from diagnosis to decision for Ra-223 treatment. Future Oncol. 2021;17:5103–18.
21. https://www.nccn.org/professionals/physician_gls/pdf/testicular.pdf

16 Work-Related Issues in Adolescents and Young Adults with Cancer

Chikako Shimizu

Abstract

Cancer diagnosis and treatment in adolescents and young adults (AYAs), the age group between 15 and 39 years, have tremendous psychosocial and economic impacts on AYA lives. Career and employment-related issues have unique aspects in this life stage, because many AYAs are in preparation of or in the early stage of their careers, and thus work-related issues are closely related to their future financial well-being, self-esteem, and relationships. Socioeconomic status at the time of diagnosis and the cancer diagnosis itself affect the post-treatment employment status. Access to a multidisciplinary support system providing psychological and physical support, as well as cancer survivor-oriented career counseling, work placement, and employment sustenance support, is desired, but the establishment and coordinated implementation of such a system remains a challenge. Effective identification of AYAs with cancer in the healthcare setting, thorough assessment of their physical condition and cognitive function, timely referral to appropriate supporting services such as social-welfare counselors and career and employment services, workplace improvements to accommodate return-to-work, and the comprehensive education of AYAs themselves and professionals in the healthcare, education, and employment sectors are important components in overcoming the stigma and work-related concerns of AYA cancer survivors and will help them reach their potential.

Keywords

Adolescent and young adults with cancer · Career support · Stigma · Workplace accommodation · Work-related issues

C. Shimizu (✉)
Department of Breast and Medical Oncology, Japan Institute of Health Security-National Center for Global Health and Medicine, Tokyo, Japan
e-mail: shimizu.c@jihs.go.jp

16.1 Introduction

The definition of adolescents and young adults (AYAs) varies by country and context, but it generally refers to the age group between 15 and 39 years [1]. Approximately 1.2 million cancer cases and 400,000 cancer-related deaths were estimated to occur among AYAs worldwide in 2018. Its incidence is significantly increasing [2], but it accounts for only a few percent of all newly diagnosed cancers. Distribution of cancer types varies across AYA age groups and sexes [2], which makes each individual cancer experience very different.

Regardless of age, diagnosis, or nationality, however, cancer and its treatments have tremendous psychosocial and economic impacts on the lives of AYAs. Among various concerns that AYAs with cancer may encounter, the work-related issues have unique aspects in this life stage, because many AYAs are in preparation for or in the early stage of their careers. Focusing on employment or career development may oversimplify the difficulties of cancer survivorship in AYAs with cancer, as work-related issues are closely related to financial well-being, self-esteem, and relationships.

In this chapter, I will describe the work-related issues of AYAs with cancer, AYAs' concerns related to employment and career development, and how adequate support by healthcare providers and others could help overcome these issues.

16.2 Work-Related Issues in AYAs with Cancer

Work-related issues in AYAs can be classified into two categories: one is the continuation of work for those who already have a job, and the other is obtaining the first job for those who have never been employed. The latter is typical in adolescents who are still receiving education and just started to think about their future job and career.

© The Author(s), under exclusive license to Springer Nature Singapore Pte Ltd. 2026
M. Endo et al. (eds.), *Cancer and Work in Asia Volume 2*, https://doi.org/10.1007/978-981-95-6537-5_16

Socioeconomic status at the time of diagnosis of cancer and cancer diagnosis itself can affect the post-treatment employment status in people in their early career, especially in those who are uninsured or have an unstable employment status. In the AYA Hope Study, an observational cohort study done in the United States in 2008, more than 70% of patients who were working or went to school full-time before diagnosis had a full-time job at 15–35 months post-diagnosis, while only 34% of former part-time workers/students had a full-time job post-diagnosis [3]. Patients who were uninsured before diagnosis were significantly less likely to be working full-time at follow-up compared with those whose insurance was provided by their employer or school. In another study examining the employment and financial outcomes of Dutch AYA cancer survivors using nationwide population-based cancer registry data, AYA cancer survivors were significantly less often employed compared with their controls at 1 year and 5 years after diagnosis [4]. In a systematic review of 26 studies reporting on the social well-being of patients and survivors diagnosed between the ages of 15 and 39 years published between 2000 and 2014, AYAs with cancer reported difficulties related to employment, educational attainment, and financial stability [5]. Moreover, uninsured AYAs with cancer were more likely to present with advanced disease and to have poor prognoses [6]. These studies highlight the importance of career support for AYAs with cancer.

Stone et al. conducted a narrative review of the literature to identify work-related issues of AYAs with cancer [7]. Their findings included the following:

1. The cycle of functional ability impacting work productivity on employment is a strong source of distress affecting not only acquiring and maintaining a job but also financial security, access to healthcare, relationships, and quality of life.
2. Survivors may initially experience delays in obtaining education and employment due to cancer diagnosis and treatment but may become equal to healthy controls overall in achieving a successful career.
3. Many young adult cancer survivors continue working throughout the treatment phase, although treatment schedules and side effects sometimes interfere with productivity.
4. Physical or cognitive consequences occasionally prompted a change in occupation.
5. Coping style, support systems, and changing perspectives about work and life in general were also influential on career decisions among young adult cancer survivors.

As described by Stone et al., the work issues of AYAs are multi-dimensional and complex. They involve physical and cognitive functional ability, coping style, and support systems. It should be noted that perspectives about work and life may change along the journey after a cancer diagnosis. Compared to AYAs without cancer, AYA cancer survivors are at higher risk of mortality and severe and life-threatening chronic health conditions and at increased risk of developing cardiac, endocrine, and musculoskeletal conditions [8, 9]. Therefore, continuous support not only in the acute phase but also in the survivorship phase is necessary from the healthcare environment, the workplace, and the society.

16.3 Concerns About Work-Related Issues from the AYA Perspective

AYA cancer survivors are eager to enter or return to the workforce after achieving disease remission to resume their previous roles and career trajectories, but they often lack appropriate career development skills and are disconnected from the labor market [10].

Stigma and fear of workplace discrimination have been identified as prominent challenges faced by AYA cancer survivors, whereas a supportive workplace, a desire to be open with co-workers, and a willingness to request support and manage expectations are regarded as positive reasons for disclosure [9]. In the aforementioned AYA Hope Study, a belief that cancer negatively influenced plans for work/school was associated with quitting work or school, and those who looked for work after completing treatment were often concerned that their medical history would be seen as a disadvantage during the hiring process [11]. To overcome such stigma, patient education, psychological support, and communication support between the patient and the workplace will be needed. In addition, professional support such as appearance care, rehabilitation, and job training may be helpful, but only a few interventions aimed at enhancing work participation of unemployed or work-disabled cancer survivors have been evaluated [12].

It is important for patients to find jobs that match not only their wishes but also their capabilities. Diminished cognitive function, concentration problems, and physical symptoms such as fatigue and pain can make it difficult for AYA cancer survivors to return to school [13]. These symptoms are often overlooked or neglected in survivorship care. It is important to conduct a thorough assessment and clarify any impairments in the physical condition or cognitive function before referring patients to supporting services such as social-welfare counselors and employment services.

Academic continuation for high school and college students may be important for those who are receiving higher education. However, continuation of higher education is merely a short-term goal from the perspective of lifelong career development. Providers in higher education should be equipped with knowledge of cancer and survivorship care to better engage in longitudinal support for vulnerable young students who are worried about their future job and career [14].

16.4 Support for Work Issues from Healthcare Professionals

A tailored, patient-centered approach is required because career support should be personalized according to the patient's developmental stage, socio-economic environment, past education, career plan, cancer experience, and its impact on daily life. For the patient, being aware of and able to express his/her own health condition, capabilities, and limitations will be advantageous when searching for a job or negotiating employment conditions in the workplace.

For healthcare providers who directly provide active cancer care, it is especially important to provide primary care for work-related issues. A multidisciplinary team in the institution providing cancer care should provide customized and coordinated care based on careful screening and assessment of the needs of each AYA. Physicians treating AYAs have the responsibility to inform them about the cancer diagnosis and prognosis so that patients can envision their life after cancer. Psychological support should be provided from nurses and/or psychologists who are familiar with development and communication specific to AYAs. A referral to a social worker to manage work issues should be considered as needed. Social workers may be able to liaise with employers and/or refer to other resources to support employment. They may communicate with school principals, school counselors, or coordinators to enable continuous education, including career education. Rehabilitation services may be better involved for those who have functional impairments. Evaluation of cognitive function and counseling by experts may be helpful for patients who have impaired cognitive function.

Although healthcare professionals such as physicians and nurses are in the closest position to grasp the work needs of AYAs with cancer, these needs are often overlooked. The primary interest of healthcare professionals may well be to cure and/or to relieve the symptoms of cancer. Not being specialists in work issues may make them hesitate to bring up work-related issues in the conversation with patients. Many healthcare providers may feel that they are too inexperienced to provide adequate care for AYAs because of the rare encounter with patients in the clinic. In addition, because healthcare providers have their own unique career paths, it is natural that they feel inadequate to provide professional advice if the career paths that AYAs want to pursue are unfamiliar to them.

In a recent qualitative study, emotional confrontation (e.g., feeling helplessness and experiencing a greater sense of empathy), questioning one's own professional attitude and skills, navigating uncertainty (e.g., discussing prognosis and end of life), and obstacles in the health care organization (e.g., lack of knowledge and clarity about responsibilities) have been identified as challenges of care for health care professionals facing AYAs with unknown and poor prognoses [15]. Primary providers should closely cooperate with social support services, which can give professional advice regarding the continuation of education, career development, and employment. Finally, there must be education for healthcare providers and a system that secures identifying the needs and coordinating the care of AYAs.

16.5 Ingenuity of Care Delivery Within the Healthcare System

With the exception of younger adolescents treated in pediatric departments, most cancer patients in the AYA generation are usually treated in adult care and are spread across multiple medical departments because of their diverse diagnoses. In the survivorship phase, their healthcare may be transitioned to a local healthcare provider. To deliver the necessary support to every patient who needs it at any time of their patient journey, an original, clever, and inventive care-delivery system should be established.

First, AYAs who potentially have support needs should be identified at the clinic or the ward where they receive active treatment for cancer. At an institution specialized in cancer, this is easy because most of the patients visiting the hospital are people with cancer. A simple age check can identify the AYA patients and refer them to a consulting service or a multidisciplinary team, if available. In contrast, in a general hospital or a university hospital, it might be more difficult to identify AYAs with cancer because there are many patients with diagnoses other than cancer. An acquisition system to efficiently manage AYAs with cancer needs to be developed at such institutions.

After identifying AYAs with potential needs, their needs should be carefully screened. Nurses or other professionals who can liaise the needs to a social work service or a multidisciplinary team may interview the patient to assess the potential needs for career development and employment. To make this process efficient, a prompt sheet may be used to screen the needs.

Hospital social workers play an important role in supporting work issues of AYAs. If a patient is treated at a pediatric hospital or ward, pediatric social workers should help patients continue their education, navigate career development, and collaborate with adult or community social workers to transition care into the adult setting where actual employment support is provided.

Social workers and other health professionals may be inexperienced in treating AYAs, particularly in regions where AYA numbers are small. Establishing an organization in which information regarding AYAs can be shared and people can network may be helpful to compensate for such lack of experience.

16.6 Evidence of Psychosocial Interventions

In contrast to established evidence of psychosocial disparities, established evidence of psychosocial interventions is rare. In a study investigating the association between the usage of vocational services and the employment of previously unemployed young adult cancer survivors aged 18–25, vocational and other training, job search assistance, job placement services, on-the-job support, and maintenance services were related to increased odds for employment.

"Recapture Life" was an Australian, psychologist-led intervention that comprised six 90-min weekly online group sessions involving peer discussion around cognitive-behavioral coping skills, such as behavioral activation, thought challenging, communication and assertiveness skill training, problem-solving, and goal setting. It was compared to both a waitlist control group and a peer-support control group in a phase II randomized controlled trial [16]. This study was underpowered, and no positive impact of intervention was identified on the quality of life of AYA cancer survivors. Rather, those who participated in the Recapture Life intervention reported higher perceived negative impacts of cancer, anxiety, and depression at follow-up compared to the peer-support control group.

Another randomized controlled study in the United States compared a self-management survivorship intervention to usual care in young adults aged 18–39 at diagnosis in the previous 1–5 years who had symptoms of cancer-related distress, insomnia, fatigue, pain, and/or depression [17]. When unmet symptom needs were addressed in self-management–focused survivorship clinic visits and follow-up calls, distress improved for 46% in the intervention arm at 6 months compared to 18% in usual care, while other symptoms did not improve. To note, in this study, a college degree predicted a greater likelihood of completing the clinic visit, suggesting that a lack of access to resources and support, such as among those with low socioeconomic status and less education, is a driving factor in sustaining unmet healthcare and symptom needs.

The above-mentioned studies were mainly focused on psychological outcomes, and it is unclear whether and how much work-related issues were addressed during the intervention. How best to engage AYA cancer survivors in psychological support and relate it to work support remains a challenge.

16.7 Potential Needs for Support in the Workplace

In a cross-sectional survey addressing colleagues' perceptions of return-to-work cancer survivors, inadequate return-to-work opportunities were associated with low workplace social support, low levels of job control, and no prior experience working with a cancer survivor [18]. To ensure continuous employment, it is suggested that AYAs require improvements in the workplace environment rather than consultation services at hospitals [19]. Workplace accommodations such as a modified workspace, a modified work schedule, and/or reduced hours may have a positive effect on cancer survivors who return to work from a sick leave [20]. In a semi-structured interview for AYA cancer survivors and occupational and environmental health professionals (OEHPs) within the workplace, self-disclosure of being a cancer survivor, sustainable working ability, gatekeeping of employment and return-to-work opportunities, and accessing support were the processes that influenced the work of AYA cancer survivors [21]. Education in the workplace to raise awareness of the needs of AYAs with cancer may help provide colleagues with a more comprehensive understanding of cancer survivors who seek new employment or return to work.

16.8 Conclusions

AYAs with cancer face numerous work issues as sequelae of cancer diagnosis and treatment. Work issues are closely related with psychological and economic well-being not only during active treatment but also beyond it. Healthcare providers and other stakeholders should understand the attributes and consequences of these work issues throughout the cancer trajectory and serve as the first point of contact for connecting patients to social workers and other occupational and career-support professionals. Raising awareness of and providing education about work issues of AYAs with cancer in the healthcare, workplace, and educational settings are important to reduce AYAs' concerns about career and work. It is also important to secure the delivery of information and support to AYAs who have work-related concerns. Structured intervention, which fulfills vocational needs and also provides both psychological and physical support, remains a challenge.

References

1. U.S. Department of Health and Human Services. Closing the Gap: Research and Care Imperatives for Adolescents and Young Adults with Cancer—Report of the Adolescent and Young Adult Oncology—Progress Review Group. National Cancer Institute of the National Institutes of Health; 2006.
2. Gupta S, Harper A, Ruan Y, Barr R, Frazier AL, Ferlay J, et al. International trends in the incidence of cancer among adolescents and young adults. JNCI J Natl Cancer Inst. 2020;112(11):1105–17. https://doi.org/10.1093/jnci/djaa007.
3. Parsons HM, Harlan LC, Lynch CF, Hamilton AS, Wu X, Kato I, et al. Impact of cancer on work and education among adolescent and young adult cancer survivors. J Clin Oncol. 2012;30:2393–400.
4. Janssen SHM, van der Meer DJ, van Eenbergen MCHJ, et al. Short- and long-term impact of cancer on employment and financial outcomes of adolescents and young adults (AYAs): a large population-based case-control registry study in The Netherlands. ESMO Open. 2022;7(4):100521. https://doi.org/10.1016/j.esmoop.2022.100521.
5. Warnder EL, Kent EE, Trevino KM, et al. Social well-being among adolescents and young adults with cancer: a systematic review. Cancer. 2016;122(7):1029–37. https://doi.org/10.1002/cncr.29866.
6. Roth M, Berkman A, Anderson CA, et al. Improved survival of young adults with cancer following the passage of the affordable care act. Oncologist. 2022;27(2):135–43.
7. Stone DS, Ganz PA, Pavlish C, Robbins WA. Young adult cancer survivors and work: a systematic review. J Cancer Surviv. 2017;11(6):765–81.
8. Chao C, Bhatia S, Xu L, Cannavale KL, Wong FL, Huang PS, Cooper R, Armenian SH. Chronic comorbidities among survivors of adolescent and young adult cancer. J Clin Oncol. 2020;38(27):3161–74.
9. Suh E, Stratton KL, Leisenring WM, Nathan PC, Ford JS, Freyer DR, et al. Late mortality and chronic health conditions in long-term survivors of early-adolescent and young adult cancers: a retrospective cohort analysis from the Childhood Cancer Survivor Study. Lancet Oncol. 2020;21(3):421–35.
10. Tan CJ, Ke Y, Ng T, Tan IMJ, Goh WL, Poon E, Farid M, Neo PSH, Srilatha B, Chan A. Work- and insurance-related issues among Asian adolescent and young-adult cancer survivors: a qualitative study. Support Care Cancer. 2020;28(12):5901–9.
11. Rabin C. Cancer-related self-disclosure in the workplace/school by adolescent and young adult cancer survivors. J Adolesc Young Adult Oncol. 2020;9(4):528–33.
12. van Ommen F, Coenen P, Malekzadeh A, de Boer AGEM, Greidanus MA, Duijts SFA. Interventions for work participation of unemployed or work-disabled cancer survivors: a systematic review. Acta Oncol. 2023;62(7):753–64.
13. Vetsch J, Wakefield CE, McGill BC, Cohn RJ, Ellis SJ, Stefanic N, et al. Educational and vocational goal disruption in adolescent and young adult cancer survivors. Psychooncology. 2018;27(2):532–8.
14. Psihogios AM, Pauly-Hubbard H, Schwartz L, Ginsberg JP, Hobbie W, Szalda D. Understanding and improving knowledge of cancer survivorship care among college providers. J Cancer Educ. 2018;33(5):1075–81.
15. Burgers VWG, van den Bent MJ, Darlington AE, Gualthérie van Weezel AE, Compter A, Tromp JM, et al. A qualitative study on the challenges health care professionals face when caring for adolescents and young adults with an uncertain and/or poor cancer prognosis. ESMO Open. 2022;7(3):100476.
16. Sansom-Daly UM, Wakefield CE, Ellis SJ, McGill BC, Donoghoe MW, Butow P, et al. Online, group-based psychological support for adolescent and young adult cancer survivors: results from the recapture life randomized trial. Cancer. 2021;13(10):2460.
17. Syrjala KL, Walsh CA, Yi JC, Leisenring WM, Rajotte EJ, Voutsinas J, et al. Cancer survivorship care for young adults: a risk-stratifed, multicenter randomized controlled trial to improve symptoms. J Cancer Surviv. 2022;16:1149–64.
18. Eguchi H, Wada K, Higuchi Y, Smith DR. Co-worker perceptions of return-to-work opportunities for Japanese cancer survivors. Psychooncology. 2017;26(3):309–15.
19. Tsuchiya M, Takahashi M, Shimizu C, Ozawa M, Higuchi A, Sakurai N, Horibe K. Perceptions toward employment and support needs in medical institutions and workplace among AYA cancer survivors. Gan To Kagaku Ryoho. 2019;46(4):691–5. (In Japanese)
20. Alleaume C, Paraponaris A, Bendiane MK, Peretti-Watel P, Bouhnik AD. The positive effect of workplace accommodations on the continued employment of cancer survivors five years after diagnosis. Support Care Cancer. 2020;28(9):4435–43.
21. Stone DS, Pavlish CL, Ganz PA, Thomas EA, Casillas JN, Robbins WA. Understanding the workplace interactions of young adult cancer survivors with occupational and environmental health professionals. Workplace Health Saf. 2019;67(4):179–88.

17 The Basics of Cancer Pharmacotherapy

Junichiro Watanabe

Abstract

Recent advances in cancer pharmacotherapy, especially in targeted therapy based on specific biomarkers, have significantly improved the patients' outcomes. However, new problems such as never-before-experienced physical toxicity and financial toxicity have arisen as well. In order to minimize these problems, the purpose of anticancer pharmacotherapy should be clarified, and appropriate use must be considered.

Keywords

Cancer pharmacotherapy · Anticancer agent · Molecular target therapy · Side effects · Adjuvant therapy · Palliative therapy

17.1 Introduction

Although drug therapy is almost the only therapeutic modality in hematologic malignancies, e.g., leukemias, lymphomas, or myelomas, the importance of drug therapy is rapidly increasing in other solid tumors as well. Details of anticancer drug therapy for the disease will be left to other chapters, and this chapter describes the mechanism of action, side effects, purpose, and problems of anti-cancer agents.

J. Watanabe (✉)
Department of Breast Oncology, Graduate School of Medicine, Juntendo University, Bunkyo-ku, Tokyo, Japan
e-mail: j.watanabe.vq@juntendo.ac.jp

17.2 Mechanism of Action and Side Effects of Anticancer Agents

17.2.1 Cytotoxic Agents (So-Called "Anticancer Drugs")

It is the oldest but is still the mainstay of anti-cancer treatment. The mechanism of action (MoA) of such cytotoxic agents is based on the theory that "Malignant cells generally undergo more frequent cell proliferation than normal cells. Therefore, the MoA is focused on the cell-proliferation process, namely the duplication of deoxyribonucleic acid (DNA) and the elongation or shortening of microtubules. By impairing it, it is possible to more selectively bring about cell death of malignant cells." The Gompertzian model (Fig. 17.1) is well known for showing the development, growth, and outcome of malignancies; however, this model is based on the following three assumptions: all malignant cells are equally responsive to the agent, drug resistance does not establish, and malignant cells do not metastasize to other organs. Therefore, the theory and practice do not always match.

Cytotoxic agents can be generally classified into two types according to their pharmacological MoA: those that damage DNA and those that damage microtubules. Furthermore, those that target DNA can be divided into three types: those that directly damage DNA, those that inhibit DNA duplication, and those that damage DNA synthesis. Such cytotoxic agents are used in a wide range of malignant diseases, including hematologic malignancies. Table 17.1 summarizes typical cytotoxic anticancer agents and their main target diseases. (Note: Please check the websites of regulatory agencies in each country for the latest approval status.)

The side effects (harms) of cytotoxic drugs are somewhat a mirror image of their effects (benefits). I.e., according to Simon and Norton's theory, it is designed to be more effective for malignant tumor cells, but normal cells are also damaged to some extent. In particular, side effects are likely to appear in organs that contain cells that are constantly

© The Author(s), under exclusive license to Springer Nature Singapore Pte Ltd. 2026
M. Endo et al. (eds.), *Cancer and Work in Asia Volume 2*, https://doi.org/10.1007/978-981-95-6537-5_17

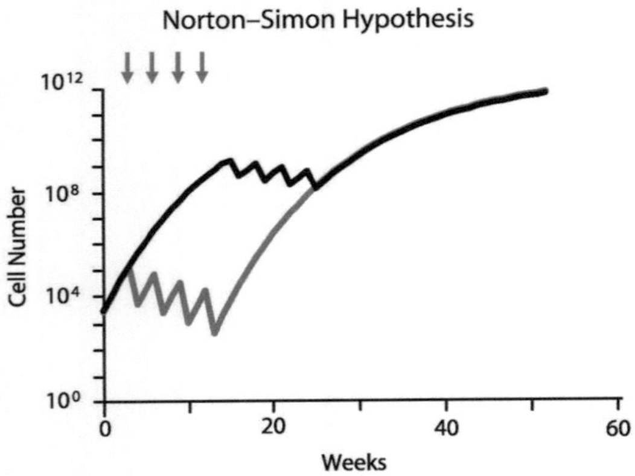

Fig. 17.1 The Norton–Simon hypothesis states that the rate of tumor volume regression is proportional to the rate of growth. (Adapted from Schmidt C. The Gompertzian view: Norton honored for role in establishing cancer treatment approach. J Natl Cancer Inst. 2004,20;96(20):1492–3. https://doi.org/10.1093/jnci/96.20.1492. PMID: 15494594)

Table 17.1 Purpose of the cancer pharmacotherapy by types of malignancies

Curative intent (chemotherapy only)
Leukemias and lymphomas (includes recurrent cases)
Testicular cancer (germ cell tumor)
Adjuvant (postoperative, curative intent)
Breast cancer
Colorectal cancer
Gastric cancer
Lung cancer
Pancreatic cancer
Sarcomas (Ewing sarcoma, osteosarcoma)
Ovarian cancer
Neoadjuvant (preoperative, curative intent, and/or function-preserving)
Anal cancer
Bladder cancer
Breast cancer
Cervical cancer
Esophageal cancer
Germ cell tumor
Head and neck cancer
Sarcomas (osteosarcoma, soft tissue sarcoma)
Rectal cancer
Palliation
Inoperable or recurrent malignancies

undergoing cell proliferation among normal cells. Specifically, it includes hematopoietic cells represented by leukocytes, hair matrix cells, gastrointestinal mucosal cells, etc., and they appear as leukopenia, hair loss, and nausea/diarrhea, respectively. In addition to this acute and subacute toxicity, accumulative toxicity to tissues and organs having cells with less vigorous cell division is also observed. For example, peripheral neuropathy due to persistent damage to nerve cells, myocardial toxicity, pulmonary toxicity, nephrotoxicity, etc. In general, these organs or tissues do not proliferate in adults; thus, they are less sensitive to anticancer agents and do not lead to cell death, but on the other hand, drugs themselves or cell damage by drugs accumulate, and, as a result, side effects are gradually established. These accumulative side effects, such as sensory neuropathy, gradually improve or disappear with the removal of anticancer agents; however, some cumulative toxicities, such as myocardial damage or interstitial pneumonitis, may become fatal or will remain as sequelae.

The details of the side effects of cytotoxic agents have sufficient evidence from their historical background, and in many cases, preventive and therapeutic methods have been established. See other sections for specific supportive care for side effects related to cytotoxic agents.

17.2.2 Endocrine Therapeutic Agents (So-Called "Hormone Therapy")

For cancers with sex hormone dependence, such as estrogen receptor-positive breast cancer or prostate cancer, drugs that inhibit actions of estrogen (female sex hormone) or androgen (male sex hormone) may be an option. Surgical castration (oophorectomy or extirpation) is also a type of endocrine therapy. The MoA of endocrine therapy is considered to be cytostatic rather than cytocidal. Therefore, it is often applied as palliative therapy in advanced cancer or postoperative therapy to reduce the risk of recurrence in early-stage breast cancer.

The main side effect of endocrine therapies is symptoms related to hormone deficiency, i.e., symptoms included in postmenopausal syndrome. In addition to hot flashes and palpitations, there are decreased bone minerals (osteoporosis), arthralgia, hair loss, decreased libido, vaginal dryness (in female)/erectile dysfunction (in male), and cognitive dysfunction.

17.2.3 Molecular-Targeted Therapeutic Agents

The definition of a molecular-targeted therapeutic agent is "a drug that acts on a specific molecule associated with the growth, invasion, or metastasis of malignant cells, that is, a protein or gene, and directly or indirectly exhibits an antitumor effect." Therefore, unlike cytotoxic agents, i.e., "authentic" anticancer drugs, molecular targeted agents have a more selective effect on malignant cells, so-called "pinpointed." However, the targeted molecules are only quantitatively or qualitatively minored than malignant cells and are also present in normal cells. Therefore, the understanding that "molecular-targeted therapies make a pinpoint attack on malignant cells, so they have few (or no) side effects" is a misunderstanding.

17.2.4 Monoclonal Antibody

Monoclonal antibodies that target specific proteins related to tumor cell growth are fully or partially humanized immunoglobulin G (IgG) by gene recombination technology. The agents are administered via drip infusion or subcutaneous injection. These monoclonal antibodies exhibit anticancer activity by binding to specific proteins on the cell membrane surface (mainly growth factor receptors), stopping the growth of cancer cells, and inducing tumor cell death (apoptosis). Some monoclonal antibodies bind to Fc receptors on natural killer (NK) cells and also have a cytotoxic effect due to antibody-dependent cell-mediated cytotoxicity (ADCC) activity. In addition, a novel monoclonal antibody (margetuximab) with higher ADCC activity has been developed by Fc-engineering.

It is known that vascular endothelial growth factor (VEGF), which is a growth factor, also causes tumor growth by binding to the VEGF receptor (VEGF-R). Monoclonal antibodies that targeted VEGF or VEGF-R include the anti-VEGF antibody, bevacizumab; the anti-VEGF-R2 antibody, ramucirumab; and the "decoy" of VEGF-R1/2, aflibercept.

17.2.5 Immunoradiotherapeutic Agent

Used in a certain type of malignant lymphoma. A radioisotope bound to an anti-CD20, commonly observed in lymphoma cells, is a monoclonal antibody that produces an antitumor effect due to an immune reaction and an antitumor effect due to beta-ray irradiation from a close distance.

17.2.6 Antibody-Drug Conjugate (ADC)

Currently, it is the most rapidly evolving type of molecular-targeting therapy. It is a monoclonal antibody combined with a cytotoxic compound as a payload. It binds to a target protein, often a growth factor receptor, and undergoes encapsulation (internalization), and the payload is released into the cell by lysosomal degradation. Gemtuzumab ozogamicin, introduced in 2000, bound ozogamicin as a payload to the anti-CD33 monoclonal antibody, which is commonly expressed on the surface of myeloid progenitor cells was the first ADC, but it did not become a standard of care (SoC) for acute myeloid leukemia. The first ADC accepted as SoC is trastuzumab emtansine (T-DM1), which is an anti-HER2 ADC approved for HER2-positive breast cancer. Trastuzumab deruxtecan (T-DXd), which has an enhanced payload, is considered to be the mainstay of anti-HER2 therapy because of its increased antitumor activity, including the bystander killing effect (Fig. 17.2). Currently, T-DXd is approved for advanced breast cancer and gastric cancer with HER2 overexpression. In addition, ADCs targeting trophoblast cell-surface antigen-2 (TROP-2), which is frequently expressed in various solid cancers, including triple-negative breast cancer, are under development, and one of the anti-TROP-2 ADCs, sacituzumab govitecan, is approved for advanced triple-negative breast cancer in the United States.

ADC targets proteins that are overexpressed on the tumor cell surface and is expected to have mild systemic toxicity due to the process of encapsulation; however, there exist systemic toxicities due to the release of payload into the blood. Thrombocytopenia and hepatic dysfunction are typical side effects of T-DM1; however, hair loss and gastrointestinal symptoms are rarely seen. On the other hand, T-DXd has the side effect of interstitial pneumonia in addition to hair loss and gastrointestinal symptoms; therefore, careful follow-up is required.

17.2.7 Tyrosine Kinase Inhibitors

Cells, regardless of whether they are normal cells or malignant cells, use a method called phosphorylation for intracellular signal transduction for their metabolism, proliferation, and even for the cell-death process. The protein involved in this phosphorylation is called tyrosine kinases (TKs), and inhibition of the activity of TK involved in cell proliferation/survival leads to suppression of proliferation or to the induction of apoptosis of malignant cells. The oldest in this category is imatinib, approved in the United States for chronic myeloid leukemia (CML) in 2001. On the other hand, in the area of non-hematologic malignancies, e.g., carcinomas and sarcomas, the development of TK inhibitors (TKIs) targeting epidermal growth factor (EGFR) and HER2 has progressed. That is, continuous phosphorylation, i.e., persistent activation in the absence of ligand, of the receptor-type TK caused by gene alterations such as base substitution in the gene (e.g., *EGFR*), gene fusion (*ALK/EML4*), or gene amplification (*HER2*), is considered the main cause of oncogenesis. These TKIs competitively bind to the phosphorylating site of TK and exhibit inhibitory effects.

A ROS1 inhibitor for *ROS1/RET* gene-fusion positive non-small cell lung cancer (NSCLC) has also been shown to be effective against papillary thyroid cancer. Several ROS1 TKIs have an antitumor effect on NSCLC with the *MET* exon 14 skipping mutation. TKIs for the HER2 TK domain also have several options. Lapatinib, neratinib, and tucatinib can be used for breast cancer with HER2 receptor overexpression. Drugs that interfere with the kinase activity of VEGF-R include sorafenib (approved by the FDA in 2005 for renal cell carcinoma [RCC], hepatocellular carcinoma [HCC], and thyroid carcinoma), sunitinib (2006, RCC, gastrointestinal stromal tumor [GIST], pancreatic neuroendo-

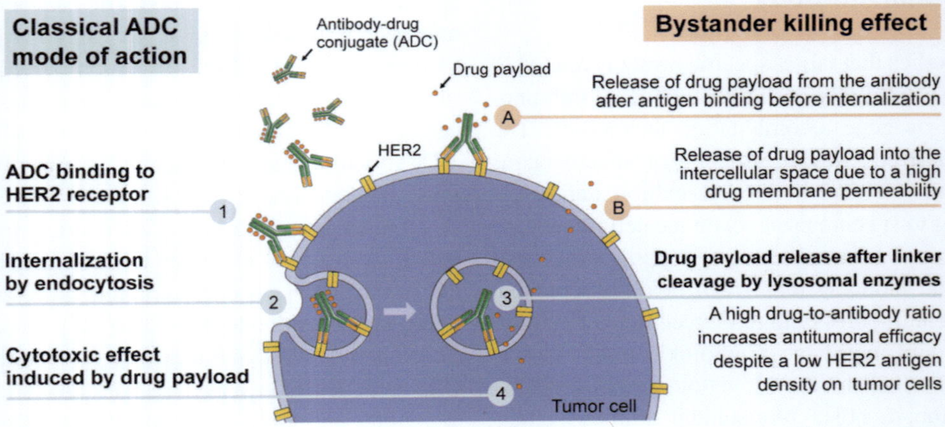

Fig. 17.2 Mode of action of HER2-directed ADCs in HER2-low tumors. Classical mode of action of ADCs with cleavable linkers: (1) After binding of the monoclonal anti-HER antibody component to HER2 expressed on the cell surface of tumor cells, (2) the ADC-HER2 complex is internalized by endocytosis. (3) After linker cleavage by lysosomal proteases, the drug payload is released and (4) can induce the cytotoxic effect leading to tumor cell death. A high drug-to-antibody ratio can increase antitumoral efficacy despite a low HER2 antigen density on tumor cells. Bystander killing effect: Using cleavable linkers, ADCs can be designed to promote drug release from the target cell to the extracellular space. Thereby, surrounding and bystander cells, which may or may not express the ADC target antigen, can be killed by taking up the cytotoxic drug. (**a**) This bystander killing can occur if the cytotoxic drug is released from the antibody after antigen binding before internalization. (**b**) Additionally, the drug payload can be released from the tumor cell into the intracellular space due to a high membrane permeability of the ADC drug payload. (Adapted from Rinnerthaler G, Gampenrieder SP, Greil R. HER2 directed antibody-drug-conjugates beyond T-DM1 in breast cancer. Int J Mol Sci. 2019,5;20(5):1115. https://doi.org/10.3390/ijms20051115. PMID: 30841523; PMCID: PMC6429068. This figure was created using Servier Medical Art templates, which are licensed under a Creative Commons Attribution 3.0 Unported License)

crine tumor [PNET]), pazopanib (2009, RCC, soft tissue sarcoma), axitinib (2012, RCC), regorafenib (2012, mCRC, HCC), cabozantinib (2012, thyroid cancer, RCC, HCC), lenvatinib (2015, thyroid cancer, HCC, thymic cancer, endometrial cancer, RCC), etc. have been developed. Many of these have a kinase activity inhibitory effect other than VEGF-R (e.g., Kit, platelet-derived growth factor receptor [PDGF-R]) and are therefore called multikinase inhibitors, including imatinib mentioned above.

Small molecule compounds with kinase inhibitory activity that do not target receptor-type TK include PI3K inhibitors, AKT inhibitors, MEK inhibitors, BRAF inhibitors, and mTOR inhibitors. Some of those inhibitors are approved for clinical use.

17.2.8 Other Small Molecule Compounds

Inhibitors of cyclin-dependent kinase 4 and 6 (CDK4/6), which are proteins that regulate the cell cycle, palbociclib, abemaciclib, and ribociclib can be used. These compounds dormant cells and induce apoptosis by inhibiting the transition of the cell cycle from G1 (Gap 1) to S (Synthesis) phases. At present, it is mainly used in combination with endocrine therapy for estrogen receptor-positive, HER2-negative advanced breast cancer.

Bortezomib is used in the treatment of multiple myeloma and rare types of lymphoma (mantle cell lymphoma) due to its ability to inhibit the proteolytic enzyme proteasome.

The chromatin contains DNA and histone protein. The DNA is wrapped by histones, and gene expression is regulated by the histone acetylation/de-acetylation process. These are called epigenome (epi + genome = over + gene) regulation, and the function of genes is turned on/off. Histone deacetylase (HDAC) inhibitors (vorinostat, panobinostat, and tucidinostat) that intervene in this epigenome regulation are mainly used in refractory blood disorders. Mutations in the *BRCA1* or *2* genes cause a variety of solid cancers, characterized by hereditary breast cancer and ovarian cancer (HBOC) syndrome. In breast cancer, ovarian cancer, prostate cancer, pancreatic cancer, etc., that show deleterious germline mutation of the *BRCA1/2* gene, it inhibits poly (ADP-ribose) polymerase (PARP), which is one of the DNA repair enzymes, and brings synthetic lethality. Such PARP inhibitors (olaparib, talazoparib, and niraparib) have been approved for clinical use.

Side effects of molecular-targeted therapies basically depend on the target molecule (e.g., side effects of the vascular system, such as hypertension or bleeding tendency, are typical for VEGF inhibitors). Details are given in the chapter by disease. However, regardless of the target molecule, some side effects might be commonly observed at a certain frequency. Interstitial lung disease (ILD) is one of the most well-known side effects of molecular-targeted therapies. The interstitium is the part involved in gas exchange, i.e., O_2 and CO_2 in the lung, and when inflammation caused by a drug occurs, the gas exchange capacity decreases, resulting in hypoxemia. Since there is no SoC for ILD, the prognosis of drug-induced ILD varies depending on the causative drug or other intrinsic/extrinsic factors.

17.2.9 Immune Checkpoint Inhibitors

Currently, it is the fastest-developing type of drug for malignancy. Immunity is a mechanism that distinguishes between self (body) and non-self (pathogen) and eliminates non-self to protect the organism. This immunity is composed of an immune system centered on T lymphocytes and B lymphocytes and is subject to monitoring and elimination by the immune system not only for pathogens such as bacteria and viruses but also for tumor cells. Immunity is an essential mechanism for protecting an individual in this way, but there is a risk that the host will be the target of an attack due to the overreaction of the immune system. In order to avoid this immune overreaction, there is a mechanism called an immune checkpoint, i.e., the "immune-brake system." The most studied immune checkpoints are the suppression of the activation of effector T cells by the binding of programmed death receptor-1 (PD-1) expressed on the surface of T cells and programmed death ligand-1 (PD-L1) to it. As shown in Fig. 17.2, tumor cells skillfully utilize this immune checkpoint. Once in the equilibrium phase of the escape phase, the tumor immune system becomes tolerant of tumor cells, leading to tumor growth. It is the anti-PD-1/-L1 monoclonal antibody that inhibits this PD-1/-L1 binding. The anti-PD-1/-L1 monoclonal antibody inhibits immune checkpoints and results in rebooting anti-tumor immunity, i.e., reactivation of cytotoxic T cells. The effectiveness of immune checkpoint inhibitors (ICIs) mainly depends on the antigenicity of the tumor. Although tumor cells are originally self-produced, they produce abnormal proteins that are not found in normal cells due to the genetic antigenicity of the tumor. That is, the recognition of abnormal proteins by the immune system as "non-self" leads to activation of tumor immunity. In other words, it is easy to show the effect of ICI when tumor immunity is suppressed by tumor-derived PD-L1, although the tumor cell has many gene mutations and, as a result of the abnormal gene, many abnormal proteins will be expressed. Tumors with high antigenicity include malignant melanoma, squamous cell carcinoma (lung cancer, esophageal cancer, etc.), and urothelial carcinoma; on the contrary, most breast carcinoma is a representative tumor with low antigenicity. Since the ICI is a monoclonal antibody (anti-PD-1, anti-PD-L1, or anti-cytotoxic T-lymphocyte-associated antigen [CTLA]-4), it is used by intravenous drip infusion. Depending on the type of malignancy or treatment setting (curative intent or palliative), ICI alone or in combination with cytotoxic agents is used. The side effects of ICIs are the flip side of action. That is damage to normal cells due to immune "runaway." Typical immune-related side effects are skin disorders (rash, erythema, etc.), endocrine disorders (thyroid dysfunction, diabetes, pituitary dysfunction, etc.), ILD, etc. As long as there are tissues where lymphocytes are present, immune-related side effects can occur in any organ, theoretically. To manage immune-related side effects, ICIs should be suspended or discontinued, and immunosuppressive agents such as corticosteroid hormones may be used. Since ICIs have a short history after the approval for clinical use, the actual frequency and, more importantly, extent of sequelae are still unclear.

17.3 Aim of Cancer Pharmacotherapy

In hematologic malignancies, it is clear that drug therapy is the mainstay of treatment because of its pathological characteristics, that is, it is a systemic disease from the onset. In some types of hematologic malignancies, systemic treatment with curative intent could be possible even in recurrent cases. However, in most solid malignancies, a curative approach is possible when the cancer is limited to the primary site and its locoregional area. It is expected that a multimodal approach, pharmacotherapy and radiation therapy, will be combined appropriately with surgical removal of cancer. On the other hand, when the patient develops distant metastasis or unresectable local recurrence, no matter how developed cancer pharmacotherapy is, a curative approach cannot be expected. Therefore, in the treatment of solid tumors, anticancer agents will be given for a certain period of time as perioperative (neoadjuvant, adjuvant, or both) systemic therapy in the early stage of cancer, if it is operable. In the case of advanced-stage or recurrent cancer, anticancer drugs are given for an indefinite period to prolong life and maintain the quality of life of the patient.

Of the perioperative drug therapies, postoperative drug therapy has established evidence for many carcinomas. For some types of lung cancer, colorectal cancer, breast cancer, gastric cancer, esophageal cancer (including pharyngeal cancer), and gynecological cancer. Such postoperative (i.e., adjuvant) anticancer therapy is performed to reduce the risk of recurrence after surgery. Breast cancer has the richest evidence of preoperative (i.e., neoadjuvant) anticancer therapy, which is equivalent to postoperative chemotherapy in terms of reducing the risk of recurrence and has the advantage of increasing the opportunity to undergo breast-conserving surgery. In addition, preoperative chemoradiation therapy is performed for esophageal cancer (including head and neck cancer), part of lung cancer, bladder cancer, osteosarcoma, germ cell tumor, etc., with the goal of downstaging, i.e., making surgery easier. In addition, there is no strong evidence of perioperative drug therapy for relatively rare carcinomas.

17.4 Conclusion

Anticancer pharmacotherapies are evolving day by day, and the best available treatment changes over a cycle of several years. On the other hand, drug costs are incredibly increasing, and such financial toxicity for individuals and society has not been well discussed.

Thus, when a patient is proposed anticancer drug therapy by his/her doctor, the best choice should be made by considering such aspects of anticancer pharmacotherapy in addition to the purpose, expected benefits, and expected harm of the therapy proposed.

18 Radiation Therapy for the Treatment of Cancer in Asia

Masaru Wakatsuki and Takashi Nakano

Abstracts

Radiation therapy is one of the main treatment methods for cancer. Although radiation therapy is widely used in high-income Asian countries, its use is not sufficiently widespread in low- and middle-income countries in the region. Large discrepancies are also observed between the estimated need for radiation therapy and its supply in most Asian countries, especially in low-and middle-income countries. Various radiation therapy projects have been conducted under the IAEA/RCA framework for more than 30 years. In addition, FNCA has contributed to improving the quality of radiation therapy and to improving treatment outcomes for predominant cancers in Asia. The IAEA and Japan have been taking the lead in promoting radiation therapy in Asia for the past 30 years. Improving the imbalance in the use of radiation therapy within each country is an important issue for the future. To achieve this, human resource exchange across countries and human resource development need to be continued through activities such as FARO and IAEA/RCA. Regarding radiation therapy equipment, which is still expensive, we hope that companies will develop radiation therapy equipment that is easier to introduce by optimizing its functions to suit the real-world conditions in Asia.

Keyword

Radiation therapy · Low- and middle-income country · Asia · Developing country · IAEA

M. Wakatsuki (✉)
QST Hospital, National Institutes for Quantum Science and Technology, Chiba, Japan
e-mail: wakatsuki.masaru@qst.go.jp

T. Nakano
National Institutes for Quantum Science and Technology, Chiba, Japan
e-mail: nakano.takashi2@qst.go.jp

18.1 Background

Population aging has become an issue in developed countries such as Japan, Europe, and the United States. According to World Population Prospects 2019, populations in Asian regions are projected to age significantly over the next several decades [1]. In the past, countermeasures against infectious diseases, such as sanitation and hygiene, were priorities for low- and middle-income countries in the Asian region. However, the aging of the population in the region likely means that a shift to cancer control is necessary. It is widely known that the number of patients with cancer in Asia has been on the rise in recent years. Thus, it is becoming increasingly important to establish strategies against this trend, just as in developed countries. GLOVOCAN 2020 showed that of the 19.29 million new cancer cases and 9.96 million cancer deaths recorded worldwide, 9.5 million new cancer cases and 5.8 million cancer deaths occurred in Asia. This indicates that nearly half of all cancer cases occur in Asia [2].

The main treatment methods for cancer are surgery, chemotherapy, and radiation therapy. However, unlike other treatment methods, radiation therapy is limited by the need for specialized radiation therapy equipment. Many barriers, such as a shortage of medical staff, including radiation oncologists, medical physicists, and radiation therapy technologists, and a shortage of radiation therapy facilities, prevent easy access to radiation therapy services in many Asian regions. Although radiation therapy is widely used in high-income Asian countries, such as Japan, South Korea, and Singapore, its use is not sufficiently widespread in low- and middle-income countries in the region. In addition, as radiation therapy is quite expensive, the disparity between its use in high-income and low-/middle-income regions is greater than that for other types of cancer treatment. Large discrepancies are also observed between the estimated need for radiation therapy and its supply in most Asian countries, especially in low- and middle-income countries. In addition, even though there are many patients who would normally be eligible for radiation therapy, the number of radiation ther-

© The Author(s), under exclusive license to Springer Nature Singapore Pte Ltd. 2026
M. Endo et al. (eds.), *Cancer and Work in Asia Volume 2*, https://doi.org/10.1007/978-981-95-6537-5_18

apy units per population is low. Furthermore, there are problems with accessibility of care due to limitations in transportation infrastructure. Thus, it is clear that limited use of radiation therapy in Asia is an important issue. Fortunately, various international activities are being carried out.

18.2 Current Status of Radiation Therapy in Asia According to IAEA/RCA Activities

The International Atomic Energy Agency (IAEA) has concluded the Regional Cooperative Agreement for Research, Development, and Training Related to Nuclear Science and Technology for Asia and the Pacific (RCA). Various radiation therapy projects have been conducted under the RCA framework for more than 30 years. The IAEA/RCA's RAS6086 project "Strengthening cancer management programmes in RCA Government Parties through collaboration with Asia Pacific National/Regional Radiation Oncology Societies" included a survey on the status of the use of radiation therapy in Asia and the Pacific. Table 18.1 shows the status of the use of radiation therapy in each country. These data were reported to the RAS6086 project of the IAEA/RCA and cover 19 countries, including Australia, Bangladesh, Cambodia, China, India, Indonesia, Japan, the Republic of Korea, Laos, Malaysia, Mongolia, Nepal, New Zealand, Pakistan, the Philippines, Singapore, Sri Lanka, Thailand, and Viet Nam (Table 18.1). (This data includes data from Australia and New Zealand.) The proportion of the elderly (65 years old and over) in the general population in 2020 [3], the incidence of cancer per year (per million people), and the percentage of patients with cancer treated with radiation therapy (number of patients who received radiation therapy per year/total incidence of cancer per year) in each country are shown in Figs. 18.1 and 18.2. The proportion of the elderly in the general population and the incidence rate of cancer show that as the rate of aging increases, the incidence rate of cancer increases (Fig. 18.1). This is similar to the trend in developed countries, suggesting that the number of patients with cancer in Asian countries, where aging populations have been projected, will increase further. The proportion of the elderly in the general population and the percentage of patients with cancer treated with radiation therapy are shown in Fig. 18.2. The data shows that the higher the proportion of elderly people, the higher the rate of administration of radiation therapy (Fig. 18.2). This is partly due to the high-income countries with an aging population. This suggests that it may be more difficult to choose other treatment options, such as surgery and chemotherapy, for the elderly than for the young due to age-related complications, and that radiation therapy may be chosen more often for the elderly than for the young. As the aging of the population of the Asian region is projected to

Table 18.1 The status of the use of radiation therapy in each country (IAEA/RCA RAS6086 project)

	Population (thousands)	Number of total cancer incidence per year	Number of total cancer deaths per year	Number of radiation oncologists	Number of medical physicists	Number of radiation therapy technologists	Number of radiation therapy facilities	Number of patients who received radiation therapy per year
Australia	25,499.881	150,782	49,221	404	362	2659	93	74,199
Bangladesh	164,689.383	156,775	108,990	180	50	200	23	20,000
Cambodia	16,718.971	18,375	12,638	11	4	17	2	675
China	1,439,323.774	4,569,000	3,003,000	19,002	4475	9673	1538	1,370,000
India	1,380,004.385	1,324,413	851,678	2083	1920	4281	530	
Indonesia	273,523.621	369,914	234,511	135	125	369	47	23,315
Japan	126,476.458	980,856	376,425	1355	689	4014	851	277,000
Rep. of Korea	51,269.183	243,837	81,203	321	180	750	99	81,818
Laos	7275.556	NA	NA	3	2	2	1	NA
Malaysia	32,365.998	48,639	29,530	130	134	473	34	15,330
Mongolia	3278.292	6702	4260	9	4	9	1	812
Myanmar	54,409.794	70,000	51,000	NA	NA	NA	NA	NA
Nepal	29,136.808	29,000	15,000	42	15	30	5	5000
New Zealand	4822.233	26,158	9818	93	80	280	10	8320
Pakistan	220,892.331	178,388	117,149	268	172	290	32	NA
Philippines	109,581.085	153,751	92,606	105	150	205	51	10,000
Singapore	5,850.343	14,907	5627	65	55	187	9	8000
Sri Lanka	21,413.25	31,834	16,691	60	38	80	9	16,700
Thailand	66,186	139,206	84,073	157	141	335	45	49,704
Viet Nam	97,338.583	353,826	122,690	318	151	356	44	34,580

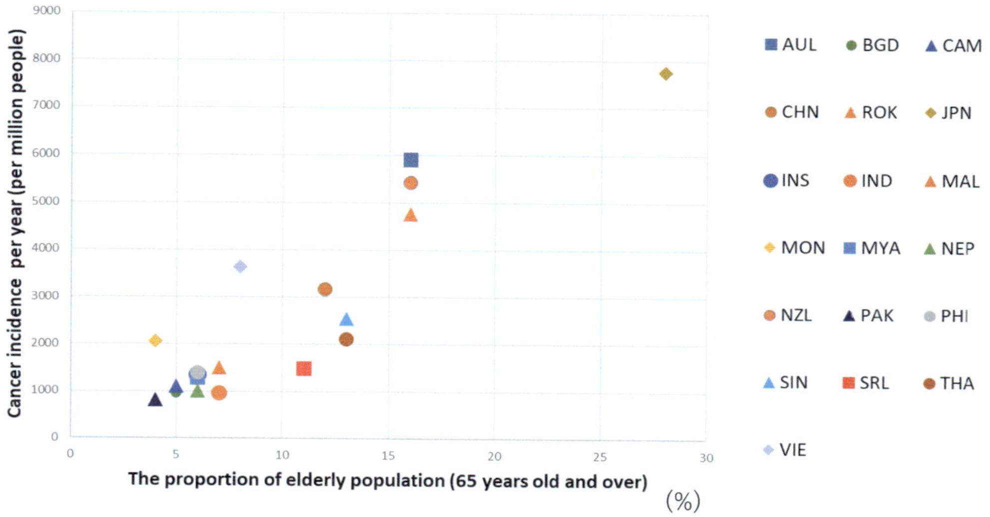

Fig. 18.1 The proportion of the elderly in the general population and the incidence rate of cancer (IAEA/RCA RAS6086 project): The Y-axis is cancer incidence per year, and the X-axis is the proportion of the elderly population (65 years old and over). Australia (AUL), Bangladesh (BGD), Cambodia (CAM), China (CHN), India (IND), Indonesia (INS), Japan (JPN), Republic of Korea (ROK), Laos (LAO), Malaysia (MAL), Mongolia (MON), Nepal (NEP), New Zealand (NZL), Pakistan (PAK), Philippines (PHI), Singapore (SIN), Sri Lanka (SRL), Thailand (THA), and Viet Nam (VIE)

Fig. 18.2 The proportion of the elderly in the general population and the percentage of patients with cancer treated with radiation therapy (IAEA/RCA RAS6086 project): The Y-axis is the percentage of cancer patients treated with radiation therapy, and the X-axis is the proportion of the elderly population (65 years old and over)

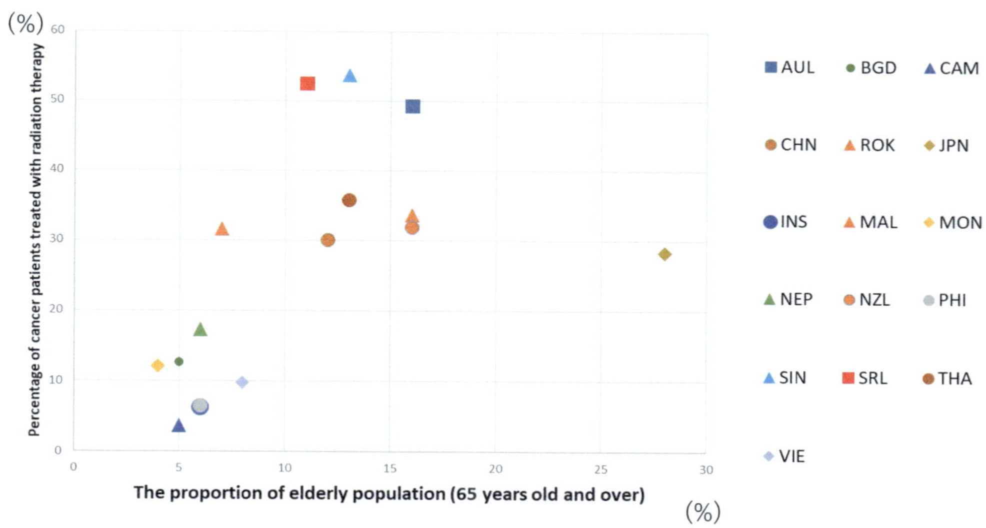

progress further, the development of radiation therapy infrastructure is considered a stuttering issue.

Other major issues regarding the development of radiation therapy infrastructure include the training of human resources who will be responsible for the administration of radiation therapy and the installation of radiation therapy facilities and equipment. Table 18.2 shows the number of medical staff and radiation therapy facilities per population (per million people) according to the report of the RAS6086 project of the IAEA/RCA. Only China, Japan, and Singapore have more than 10 radiation oncologists per million people in Asian countries (Table 18.2). The countries with less than 3 radiation oncologists per million people are Bangladesh, Cambodia, India, Indonesia, Laos, Mongolia, Nepal, Pakistan, the Philippines, Sri Lanka, and Thailand. Among them, Cambodia, Indonesia, Laos, and the Philippines have a particularly low number of radiation oncologists (less than one per million population). Regarding medical physicists, only Japan and Singapore have more than five medical physicists per million people, whereas four countries have less than one per million people. For radiation therapy technologists, only Japan and Singapore have more than 30 per million people, whereas 11 countries have less than 5 per million people. This lack of medical staff, which is essential for the widespread use of radiation therapy, is a problem in many Asian countries. Figure 18.3 shows the percentage of patients

Table 18.2 The number of medical staff and radiation therapy facilities per population (IAEA/RCA RAS6086 project)

	The number of radiation oncologists per million people	The number of medical physicists per million people	The number of radiation therapy technologists per million people	The number of radiation therapy facilities per million people	Percentage of cancer patients treated with radiation therapy
Australia	15.84	14.20	104.27	3.65	49.21
Bangladesh	1.09	0.30	1.21	0.14	12.76
Cambodia	0.66	0.24	1.02	0.12	3.67
China	13.20	3.11	6.72	1.07	29.98
India	1.51	1.39	3.10	0.38	0.00
Indonesia	0.49	0.46	1.35	0.17	6.30
Japan	10.71	5.45	31.74	6.73	28.24
Rep. of Korea	6.26	3.51	14.63	1.93	33.55
Laos	0.41	0.27	0.27	0.14	NA
Malaysia	4.02	4.14	14.61	1.05	31.52
Mongolia	2.75	1.22	2.75	0.31	12.12
Myanmar	0.00	0.00	0.00	0.00	0.00
Nepal	1.44	0.51	1.03	0.17	17.24
New Zealand	19.29	16.59	58.06	2.07	31.81
Pakistan	1.21	0.78	1.31	0.14	NA
Philippines	0.96	1.37	1.87	0.47	6.50
Singapore	11.11	9.40	31.96	1.54	53.67
Sri Lanka	2.80	1.77	3.74	0.42	52.46
Thailand	2.37	2.13	5.06	0.68	35.71
Viet Nam	3.27	1.55	3.66	0.45	9.77

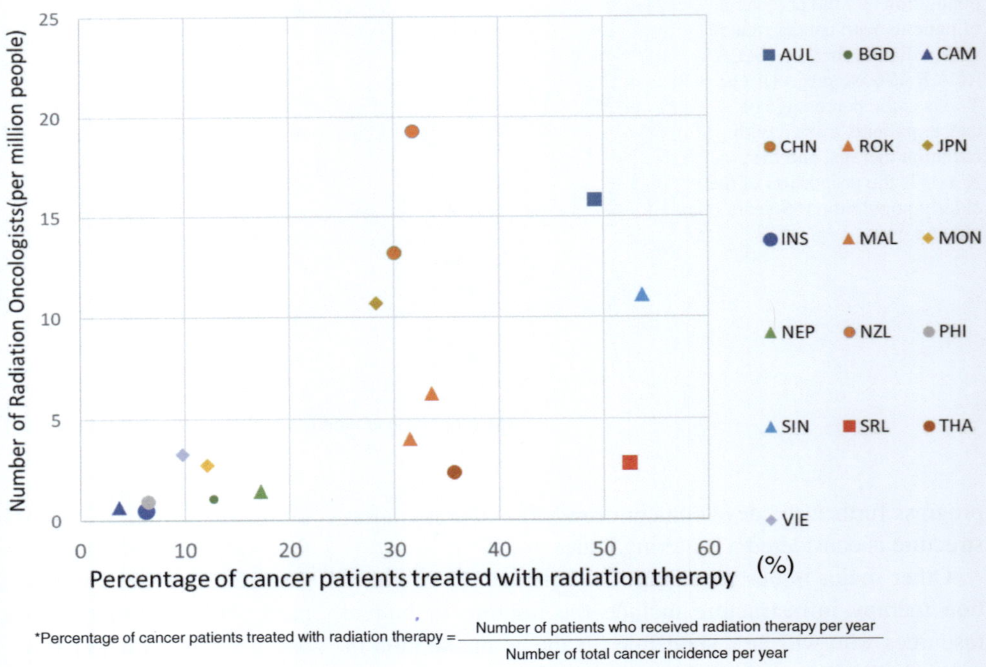

Fig. 18.3 The percentage of patients with cancer treated with radiation therapy and the number of radiation oncologists per million people in each country (IAEA/RCA RAS6086 project): The Y-axis is number of radiation oncologist (per million people), and the X-axis is the percentage of cancer patients treated with radiation therapy

with cancer treated with radiation therapy and the number of radiation oncologists per million people in each country (Fig. 18.3). The data shows that as the number of radiation oncologists increases, the number of patients treated with radiation therapy increases, suggesting a moderate correlation. The same trend is observed for medical physicists and radiation therapy technologists, suggesting that an increase in the number of medical staff and facilities is essential for the widespread use of radiation therapy.

Owing to advancements in the development of radiation therapy equipment, remarkable progress has been made in the use of high-precision radiation therapy, such as image-guided brachytherapy, intensity-modulated radiation therapy (IMRT), stereotactic body radiation therapy, and stereotactic radiation therapy (SRT). However, these treatment methods require training of medical staff, which is also important. The IAEA/RCA's RAS6086 survey showed that many countries have already introduced these treatments. This suggests that even in low- and middle-income countries, central facilities are already equipped with advanced radiation therapy equipment.

18.3 Activities of the Forum for Nuclear Cooperation in Asia

The Forum for Nuclear Cooperation in Asia (FNCA) is a Japan-led cooperation framework for the peaceful and safe use of nuclear science and technology in Asia. Eight projects, including a radiation oncology project, are currently underway under this framework. The radiation oncology project was launched in 1993, and 11 countries, including Bangladesh, China, Indonesia, Japan, Kazakhstan, the Republic of Korea, Malaysia, Mongolia, the Philippines, Thailand, and Viet Nam, have recently participated in the project. The purpose of the project is to establish optimal radiation therapy and chemotherapy treatment protocols for predominant cancers in Asia, to improve the quality of radiation therapy in FNCA member countries, and to improve treatment outcomes for predominant cancers in Asia. For these purposes, several activities, including international multi-institutional clinical studies of radiation therapy (RT) or chemoradiotherapy (CRT) for various cancers and physical quality assurance and quality control of radiation therapy, are being conducted. When completed, the programs of the FNCA will be introduced to increase the use and quality of radiation therapy across the Asian region.

Since the radiation therapy project commenced in 1993, FNCA has conducted four multi-institutional clinical studies of RT or CRT for advanced cervical cancer in the FNCA member countries. In the first study (Cervix-I, 1996–2003), RT was standardized for cervical cancer because there are differences in the RT techniques used in the member countries [4]. Patients with locally advanced cervical cancer were treated according to a standardized protocol, and they achieved favorable treatment outcomes. In the second study (Cervix-II, 1999–2006), the toxicity and efficacy of a protocol of accelerated hyperfractionated RT was evaluated because it was difficult to use CRT in some developing countries at the time due to technical and socio-economic constraints [5]. In the third study (Cervix-III, 2003–2010), a phase II clinical study of CRT for locally advanced cervical cancer was conducted. Patients with locally advanced cervical cancer were treated using concurrent RT and weekly cisplatin chemotherapy. The results showed that the treatment achieved favorable outcomes with acceptable toxicities [6, 7]. In the fourth study (Cervix-IV, 2009–2018), a phase II clinical study of concurrent extended-field RT and weekly cisplatin chemotherapy for node-positive locally advanced cervical cancer was conducted [8].

We encountered many problems and difficulties while conducting the first study. There were wide differences in cultural and socio-economic statuses among countries, which may have resulted in a large imbalance in patient enrollment. We also noted wide differences in the use of cancer imaging among institutions, which may have resulted in staging errors. Furthermore, poor compliance with the treatment protocol and poor follow-up rate posed considerable challenges. However, these problems were solved through the dedicated efforts of the physicians in the study group. Thus, the qualities of the recent Cervix-III and IV studies were improved, with excellent compliance with the protocols and satisfactory follow-up rates being recorded. The Cervix-III protocol has become one of the standard treatment protocols for CRT for cervical cancer in FNCA member countries. Radiation oncologists and medical physicists in FNCA member countries have been trained based on the results of these clinical studies. The network established by the FNCA project has the potential to promote and strengthen international cooperation in the field of radiation oncology in Asia. Currently, a clinical study of 3D image-guided brachytherapy for cervical cancer is being conducted by FNCA.

18.4 The Future of Radiation Therapy in Asia

There is no doubt that the use of radiation therapy in the Asian region has been spreading rapidly in recent years. Several initiatives/projects have facilitated this trend. The first is the Federation of Asian Organizations for Radiation Oncology (FARO). FARO was established in 2014 with the participation of radiation oncology societies in 11 countries (Bangladesh, China, India, Indonesia, Japan, Korea, Malaysia, the Philippines, Singapore, Sri Lanka, and Thailand). Currently, FARO consists of 14 countries, including the original 11 countries and Pakistan, Myanmar, and Mongolia. FARO is intended to function as a federation of radiation oncology societies in Asia and aims to foster the role of radiation oncology in improving the basic level of radiation therapy for the benefit of patients with cancer in the Asian region. In addition to organizing annual meetings, FARO has started initiatives for the future, such as launching a leadership development program to foster new leaders. Furthermore, since a requirement for participation in FARO is the organization of radiation oncology societies in each country, FARO has contributed to the development of regional organizations, such as the establishment of radiation oncology societies in Myanmar and Mongolia. In the future, further development of FARO is expected as a counterpart to the academic societies in developed countries, such as the American Society for Radiation Oncology and the European Society for Radiotherapy and Oncology. The second initiative is the IAEA/RCA. RAS6086 was a project of the IAEA/RCA established to strengthen collaboration among radiation oncologists in the Asia-Pacific region, including collaboration with FARO and other organizations. Previous projects have focused on the spread of advanced radiation therapy, such as image-guided brachytherapy, IMRT, and SRT, and their results have led to the widespread use of such advanced radiation therapy methods at representative facilities in various countries. Regarding medical physicists, there are ongoing projects for their training. As of 2022, projects related to radiation therapy, such as the Virtual Tumor Board project and the project on the standardization of palliative radiation therapy, are underway. Further, activities established to equalize the use of radiation therapy across Asia are in progress.

The IAEA and Japan have been taking the lead in promoting radiation therapy in Asia for the past 20–30 years. As a result, the use of radiation therapy is gradually expanding and progressing. However, the use of radiation therapy is still insufficient, especially in low- and middle-income countries. Thus, improving the imbalance in the use of radiation therapy within each country is an important issue for the future. To achieve this, human resource exchange across countries and human resource development need to be continued through activities such as FARO and IAEA/RCA. Regarding radiation therapy equipment, which is still expensive, we hope that companies will develop radiation therapy equipment that is easier to introduce by optimizing its functions to suit the real-world conditions in Asia.

Acknowledgements The authors thank Prof. Nakano, who is the National Representative of Japan to the IAEA/RCA; Prof. Tamaki and Dr. Kubo, who are members of the National Response Committee to the IAEA/RCA; and the members of the radiation oncology project in FNCA.

References

1. The United Nations. The 2019 revision of world population prospects. https://populationunorg/wpp/.
2. Sung H, Ferlay J, Siegel RL, Laversanne M, Soerjomataram I, Jemal A, et al. Global Cancer Statistics 2020: GLOBOCAN Estimates of Incidence and Mortality Worldwide for 36 Cancers in 185 Countries. CA Cancer J Clin . 2021;71(3):209–49
3. The World Bank. Population ages 65 and above (% of total population). https://www.worldbank.org/en/home
4. Nakano T, Kato S, Cao J, Zhou J, Susworo R, Supriana N, et al. A regional cooperative clinical study of radiotherapy for cervical cancer in east and south-east Asian countries. Radiother Oncol. 2007;84(3):314–9.
5. Ohno T, Nakano T, Kato S, Koo CC, Chansilpa Y, Pattaranutaporn P, et al. Accelerated hyperfractionated radiotherapy for cervical cancer: multi-institutional prospective study of forum for nuclear cooperation in Asia among eight Asian countries. Int J Radiat Oncol Biol Phys. 2008;70(5):1522–9.
6. Kato S, Ohno T, Thephamongkhol K, Chansilpa Y, Cao J, Xu X, et al. Long-term follow-up results of a multi-institutional phase 2 study of concurrent chemoradiation therapy for locally advanced cervical cancer in east and Southeast Asia. Int J Radiat Oncol Biol Phys. 2013;87(1):100–5.
7. Kato S, Ohno T, Thephamongkhol K, Chansilpa Y, Yuxing Y, Devi CR, et al. Multi-institutional phase II clinical study of concurrent chemoradiotherapy for locally advanced cervical cancer in east and Southeast Asia. Int J Radiat Oncol Biol Phys. 2010;77(3):751–7.
8. Wakatsuki M, Kato S, Ohno T, Banu PA, Hoang NC, Yadamsuren E, et al. A multi-institutional observational study of prophylactic extended-field concurrent chemoradiation therapy using weekly cisplatin for patients with pelvic node-positive cervical cancer in east and Southeast Asia. Int J Radiat Oncol Biol Phys. 2019;105(1):183–9.

19 Psycho-Oncology

Maiko Fujimori

Abstract

Psycho-oncology is a subspecialty of oncology that deals with the behavioral science aspects of cancer, including psychiatry, psychology, and sociology. Psycho-oncology research and clinical practice address a better understanding of, and the care for, the psychological response and the adaptation to cancer-related issues in patients and caregivers.

Communication with patients is an essential clinical practice for all healthcare professionals. In particular, the clinical importance of advance care planning, in which patients share in advance with caregivers and healthcare professionals about their preferences and values-based care, has been increasingly recognized in recent decades. Communication skills training using behavior-change techniques is effective for healthcare professionals in acquiring desirable communication behaviors. An effective patient-centered approach is the question prompt list, a comprehensive list of questions that patients frequently ask healthcare professionals.

Patients develop various psychological symptoms throughout their cancer journey. Depression is one of the major psychological symptoms. It is critical to promptly conduct appropriate screening for psychological distress and provide medication and psychotherapy by mental health professionals.

Progress in psycho-oncology has been closely linked to the development of cancer medicine and its surrounding social environment. This progress has expanded in recent years in Asian countries as well.

M. Fujimori (✉)
Division of Survivorship Research, National Cancer Center Institute for Cancer Control, Tokyo, Japan
e-mail: mfujimor@ncc.go.jp

Keywords

Psycho-Oncology · Communication between patients and healthcare professionals · Bad News · Advance care planning · Psychological distress · Depression · Screening

19.1 Introduction

Psycho-oncology is a subspecialty of oncology that deals with the behavioral science aspects of cancer, including psychiatry, psychology, and sociology. Since the addition of drug therapy to anti-cancer treatment, which was previously limited to surgery and radiation therapy in the 1940s, dramatic progress in anti-cancer treatment has led to the need for supportive care and palliative therapy since the 1960s. Consequently, attention has also been paid to psychosocial care. In the 1970s, as Western countries adopted informed consent-based treatment as standard cancer care, most cancer centers and hospitals began to provid psycho-oncology care for severely distressed patients, their caregivers, and healthcare professionals [1]. Under these circumstances, psycho-oncology research has steadily led to a better understanding of the psychosocial effects of a broader range of cancers, including adaptation to cancer and treatments, the prevalence of psychiatric disorders of patients, their caregivers, and healthcare professionals; psychosocial and behavioral variables that contribute to cancer risk and survival; psychotherapeutic and psychopharmacologic interventions for inproving quality of life (QOL); cancer prevention; advance care planning; survivorship care planning; and communication between patients, their caregivers, and healthcare professionals, including shared decision-making in oncology.

The clinical practice of psycho-oncology addresses a variety of issues, including care for psychological responses after cancer-related truth-telling; support in adapting to cancer; assessment and management of psychiatric disorders

© The Author(s), under exclusive license to Springer Nature Singapore Pte Ltd. 2026
M. Endo et al. (eds.), *Cancer and Work in Asia Volume 2*, https://doi.org/10.1007/978-981-95-6537-5_19

and symptoms such as depression, cancer-related fatigue, cognitive impairment, and interpersonal relationships with families, healthcare professionals, and society in patients with cancer; and psychosocial care for caregivers, bereavement, and healthcare professionals caring for patients with cancer. Although psycho-oncological issues need to be managed by multidisciplinary healthcare professionals depending on severity, these issues are highly prevalent, diverse, and challenging for healthcare professionals to manage. Therefore, psycho-oncologists worldwide have begun to train an increasing number of social workers, psychologists, nurses, and psychiatrists who can provide consultative services in support of the psychosocial oncology care of patients with cancer and their caregivers at all stages of the cancer trajectory, including cancer survivorship, to meet their specific needs. A growing body of literature has produced reliable screening and assessment methods for psychological distress and unmet psychosocial support needs, as well as interventions for treatment and management, and accumulated evidence regagrding their efficacy and effectiveness.

19.2 Communication Between Patients and Healthcare Professionals

19.2.1 Communication in an Oncology Setting

Communication between patients and their caregivers is an essential clinical practice for all healthcare professionals because it is similar to that in other complex medical intervention procedures, as it requires careful planning and execution. In addition to essential communication in routine medical care, patients and healthcare professionals are often required to have difficult communication to discuss bad news, such as diagnosing incurable cancer, identifying recurrence or progression of cancer, and discussing prognosis. Such difficult communication is called "bad news," which is defined as any information likely to drastically alter a patient's view of his or her future (whether at the time of diagnosis or when facing the failure of curative intention) in an oncology setting [2]. When bad news is provided, the patient becomes upset and experiences psychological distress. Active listening and eliciting patients' anxieties and concerns help screen for psychological distress. After providing bad news, it is common to discuss treatment strategies and make optimal treatment decisions for patients simultaneously. In oncology practice, based on informed consent, adequate information and emotional support are provided to the patient, followed by a treatment alliance. With the development of cancer medicine, communication will become increasingly crucial as treatment becomes more complicated, including precision treatments based on comprehensive cancer genetic profiling testing.

19.2.2 Patient-Centered Communication

It is crucial to consider and understand the patient's perspective on communication because the patient is the one whose life is directly affected by the bad news [3]. Patients' preferred communication behaviors by healthcare professionals have been shown to be related to lower levels of psychological distress and higher levels of patient satisfaction [4]. Patients' preferred communication behaviors by oncologists are summarized in the following four elements [5]: "Supportive environment: spend sufficient time to communicate." "How to deliver the bad news: clearly communicate so that the patient fully understands it." "Additional information: give a variety of appropriate and sufficient information." "Reassurance and emotional support: encourage and empathize with the patients' emotional expression." There is a perspective that seeks to understand the medical and psychosocial background variables that predict patient's communication preferences. For example, younger, female, and more educated patients as well as patients with a higher level of distress, value receiving emotional support [6]. However, patients' preferences are highly individual because the contribution of background variables to these preferences is low [5]. Therefore, the value of providing personalized and optimized communication for each patient has been recognized.

19.2.3 Learning Communication by Healthcare Professionals

Communication has often been viewed as innate or human and has not been incorporated into medical education. However, communication behaviors do not automatically improve with the clinical experience and knowledge of healthcare professionals. Learning using behavior-change techniques is effective for acquiring desirable communication behaviors. Many studies suggest that well-designed training programs using validated behavior-change techniques to teach communication skills can improve the communication skills of healthcare professionals and enhance patient-reported outcomes related to communication behaviors of healthcare professionals and patient health outcomes [7, 8]. "Communication skill training (CST)" includes experiential learning centered on skill practice, such as role-playing with simulated patients using scenarios. Facilitators of CST need to have sufficient theoretical knowledge and experience to effectively teach the desired communication skills through lectures and experiential learning exercises [9]. A CST program based on patient preferences is effective in enabling oncologists to acquire preferred communication skills and in reducing psychological distress in patients with cancer [10]. Therefore, CST is highly recommended for healthcare professionals [9].

19.2.4 Promote Communication with Patients

A question-asking prompt list (QPL) has been proposed as a patient-centered approach. A QPL is a structured list of questions covering the items a patient may want to ask their oncologist about their illness and treatment [11]. Before their consultation, patients were given a QPL to read and determine which questions they would like to ask. In a cancer setting, QPLs have been shown to encourage patients to obtain more information related to their cancer, its treatment, and life with cancer, and to share their life values and treatment preferences with healthcare professionals, regardless of cancer stage. Patients who received a QPL asked more questions [12, 13] and rated the QPL as significantly more helpful for caregivers [12], as well as more helpful in facilitating communication with their physician [14]. QPLs used in important discussions such as decision-making related to first-line anti-cancer treatment, end-of-life care, and prognosis have been developed [13, 15, 16]. As a new challenge, the effectiveness of an integrated intervention combining CST for physicians and coaching with QPL for patients has been demonstrated [17, 18].

19.2.5 Advance Care Planning

Recently, the clinical importance of end-of-life communication and formal advance care planning (ACP) in cancer care has been reported [19]. Interventions that provide patients with coaching on communication with their caregivers and healthcare professionals in advance and provide oncologists with communication skill training, including the delivery of particularly bad news, facilitate opportunities for communication among patients, caregivers, and healthcare professionals [17]. Guidelines and protocols for communication provide recommendations on the timing, content, and structure of conversations [20, 21].

End-of-life discussions are drawing attention because they are associated with quality of life and death. In end-of-life discussions and prognostic disclosure discussions, patients prefer that oncologists provide additional reassurance statements and "hope for the best, and prepare for the worst" statements in addition to being explicitly informed [22–24]. Patient autonomy is regarded as one of the top priorities across countries, cultures, and religions, and the concept of a "good death" has been proposed and considered. From a policy perspective, ACP advocacy is a means of honoring patient autonomy [25]. Through international Delphi consensus studies conducted in the Western countries, ACP was defined as the process that enables individuals to define goals and preferences for future medical treatment and care, to discuss these goals and preferences with caregivers and healthcare professionals, and to record and review these preferences if appropriate [26, 27]. In addition, the effectiveness of web-based tools that facilitate ACP implementation has been previously demonstrated [28]. In Asian countries, the definition and recommendations of ACP by the International Delphi consensus study are currently under consideration [19]. Further evidence of the efficacy and effectiveness of ACP is expected to accumulate, with clinical practice guidelines being published, and clinical implementation promoted.

19.3 Psychological Distress

19.3.1 Impact of Cancer on Psychological Distress

Patients with cancer develop various psychological symptoms throughout their cancer journey. Depression, including major depression and adjustment disorders, is one of the main psychological symptoms. Depression is a major complication in patients with cancer. Its prevalence is 30–40%, which is higher than that in the general population [29]. Despite its high prevalence, it has often been overlooked. Because they are undergoing physical treatment, both patients themselves and healthcare professionals tend to interpret depression-related symptoms, such as sleep disturbance, appetite changes, and fatigue, as physical symptoms related to cancer and adverse events of cancer treatment. Biological factors associated with cancer are also involved in this process. For example, it has been suggested to be caused by depression, brain metastases, paraneoplastic syndromes, hypercalcemia, treatment-induced factors, steroids, interferons, whole-brain irradiation, and underlieved pain. Aging is a risk factor for depression and carcinogenesis. Older adults are less likely to be aware of depressive moods and often complain of loss of interest, cognitive decline, and indefinite physical complaints. It has also been pointed out that depression is underestimated and mishandled due to the downplaying of psychological symptoms and the hesitation of patients to express emotions.

Suicide has the gratest impact on the mental health of patients with cancer, and depression is the greatest risk factor for suicide. The suicide rate of patients with cancer is 1.6 times higher (1.7 times for men and 1.3 times for women) than that of the general population [30]. The risk is highest (4.1 times) during the first month after cancer diagnosis [31]. Depression, pain, and poor social support have been identified as significant risk factors for suicidal ideation [32, 33]. It has also been suggested that even if suicide does not occur, aggressive anti-cancer treatment may be refused because of a sense of worthlessness and self-blame. In addition, depression in patients exacerbates the mental distress of their caregivers.

19.3.2 Assessment of Psychological Distress

Cancer can cause significant psychological distress in patients with cancer and their caregivers. Therefore, it is critical to quickly and systematically identify psychological distress in patients and caregivers who require specialized psychosocial treatment, and to adress it appropriately. Given the worldwide prevalence of psychological distress in patients with cancer, the International Psycho-Oncology Society endorsed the International Psycho-Oncology Standard of Care document, which recognized distress as the sixth vital sign in June 2009, and this was endorsed by delegates at the UICC meeting in August 2010 [34]. Accordingly, screening for clinical depression in patients with cancer and their caregivers is recommended by the NCCN guidelines [35]. Systematic reviews, including meta-analyses, have reported that screening tools such as the Hospital Anxiety and Depression Scale, Beck Depression Inventory, and Center for Epidemiologic Studies Depression Scale have been applied and utilized in patients with cancer [36]. Patients with cancer and their caregivers who screened positive for distress require access to a referral system to psycho-oncologists and to treatment services. However, if this is not possible, screening alone will have no clinically meaningful impact [37].

For patients who are positively screened for distress, mental health professionals conduct diagnostic interviews based on the *Diagnostic and Statistical Manual of Mental Disorders* by the American Psychiatric Association and the *International Classification of Diseases* by the World Health Organization and provide appropriate treatment according to the psychiatric diagnosis.

19.3.3 Treatment of Psychological Distress

Typical treatments for depression in patients with cancer are medication and psychotherapy, which are essentially the same as those used for depression in the general population. However, as medication takes several weeks to take effect, it is difficult to adequately treat if the prognosis is short. Therefore, it is necessary to comprehensively evaluate the administration route, prognosis and physical condition, and to develop a treatment plan that does not impair QOL. If depression is not severe, psychotherapy alone can reduce it and does not require medication. For patients who do not have access to medication, psychotherapy alone will also treat depression. However, if depression is severe, combination therapy with medication and psychotherapy is recommended.

19.4 Conclusion

Progress in psycho-oncology has been closely linked to the development of cancer medicine and its social environment. This progress has been driven by Western countries playing a central role. However, clinical activities and research in psycho-oncology have expanded in recent years in Asian countries as well. Furthermore, if societies worldwide were to participate in cross-cultural psycho-oncological studies, our understanding of the concept of quality of life that crosses all cultural boundaries would be improved.

Asian countries are more likely to have family-centered models of medical decision-making than the patient-autonomy model favored by most Western countries. Consequently, communication-related shared decision-making between patients, their caregivers, and healthcare professionals has become increasingly complex and important in Asia. However, limited research on psycho-oncology, including communication, has hindered efforts to standardize desirable psycho-oncology care. Further expansion of research and training in psycho-oncology would provide healthcare professionals with opportunities to understand the concept of human care as individuals caring for other individuals with cancer, as well as bring significant benefits to patients receiving psycho-oncology care.

References

1. Holland JC (ed). Paycho-Oncology. New York: Oxford University Press; 1998.
2. Buckman R. Breaking bad news: why is it still so difficult? Br Med J (Clin Res Ed). 1984;288(6430):1597–9.
3. Parker PA, Baile WF, de Moor C, Lenzi R, Kudelka AP, Cohen L. Breaking bad news about cancer: patients' preferences for communication. J Clin Oncol. 2001;19(7):2049–56.
4. Schofield PE, Butow PN, Thompson JF, Tattersall MHN, Beeney LJ, Dunn SM. Psychological responses of patients receiving a diagnosis of cancer. Ann Oncol. 2003;14(1):48–56.
5. Fujimori M, Uchitomi Y. Preferences of cancer patients regarding communication of bad news: a systematic literature review. Jpn J Clin Oncol. 2009;39(4):201–16.
6. Fujimori M, Akechi T, Uchitomi Y. Factors associated with patient preferences for communication of bad news. Palliat Support Care. 2017;15(3):328–35.
7. Stein T, Frankel RM, Krupat E. Enhancing clinician communication skills in a large healthcare organization: a longitudinal case study. Patient Educ Couns. 2005;58(1):4–12.
8. Boissy A, Windover AK, Bokar D, Karafa M, Neuendorf K, Frankel RM, Merlino J, Rothberg MB. Communication skills training for physicians improves patient satisfaction. J Gen Intern Med. 2016;31(7):755–61.
9. Gilligan T, Coyle N, Frankel RM, Berry DL, Bohlke K, Epstein RM, Finlay E, Jackson VA, Lathan CS, Loprinzi CL, Nguyen LH, Seigel C, Baile WF. Patient-clinician communication: American Society of Clinical Oncology Consensus Guideline. J Clin Oncol. 2017;35(31):3618–32.

10. Fujimori M, Shirai Y, Asai M, Kubota K, Katsumata N, Uchitomi Y. Effect of communication skills training program for oncologists based on patient preferences for communication when receiving bad news: a randomized controlled trial. J Clin Oncol. 2014;32(20):2166–72.
11. Butow PN, Dunn SM, Tattersall MH, Jones QJ. Patient participation in the cancer consultation: evaluation of a question prompt sheet. Ann Oncol. 1994;5(3):199–204.
12. Butow P, Devine R, Boyer M, et al. Cancer consultation preparation package: changing patients but not physicians is not enough. J Clin Oncol. 2004;22:4401–9.
13. Clayton JM, Butow PN, Tattersall MH, et al. Randomized controlled trial of a prompt list to help advanced patients with cancer and their caregivers to ask questions about prognosis and end-of-life care. J Clin Oncol. 2007;25:715–23.
14. Bruera E, Sweeney C, Willey J, Palmer JL, Tolley S, Rosales M, Ripamonti C. Breast cancer patient perception of the helpfulness of a prompt sheet versus a general information sheet during outpatient consultation: a randomized, controlled trial. J Pain Symptom Manag. 2003;25:412–9.
15. Shirai Y, Fujimori M, Ogawa A, Yamada Y, Nishiwaki Y, Ohtsu A, Uchitomi Y. Patients' perception of the usefulness of a question prompt sheet for advanced cancer patients when deciding the initial treatment: a randomized, controlled trial. Psychooncology. 2012;21(7):706–13.
16. Sato A, Fujimori M, Shirai Y, Umezawa S, Mori M, Jinno S, Umehashi M, Okamura M, Okusaka T, Majima Y, Miyake S, Uchitomi Y. Assessing the need for a question prompt list that encourages end-of-life discussions between patients with advanced cancer and their physicians: a focus group interview study. Palliat Support Care. 2022. In Press.
17. Epstein RM, Duberstein PR, Fenton JJ, Fiscella K, Hoerger M, Tancredi DJ, Xing G, Gramling R, Mohile S, Franks P, Kaesberg P, Plumb S, Cipri CS, Street RL Jr, Shields CG, Back AL, Butow P, Walczak A, Tattersall M, Venuti A, Sullivan P, Robinson M, Hoh B, Lewis L, Kravitz RL. Effect of a patient-centered communication intervention on oncologist-patient communication, quality of life, and healthcare utilization in advanced cancer: the VOICE randomized clinical trial. JAMA Oncol. 2017;3(1):92–100.
18. Fujimori M, Sato A, Okusaka T, Yamaguchi T, Ikeda M, Ueno M, Ozaka M, Miyaji T, Mashiko T, Okamura M, Goto S, Majima Y, Uchitomi Y. A randomized controlled trial with a cluster of oncologists evaluating of an integrated communication support program for oncologists, caregivers, and patients with rapidly progressing advanced cancer on patient-centered conversation: J-SUPPORT 1704 study. 2021 ASCO Annual Meeting. 2021:12119.
19. Cheng SY, Lin CP, Chan HY, Martina D, Mori M, Kim SH, Ng R. Advance care planning in Asian culture. Jpn J Clin Oncol. 2020;50(9):976–89.
20. Bernacki RE, Block SD. Communication about serious illness care goals: a review and synthesis of best practices. JAMA Intern Med. 2014;174:1994–2003.
21. Clayton JM, Hancock K, Parker S, et al. Sustaining hope when communicating with terminally ill patients and their families: a systematic review. Psychooncology. 2008;17:641–59.
22. Mori M, Fujimori M, Ishiki H, Nishi T, Hamano J, Otani H, Uneno Y, Oba A, Morita T, Uchitomi Y. The effects of adding reassurance statements: cancer patients' preferences for phrases in end-of-life discussions. J Pain Symptom Manag. 2019;57(6):1121–9.
23. Mori M, Fujimori M, Ishiki H, Nishi T, Hamano J, Otani H, Uneno Y, Oba A, Morita T, Uchitomi Y. Adding a wider range and "Hope for the best, and prepare for the worst" statement: preferences of patients with cancer for prognostic communication. Oncologist. 2019;24(9):e943–52.
24. Mori M, Fujimori M, van Vliet LM, Yamaguchi T, Shimizu C, Kinoshita T, Morishita-Kawahara M, Inoue A, Inoguchi H, Matsuoka Y, Bruera E, Morita T, Uchitomi Y. Explicit prognostic disclosure to Asian women with breast cancer: a randomized, scripted video-vignette study (J-SUPPORT1601). Cancer. 2019;125(19):3320–9.
25. Cheng SY, Lin WY, Cheng YH, Huang CH, Chen CY, Hwang SJ, Tsai ST, Chiu TY. Cancer patient autonomy and quality of dying-a prospective nationwide survey in Taiwan. Psychooncology. 2016;25:179–86.
26. Rietjens JAC, Sudore RL, Connolly M, van Delden JJ, Drickamer MA, Droger M, van der Heide A, Heyland DK, Houttekier D, Janssen DJA, Orsi L, Payne S, Seymour J, Jox RJ, Korfage IJ. European Association for Palliative Care. Definition and recommendations for advance care planning: an international consensus supported by the European Association for Palliative Care. Lancet Oncol. 2017;18:e543–51.
27. Sudore RL, Lum HD, You JJ, Hanson LC, Meier DE, Pantilat SZ, Matlock DD, Rietjens JAC, Korfage IJ, Ritchie CS, Kutner JS, Teno JM, Thomas J, McMahan RD, Heyland DK. Defining advance care planning for adults: a consensus definition from a multidisciplinary Delphi panel. J Pain Symptom Manag. 2017;53:821–32 e1.
28. Sudore RL, Boscardin J, Feuz MA, McMahan RD, Katen MT, Barnes DE. Effect of the prepare website vs an easy-to-read advance directive on advance care planning documentation and engagement among veterans: a randomized clinical trial. JAMA Intern Med. 2017;177:1102–9.
29. Mitchell AJ, Chan M, Bhatti H, Halton M, Grassi L, Johansen C, Meader N. Prevalence of depression, anxiety, and adjustment disorder in oncological, haematological, and palliative-care settings: a meta-analysis of 94 interview-based studies. Lancet Oncol. 2011;12(2):160–74.
30. Amiri S, Behnezhad S. Cancer diagnosis and suicide mortality: a systematic review and meta-analysis. Arch Suicide Res. 2020;24(sup2):S94–S112.
31. Harashima S, Fujimori M, Akechi T, Matsuda T, Saika K, Hasegawa T, Inoue K, Yoshiuchi K, Miyashiro I, Uchitomi Y, J Matsuoka Y. Death by suicide, other externally caused injuries and cardiovascular diseases within 6 months of cancer diagnosis (J-SUPPORT 1902). Jpn J Clin Oncol. 2021;51(5):744–52.
32. Breitbart W, Rosenfeld B, Pessin H, Kaim M, Funesti-Esch J, Galietta M, Nelson CJ, Brescia R. Depression, hopelessness, and desire for hastened death in terminally ill patients with cancer. JAMA. 2000;284(22):2907–11.
33. Akechi T, Okuyama T, Sugawara Y, Nakano T, Shima Y, Uchitomi Y. Suicidality in terminally ill Japanese patients with cancer. Cancer. 2004;100(1):183–91.
34. Bultz BD, Johansen C. Screening for distress, the 6th vital sign: where are we, and where are we going? Psychooncology. 2011;20(6):569–71.
35. Riba MB, Donovan KA, Andersen B, Braun I, Breitbart WS, Brewer BW, Buchmann LO, Clark MM, Collins M, Corbett C, Fleishman S, Garcia S, Greenberg DB, Handzo RGF, Hoofring L, Huang CH, Lally R, Martin S, McGuffey L, Mitchell W, Morrison LJ, Pailler M, Palesh O, Parnes F, Pazar JP, Ralston L, Salman J, Shannon-Dudley MM, Valentine AD, McMillian NR, Darlow SD. Distress management, version 3.2019, NCCN clinical practice guidelines in oncology. J Natl Compr Cancer Netw. 2019;17(10):1229–49.
36. Wakefield CE, Butow PN, Aaronson NA, Hack TF, Hulbert-Williams NJ, Jacobsen PB, International Psycho-Oncology Society Research Committee. Patient-reported depression measures in cancer: a meta-review. Lancet Psychiatry. 2015;2(7):635–47.
37. Palmer SC, Coyne JC. Screening for depression in medical care: pitfalls, alternatives, and revised priorities. J Psychosom Res. 2003;54:279–87.

Pain Management

20

Masako Iseki

Abstract

The pains cancer patients experience

Treating pains that cancer patients suffer from requires a basic set of knowledge, including the general idea about pain, their evaluation methods, classification, mechanisms, treating strategies, and coping techniques. In recent years, people "who have been diagnosed as having cancer but survived it," including those who have had cancer before, are being treated for cancers, are under observation for the progress of cancers, and are in the terminal stages of cancer, are called "cancer survivors" in the broad sense of the term (National Cancer Institute. Facing Forward: Life after cancer treatmen. https://www.cancer.gov/publications/patient-education/facing-forward). While approximately 30–40% of the cancer survivors are said to suffer from certain types of physical pains, treatments that are appropriate for those pains vary depending on the direct cause of the pain and in which stage of the cancer the patient is suffering (Paice et al., J Clin Oncol 34: 3325–45, 2016). This article is an overview of the pains that cancer patients suffer while providing an opportunity to gain a deeper understanding about pain in general.

Keywords

Somatic pain · Visceral pain · Neuropathic pains · Opioids · Gabapentinoids · Nociceptive pain

20.1 Introduction-What Is Pain?

Unlike other sensations such as vision, hearing, taste, smell, and touch, pain is a sensation that the affected person cannot share with others. People may enjoy movies, music, food, the scent of flowers, or the touch of clothes together with others, but we can only feel sympathy for other people's pains. Pains cannot be shared together.

In addition, different people feel different pains even when they suffer from the same injury, and a person may feel different pains from the same injury depending on what circumstances the injury occurred in. Indeed, it is said that the sensation of pain is affected by various factors, including race, sex, growing process, and social circumstance, among many others.

20.2 Definition of Pain [3]

In 2020, the International Association for the Study of Pain (ISP) defined pain as "an unpleasant sensory and emotional experience associated with, or resembling that associated with, actual or potential tissue damage."

To this definition, IASP has further added the following six items as "notes":

- Pain is always a personal experience that is influenced to varying degrees by biological, psychological, and social factors.
- Pain and nociception are different phenomena. Pain cannot be inferred solely from activity in sensory neurons.
- Through their life experiences, individuals learn the concept of pain.
- A person's report of an experience as pain should be respected*.
- Although pain usually serves an adaptive role, it may have adverse effects on function and social and psychological well-being.
- Verbal description is only one of several behaviors to express pain. Inability to communicate does not negate the possibility that a human or a nonhuman animal experiences pain.

M. Iseki (✉)
Department of Anesthesiology and Pain Medicine, School of Medicine, Juntendo University, Bunkyo-ku, Tokyo, Japan
e-mail: miseki@juntendo.ac.jp

© The Author(s), under exclusive license to Springer Nature Singapore Pte Ltd. 2026
M. Endo et al. (eds.), *Cancer and Work in Asia Volume 2*, https://doi.org/10.1007/978-981-95-6537-5_20

20.3 The Roles of Pain

The sensation of pain plays an important role in our daily lives. Indeed, pain is the very necessary sensation as it provides signals for us to avoid danger, helping us to adequately cope with underlying conditions. Pain from gallstones or appendicitis, for example, allows doctors to diagnose them. Pain that is aggravated when moving the parts suffered from sprain or bone fracture forces us to rest, facilitating better recovery of the lesion. Hurting one's finger by touching thorns on a rose teaches the person to avoid doing so in the future.

Pain, on the other hand, is simply an annoyance once being properly diagnosed of its cause. If the pain is prolonged, it changes its nature from a warning sign to something that damages our quality of life through unpleasant sensational and emotional experiences.

20.4 Impacts of Pain

Prolonged pain gives rise to various physically, mentally, and socially detrimental effects. If the pain severely limits activities of daily living, the patient may suffer from disuse atrophy of muscles. Mental distress associated with pain also causes anxiety and depression. Sleep disorders such as inability to go to sleep, nocturnal awakening, early awakening, or lack of feeling refreshed after sleep may also be caused by pain [4].

These experiences may create negative feedback in the affected patient both mentally and physically. Pain also affects the patient's home, school, or work lives. Presenteeism, working while sick (under pain in our case), and absenteeism, being absent from work due to sickness (again pain in our case), are recognized as important social issues.

The International Association for the Study of Pain (IASP) and WHO define chronic pain as "pain that persists or recurs for longer than three months." In an online epidemiological survey conducted in Japan covering 20,000 ordinary people, those who experience pain that exceeds NRS = 4 at least twice weekly for longer than three months were considered to have chronic pain. In this study, 26.4% of the survey participants were suffering from chronic pain, while 6.4% suffered from neuropathic pains. Both the intensity of pain and degree of difficulties in daily lives were stronger in neuropathic pain patients than those suffering from other pains (Tables 20.1 and 20.2). For the durations of pains, more than 50% of the patients in both groups had been suffering for five or more years [5]. Studies conducted in France and Germany exhibited similar trends, i.e., the percentages of patients with chronic pains were 31.7% in France [6] and 24.9% in Germany [7, 8], and those with neuropathic pains were 6.9% and 6.5%, respectively.

Table 20.1 Strength and duration of pains found in a Japanese survey[a]

		NeP (*n* = 838)	Non-NeP (*n* = 2527)
Strength	Mild	–	–
	Moderately severe	46.8%	76.1%
	Severe	53.2%	23.9%
Duration	< 0.5 yr	15.3%	16.4%
	~ 1 yr	20.7%	13.3%
	~ 2 yrs	9.9%	9.9%
	~ 3 yrs	9.1%	8.4%
	~ 4 yrs	3.2%	4.3%
	~ 5 yrs	51.7%	47.7%

[a]OGAWA et al. [6]
NeP neuropathic pains, *non-NeP* other pains

Table 20.2 Degrees of difficulty in daily lives

	% of patients with difficulty	
Activities	NeP (*n* = 838)	Non-NeP (*n* = 2527)
Swallowing food	5.2	1.4
Defecation/urination	6.5	3.4
Sleep	33.9	18.1
Indoor walking	11.2	4.4
Outdoor walking	19.9	9.0
Ascending/descending stair	28.7	14.9
Exercise/sports	35.7	21.4
None	16.0	32.1
In all activities above, difficulties were significantly higher in NeP patients		
Work/school attendance	Nep	Non-NeP
Quit or suspended	6.5	2.4
Frequently takes off	2.6	1.1
Occasionally takes off	16.3	8.5

On the other hand, what will happen if a cancer survivor suddenly experiences a strong pain without any apparent cause? With the cause unclear, the survivor will doubtlessly be tormented not just by the physical pain but also by the fear of recurrence or metastasis of the cancer. Even if the cause is identified, the physical pain will be very detrimental to the patient's daily activities, resulting in severe psychological stress unless a series of proper pain management techniques is introduced. With good pain management, however, the quality of life of the patient may be maintained even when the patient is in the final stage of the cancer.

20.5 Causes and Mechanisms of Pains that Cancer Patients Experience

In addition to pains directly caused by cancer, patients experience various pains through the courses of their treatments or the progress of the disease stages, or by contracting painful diseases that are not related to cancer.

20.5.1 Classification of Pains by Causes (Table 20.3)

Pains directly caused by cancer include pains that are caused by invasion and/or metastasis of cancer, while pains that are not directly caused by cancer include pains caused by cancer treatments, including operation, chemotherapy, and/or radiotherapy; pains caused by immobility or prolonged bed rest; and pains that are caused by diseases not related to the cancer [9]. As the treatment strategy for pains directly caused by cancer differs from that for other pains, it is required for treatment providers that they properly diagnose the cause of the pain and then have the patient and his/her family develop an understanding of the treatment methodology by providing education to them [2].

Table 20.3 Pains cancer patients experience

Pains directly caused by cancers
Pains with progress, invasion and metastasis of cancers
Pains caused by cancer treatments
Pains caused by surgical treatments
Surgeries and other treatments
Pains caused by chemotherapy
Chemotherapy induced peripheral neuropathy (CIPN)
Pains caused by radiotherapy
Pains caused by hormonal treatments
Pains caused by marrow transplant
Pains caused by bisphosphonate-induced jaw osteonecrosis
Pains caused by consumption and debilitation
Myofascial pain syndrome and bedsore associated with prolonged bed rest
Pains not directly related to cancers
Herpes zoster associated pain, chronic hip pains, knee pains, etc.

20.5.2 Classification of Pains by Mechanisms

Pains are also classified according to their mechanisms into nociceptive pains, neuropathic pains, and mixed pains in which both of these mechanisms are combined. With nociceptive pains, nociceptors (pain receptors) produce pain signals when they are stimulated. These signals are propagated from peripheral nerves to the spinal cord and to the brain. A pain-producing substance is produced in the lesion site. Nociceptive pains are further classified into somatic pains and visceral pains (Fig. 20.1). While somatic pains derive from skin, muscle, or bone, visceral pains derive from internal organs. On the other hand, nociceptors are not involved with neuropathic pains, which are defined as pains that are caused by diseases or lesions in the components of the somatosensory nervous system, including peripheral, spinal, and brain nerves. Neuropathic pains develop when such nerves are damaged, pressurized, or degenerated [10].

To these pains, psychological and social factors may act as modifiers. For example, in the case of pains from breast cancer, while the pain caused by metastasis of the cancer to bones is manifested as movement-aggravated nociceptive pain localized in the hip region, further invasion of the cancer to the spinal nerve generates electric shock-like pains in the lower limbs as well as neuropathic pains associated with numbness and decreased sensation, resulting in the patient having both types of pains. This necessitates the treatment provider to plan a pain relief strategy that counters both mechanisms of pain.

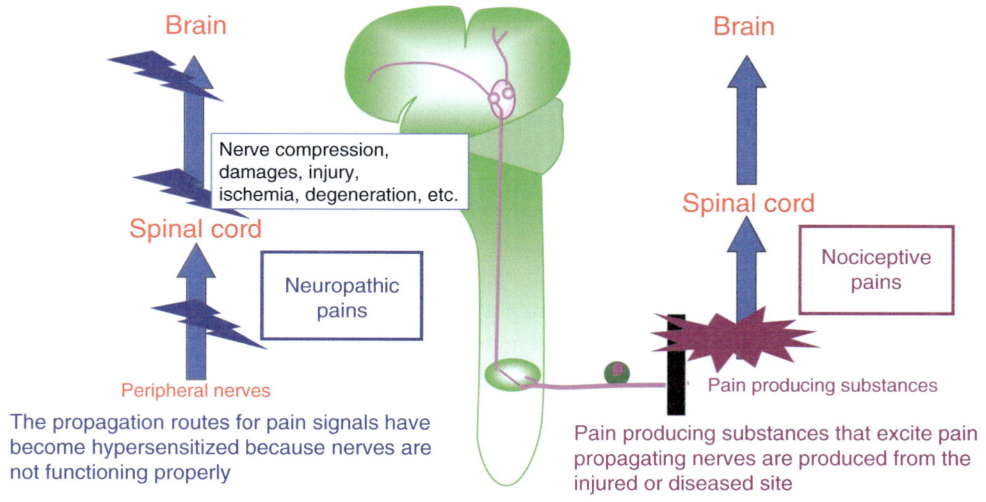

Fig. 20.1 Classification of pain mechanisms

Table 20.4 Methods for evaluating pain

Medical interview for pains	Objective findings
1. Time of onset	1. Visual/palpating/percussive examination
2. Affected region	2. Physical findings
3. Strength	3. Neurological findings
4. Pattern	4. Blood tests
5. Characteristics	5. Others
6. Exacerbating/mitigating factors	
7. Associated symptoms	
8. Degree of difficulty in daily life	
9. Psychological and social background	

20.6 Evaluation of Pain (Table 20.4)

For proper pain management, the pain must be evaluated from multiple points of view. In addition, because pain is a subjective sensation, the treatment provider must listen to the complaints expressed by the patient (Table 20.3). The Support Team Assessment Schedule (STAS) developed in the UK allows medical professionals to evaluate nine pain-related items, including pain control and anxiety, with the scale from zero to five, which is also used in Japan as the translated version STAS-J [11]. BPI (Brief Pain Inventory), [12] on the other hand, was developed as a questionnaire for cancer pain patients but is now used for not just cancer but various other pains as well.

20.6.1 Strength of Pain [13]

Strength of pain is an important indicator in deciding the treatment strategy for the affected patient, which is commonly expressed using scales such as the Numerical Rating Scale (NRS), Visual Analog Scale (VAS), and Faces Pain Scale (FPS). NRS requests each patient to evaluate his/her pain on a scale of eleven (0 to 10), with "0" being without any pain and "10" the strongest possible pain the patient can imagine. 1–3 are classified as "mild pain," 4–6 as "moderate pain," and 7–10 as "severe pain." VAS requests each patient to pinpoint how strong their pain is on a straight line with "1" and "10" on each end of the line. FPS targets infants and elderly people to evaluate his/her pain from the facial expression observed by the evaluator.

20.6.2 Patterns and Characteristics of Pain [13]

To elucidate the pattern of pain, the treatment provider interviews the patient to decide if the patient's pain is continuous or intermittent, painful at rest or only with body movements, and the presence/absence of breakthrough pains. As both nociceptive and neuropathic pains have specific characteristics, the former is often expressed as throbbing or grinding, while the latter is like electric shock or pains with numbness. The interviewer must listen to what set of words the patient uses to describe his/her pain. The treatment provider then determines the characteristics of the pain based on these findings as well as medical images and other pathological findings.

20.6.3 Difficulty in Daily Life

As one of the major objectives of pain relief is to restore normal daily lives of patients, it is important to evaluate the degree of difficulty each patient experiences in his/her daily life. WHO defines basic questions that should be included in this evaluation as (1) if the pain impairs sleep and (2) if the pain persists even at rest or only with body movements and states that at least proper sleep and alleviation of pain at rest should be obtained.

20.6.4 Psychological States

Pain often results in anxiety, and prolonged pain may lead to depression. Inversely, the presence of anxiety and/or depression acts as an enhancement factor for pain. To quickly evaluate anxiety and depression, HADS (Hospital Anxiety and Depression Scale) is useful [14]. Diagnosed cancer patients may already have anxiety or depression due to the fact that the patients are afflicted with cancer or because of adverse effects of cancer treatments. Such patients often suffer from so-called pain catastrophizing thoughts, including rumination (thinking about something repeatedly), helplessness, and/or magnification of the pain.

20.7 Treatment Methodologies for Pain [13, 15, 16]

20.7.1 Treatments for Pains that Are Directly Caused by Cancer

Pain alleviation is provided side-by-side with cancer treatments, as the treatments may itself eliminate or reduce the pain. We first identify the cause of the pain, evaluate its strength and character, and then, in many cases, start with chemotherapy. Regarding chemotherapy, there is an international consensus that depending on the strength of the pain, the treatment provider should use (1) non-opioid analgesics such as NSAIDs or acetaminophen for mild (NRS: 1–3) pains, (2) appropriate opioids for light to moderate (NRS: 4–7) pains, and (3) strong opioids for severe (NRS: 8–10) pains [15].

Based on the characteristics of the pain (Table 20.5), nociceptive pains are divided into visceral pains and somatic pains. While visceral pains are generally dull and not clearly localized, somatic pains are generally sharp and are aggravated with physical movements of the patients. Opioids are generally effective against visceral pains. In case of somatic pains, it is important to use analgesics such as opioids or other drugs when breakthrough pains appear. Neuropathic pains, on the other hand, are caused when tumors invade into or compress spinal or peripheral nerves and are characterized by numbness and/or electric shock-like pains. Because opioids are not as effective on neuropathic pains as on visceral pains, analgesics more effective on neuropathic pains are used together with opioids. For pains in specific parts of the body, other remedies and/or nerve blocks are also used. Figure 20.2 presents a general strategy for pains that are directly caused by cancers.

Table 20.5 Classification of pains based on their characteristics

Nociceptive pains	Visceral pains	Not clearly localized and dull pains, such as from abdominal tumors Heavy thudding pains	Generally opioids are effective
	Somatic pains	Localized and clearly defined pain, such as from bone metastasis Sharp penetrating pains	Using rescue medication to movement-related pains is important
Neuropathic pains		Electrifying, numbing or tingling pains, such as from invasions to nerve plexus or spinal cord	Often refractory, requiring analgesics specifically targeted to neuropathic pains

Source: Japanese Society of Palliative Medicine (JSPM) PEACE Project "Evaluation and treatment of cancer pains (Jan. 2011)"

Use of Opioids

While opioids are useful to alleviate cancer pains, they are also associated with several adverse effects, including nausea, constipation, and drowsiness. Dry mouth, oliguria (very little urine), hallucination, respiratory depression, and addiction may also be associated with opioids. When starting opioid treatments, it is common to combine an antiemetic to prevent nausea and a laxative for constipation. It has been reported that 30% of patients who are administered opioids experience nausea. While administration of antiemetics may be stopped after two weeks of opioid administration, by that time patients generally develop tolerance; nausea may reappear if the dose is increased. Constipation must be controlled throughout the opioid administration because no tolerance develops to constipation.

Among many types of opioids used in pain treatments (Table 20.6), strong opioids are used against most pains directly caused by cancer. Various dosage forms are available, including ultra-short-acting and short-acting preparations that are used for rescue administration, sustained-release

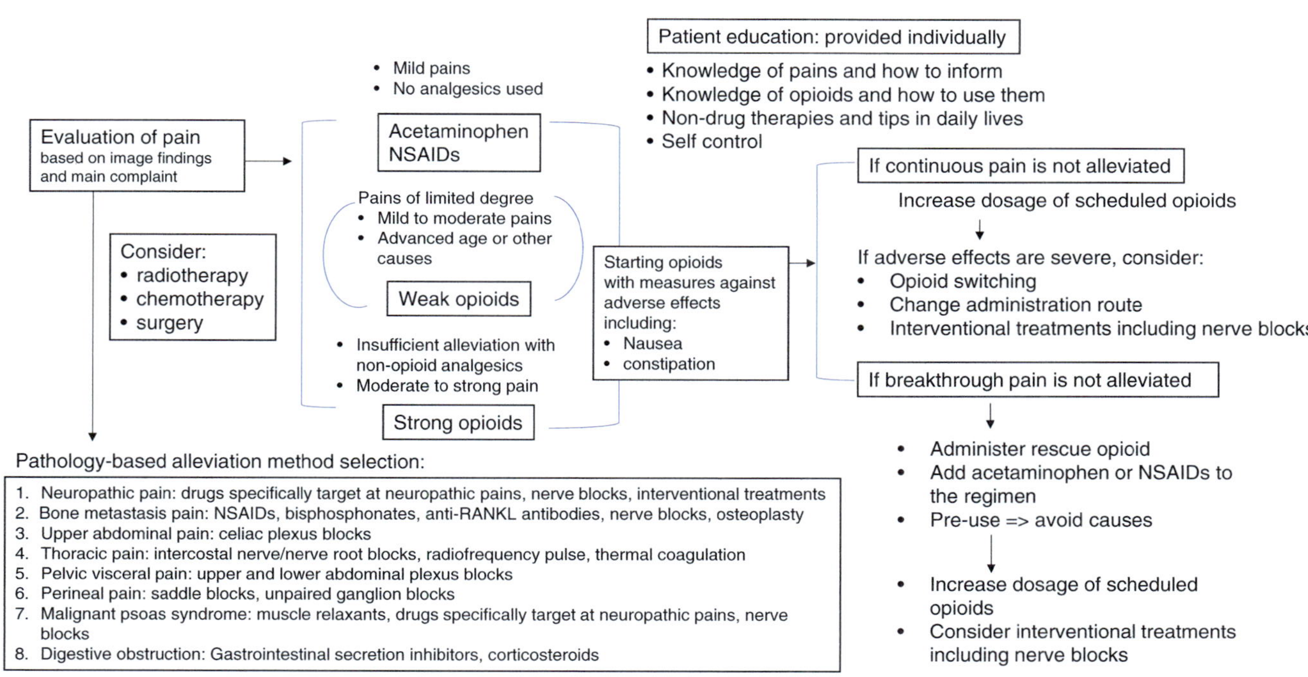

Fig. 20.2 Alleviation strategy against pains directly caused by cancers

Table 20.6 Major opioids used in pain treatments in Japan

	Name	Formulation	Regulatory classification[a]
Weak opioids	Tramadol	Orally disintegrating tablets, sustained-release tablets Twice daily formulations, combination drug with acetaminophen	Prescription drugs -
	Buprenorphine	Suppository, injection, patch Psychotropics	Psychotropics
	Pentazocine	Tablets Injection	Psychotropics
	Codeine	1% (powder, tablets) 10% (powder, tablets)	Medical narcotics
	Tapentadol	Sustained-release tablets	Medical narcotics
Strong opioids	Hydromorphone	Rapid-release formulation Sustained-release formulation Injection	Medical narcotics
	Morphine	Tablets, powder Injection Suppository, aqueous solution Sustained-release formulation (capsules, tablets)	Medical narcotics
	Oxicodone	Rapid-release formulation (fine granules), tablets TR tablets (non-chewable) Injection	Medical narcotics
	Fentanyl	Patch for 1day and 3 days Injection Buccal preparations Sublingual tablet	Medical narcotics
	Methadone	Sustained-release tablets	Medical narcotics

[a]Under Japanese Pharmaceutical Laws

preparations for regular prescriptions, suppositories, transdermal patches, and injectable preparations. Pain control is generally carried out by alleviating the continuous pain with long-acting opioids, occasionally augmented with ultra-short-acting or short-acting preparations when the pain aggravates. Opioid switching (using different type(s) of opioids) or changing the administration route may also be considered in order to reduce adverse side effects as well as to enhance the therapeutic effect.

In case the life prognosis is long, however, prolonged use of large amounts of strong opioids or an ill-planned increase of dosage must be carefully monitored, as they may lead to addiction or opioid-induced hyperalgesia.

Use of Analgesics for Neuropathic Pains

Treatments for neuropathic pains include gabapentinoids (pregabalin, gabapentin, and mirogabalin) that suppress abnormal excitation of spinal and peripheral nerves by acting on the calcium channel α2 delta in the dorsal horns of the spinal cord and tricyclic antidepressants, as well as Serotonin-Noradrenalin Reuptake Inhibitors (SNRIs) that support recovery of the descending pain inhibitory system that humans inherently have to control pain. In addition, sodium channel blockers, including lidocaine and valproic acid, are used to suppress abnormal excitation of the peripheral nerves, while NMDA receptor antagonists, including ketamine, are used to suppress abnormal excitation of the spinal nerve. Steroids are also used to control nerve inflammation and edema.

Interventional Treatments Including Nerve Blocks

For localized pains, nerve blocks are useful. Nerve block is a treatment method that blocks propagation of nerve signals in sensory, motor, and/or sympathetic nerves with topical anesthetics or neurolytic agents. Alleviation of pain in particular is obtained by blocking sensory and/or sympathetic nerves. Among various nerve block treatments, the usefulness of celiac nerve blocks against pains caused by pancreatic cancer is well recognized. Cancer-derived thoracic pains are treated with pulsed radiofrequency or thermal coagulation therapies. Using these nerve block treatments helps alleviate cancer pains, enabling reduction of opioid dosage, which in turn improves the patient's quality of life as opioid-induced drowsiness or constipation is reduced. For refractory cancer pains that are resistant to opioids and other drugs, epidural or subarachnoid continuous infusion of an opioid and a topical anesthetic may be introduced because such combined administration can achieve pain alleviation with less amount of opioids than using opioid-only systemic administration. As these interventional treatments, including nerve blocks, require specialized knowledge and techniques, patients are advised to consult anesthesiologists who are well experienced in the pain clinic practice.

Other Non-drug Therapies

Orthotic (body-supporting) devices and appropriate exercise therapies are useful against pains such as those from bone metastasis. Other physical therapies, acupuncture and/or moxibustion, aromatherapy, mindfulness, and VR glasses are also used. Team medicine, joined with various other professions, including physical therapists and clinical psychologists are also practiced.

20.7.2 Treatment for Pains that Are Associated with Cancer Treatments or Unrelated to Either Cancer or Its Treatments

Treatment for non-cancer pains, including those caused by cancer treatments or unrelated to either the cancer or its treatments, should be performed even while the cancer treatment is in progress. In particular, chronic pains such as post-surgical pains or postherpetic neuralgia should be treated independently of pains that are directly caused by cancer, incorporating non-drug therapies as much as possible. It is also desirable for patients to enhance their sense of self-efficacy while also learning to live with chronic pains. When a mood or sleep disorder is pronounced, multidisciplinary care should be provided at the same time as other treatments [17].

Strong opioids are indicated for patients who have clear physical causes of the pain and very few psychosocial factors involved. The maximum recommended dosage for opioids is 90 mg/day of morphine equivalents. It is also recommended to evaluate both the pain and efficacy of the treatment after a certain dosing period (3–6 months); at that time the possibility of dosage reduction, discontinuation, or a "drug holiday" should be evaluated. This is because it has been shown that lengthy administration of large doses of strong opioids does not improve either the pain or the quality of life of the patient. Our experiences with the so-called opioid crisis in the US have also taught us that poorly planned use of strong opioids is harmful to both the society and the patients themselves [18].

References

1. National Cancer Institute. Facing Forward: Life after cancer treatment. https://www.cancer.gov/publications/patient-education/facing-forward
2. Paice JA, Portenoy R, Lacchetti C, et al. Management of chronic pain in survivors of adult cancers: American Society of Clinical Oncology Clinical Practice Guideline. J Clin Oncol. 2016;34:3325–45.
3. Raja SN, Carr DB, Cohen M, et al. The revised International Association for the Study of Pain definition of pain: concepts, challenges, and compromises. Pain. 2020;161:1976–82.
4. Whibley D, AlKandari N, Kristensen K, et al. Sleep and pain: a systematic review of studies of mediation. Clin J Pain. 2019;35:544–58.
5. Treede RD, et al. Chronic pain as a symptom or a disease: the IASP Classification of Chronic Pain for the International Classification of Diseases (ICD-11). Pain. 2019;160:19–27.
6. Ogawa S, Iseki M, Kikuchi S. A large scale survey on chronic pain and neuropathic pain. Clin Orthop Surg. 2012;47:565–74. (Japanese)
7. Bouhassira D, Lantéri-Minet M, Attal N, et al. Prevalence of chronic pain with neuropathic characteristics in the general population. Pain. 2008;136:380–7.
8. Ohayon MM, Stingl JC. Prevalence and comorbidity of chronic pain in the German general population. J Psychires. 2012;46:444–50.
9. NCCN clinical practice guidelines in oncology (NCCN guidelines®) survivorship. Version 1. 2016. NCCN.org
10. Baron R, Binder A, Wasner G. Neuropathic pain: diagnosis, pathophysiological mechanisms, and treatment. Lancet Neurol. 2010;9:807–19.
11. Nakajima N, Hata Y, Onishi H, Ishida M. The evaluation of the relationship between the level of disclosure of cancer in terminally ill patients with cancer and the quality of terminal care in these patients and their families using the Support Team Assessment Schedule. Am J Hosp Palliat Care. 2013;30:370–6.
12. Ceeland CS, Ryan KM. Pain assessment: global use of brief pain inventory. Ann Acad Med Singap. 1994;23:129–38.
13. Fallon M, Giusti R, Aielli F, et al. Management of cancer pain in adult patients: ESMO Clinical Practice Guidelines. Ann Oncol. 2018;29(Supplement 4):iv166–91.
14. Snaith RP. The hospital anxiety and depression scale. Health Qual Life Outcomes. 2003;1:29. https://doi.org/10.1186/1477-7525-1-29.
15. NCCN clinical practice guidelines in oncology (NCCN guidelines®) adult cancer pain. Version 2. 2019. NCCN.org
16. WHO guidelines for the pharmacological and Radiotherapeutic Management of Cancer Pain in adults and adolescents. Geneva: World Health Organization; 2018. https://www.ncbi.nlm.nih.gov/books/NBK537492/
17. Clinical practice guideline for the management chronic pain. The committee for Clinical practice guideline for the management chronic pain. Tokyo: Shinko Trading Co. Ltd; 2021, pp. 453–468. (Japanese and English)
18. Guidelies for prescribing opioid analgegics for chronic non-cancer pain. 2nd.ed. The committee for the guideline for prescribing opioid analgegics for chronic non-cancer pain of JAPC. Co. Ltd. Tokyo. 2017 (Japanese and English)

21 Medical Rehabilitation of Patients with Cancer in Japan

Kazunari Abe

Abstract

This article presents a short history of the medical rehabilitation of cancer patients in Japan. The term last around 60 years, from 1962 to 2022. Rehabilitation interventions were coordinated with the treatment of cancer. The outcome of cancer rehabilitation should include improvements in Activities of Daily Living and/or Quality of Life during or after cancer treatment.

Our rehabilitation of patients with cancer now takes place in cancer centres, general hospitals, and some in-home settings.

Keywords

Activities of Daily Living · Disuse syndrome · Palliative care · Quality of life · Supportive care

21.1 Background

Cancer has been the most morbid disease in Japan, the primary cause of mortality among the Japanese from 1981 to the present – more than forty years [1]. It is said that half of the Japanese population has experienced cancer sometime during in their lives, and approximately a third of Japanese people have died of cancer.

The government of Japan established the National Cancer Centre in Tokyo in 1962. The centre consisted of two major divisions, a research institute and a hospital. But at that time there were not departments of rehabilitation for patients with cancer. The main policy of the centre must be cancer control by any means, mainly by analysing the mechanisms of cancer and seeking a cure to the extent possible. In the 1970s, around 40% of cancer patients had a 5-year survival rate.

Early in the 21st century, a small number of cancer rehabilitation centres have opened up around the country. In December 2005, a nationwide survey was carried out by the Japan Council for Quality Health Care in which questionnaires regarding cancer rehabilitation were mailed to departments associated with medical rehabilitation at 1693 healthcare institutions accredited as acute-care hospitals. The survey showed that at that time, 62% (1045/1963) of the institutions offered medical rehabilitation for patients with cancer [2].

Table 21.1 shows some major events related to national policy on cancer treatment in Japan.

Following passage of the Cancer Control Act in 2006, the health authority launched a health insurance system adding cancer rehabilitation for certain kinds of inpatients in 2010. This marks the official starting point of medical rehabilitation of cancer patients in Japanese society [3].

Table 21.1 Major events related to cancer treatment in Japan

1962	National Cancer Centre is founded
1965	*Physical Therapist and Occupational Therapist Act*
1981	Cancer becomes leading cause of death in Japan
1984	Comprehensive 10-year strategy for cancer control (until 1993)
1994	New 10-year strategy to overcome cancer (–2003)
2004	The third-term comprehensive 10-year strategy for cancer control (until 2013)
2006	Cancer Control Act
2007	Basic plan to promote cancer control programme
2010	*Inpatient cancer rehabilitation implemented within social insurance system*
2012	Basic plan to promote cancer control programme revised
2013	Cancer Registration Promotion Act
2016	Amendment and implementation of a law to partially revise Cancer Control Act
2018	Third-term basic plan to promote cancer control programme, revised (*newly included cancer rehabilitation*)

Source: Department of Health

K. Abe (✉)
Peace Nursing Station, Department of Rehabilitation,
Kurihara, Miyagi, Japan

© The Author(s), under exclusive license to Springer Nature Singapore Pte Ltd. 2026
M. Endo et al. (eds.), *Cancer and Work in Asia Volume 2*, https://doi.org/10.1007/978-981-95-6537-5_21

21.2 Cancer Treatment and Medical Rehabilitation

Cancer treatment and medical rehabilitation have constituted a good combination as opposed to a simple coordination. When cancer treatment changed, rehabilitation interventions on cancer patients was revised as well. A good example of this is the journey of an osteosarcoma patient in the field of orthopaedic oncology, which demonstrates how changes in cancer treatment affect rehabilitation interventions.

Ten years have passed since the founding of the national cancer centre; the Chiba Cancer Centre was established in the city of Chiba near Tokyo in 1972. The Chiba Cancer Centre was a pioneer among cancer hospitals run by local authorities in Japan [4].

In the 1970s, the main treatment for osteosarcoma was a resection of the malignant tumour, such as the amputation of a lower extremity, targeting mostly the knee joint. After the excision, medical rehabilitation was indicated for the patient, with treatment that included standing up at the first approach, then walking with a lower-extremity prosthesis for younger patients to rebuild their physical and mental capabilities as part of the long, arduous training for Activities of Daily Living. The treatment consisted of three phases. At that time, only 17% of patients had a 5-year survival rate.

In the 1980s, an osteosarcoma diagnosis meant surgery that usually involved replacing the knee joint with an artificial one, like Kotz's knee joint developed by Dr. Kotz of Vienna University in Austria, to excise the malignant tumour [5]. The subsequent rehabilitation intervention consisted of adapting a walking exercise with parallel bars for assistance. Although patients could return to a relatively normal daily life, they were unable to run or participate in sports to avoid damaging the artificial joint. Additional challenges included the risk of infection associated with prosthetic materials and limited durability, as the artificial knee typically required replacement every 5 to 10 years, necessitating further surgery and exposing patients to additional risk factors.

It was said that the treatment course consisted of four phases: (A) diagnosis, (B) surgery of primary site, (C) chemotherapy, and (D) rehabilitation intervention, at least to the point where the patient could walk again. This approach increased the 5-year survival rate to approximately 51% of patients, nearly three times higher than earlier treatment methods for osteosarcoma. The key factor in this improvement was the addition of chemotherapy following surgical resection of the malignant tumor, which was gradually recognized as effective at preventing lung metastasis and thereby improving patient survival.

The 1990s saw the advent of rotationplasty of the knee joint, which obviated the need for the placement of an artificial joint inside the body. Then rehabilitation intervention was modified from walking with an orthopaedic device to using one's own body with a special, small orthosis for patients who received the rotationplasty [6].

The treatment course comprised five phases: (A) diagnosis, (B) chemotherapy before surgery to reduce the tumour size, (C) surgery of the primary site, (D) chemotherapy after surgery, and, finally, (E) rehabilitation intervention, at least to the point where the patient can walk again during chemotherapy longer because of severe side-effects of chemotherapy. Finally, with this method, five years survival rate of osteosarcoma has improved up to of 83%.

The treatment of osteosarcoma at the Chiba Cancer Centre should follow more phases of the treatment journey, then shifting medical rehabilitation intervention as well. That means establishing a close relationship between cancer treatment and rehabilitation intervention of the patient with primary bone malignancy, as we noted in the preceding discussion. Thus, medical rehabilitation staff should know the details of cancer treatment. This is a crucial issue in rehabilitation intervention for fulfilling patients' wishes regarding their Activities of Daily Living and quality of life. Table 21.2 shows some phases of the treatment journey of osteosarcoma changed survival term of the patient.

We have seen similar situations in connection with other cancer treatments, such as chemotherapy or radiation therapy in addition to surgery, or a combination of them. Rehabilitation staff should know how to treat cancer because the treatment caused some effects and any adverse effects to handle by the concrete interventions of medical rehabilitation.

Table 21.2 Some phases of osteosarcoma treatment

Period	Five-year survival rate	Phase	I. Diagnosis	Pre-chemo	II. Surgery	Post-chemo	III. Rehabilitation
1970s	17%	3	Diagnosis		Surgery		Rehablilitation
1980s	51%	4	Diagnosis		Surgery	Post-chemo	Rehablilitation
1990s	83%	5	Diagnosis	Pre-chemo	Surgery	Post-chemo	Rehablilitation

Source: Department of Orthopaedics, Chiba Cancer Centre

21.3 Rehabilitation of Patients with Cancer

Unfortunately, medical rehabilitation is entire ineffective when it comes to treating cancer cells like chemotherapy or radiation therapy or surgical oncology of a specific organ, although rehabilitation aims to restore the functioning of patients during or after cancer treatment. One of the main reasons why patients with cancer need rehabilitation intervention is to prevent or reduce the adverse effects of the treatment of certain forms of cancer, such as chemotherapy, radiation therapy, or surgical oncology. Where it has been more complex situation with combination of these measures.

Chemotherapy has many side effects of varying degrees of severity. In this situation, rehabilitation interventions in support of patients in their cancer journey have to be vital to maintain Activities of Daily Living where they received to cure cancer, inpatients in particular. When patients felt severely cancer related fatigue (CRF), rehabilitation approaches reduce it [7].

When cancer patients undergo resection of the alimentary canal, the digestive tract must be reconstructed because of the impairment of the functioning of the digestive system after surgery. If the digestive system is not reconstructed, severe limitations will be imposed on daily life caused by a low level of digestive activity, following gastrectomy for gastric cancer or colorectomy for colorectal cancer. The more the 5-year survival rate improves, the more survivors will require rehabilitation to reduce these limitations on daily life. Gastric cancer and colorectal cancer are widespread, ranking second or third in terms of morbidity among the Japanese; however, several articles have been published on rehabilitation following digestive cancer treatment in Japanese cancer centres or general hospitals. Stoma rehabilitation by nursing staff was an exception to that [8]. Interventions mostly by oncology nurses date back to the 1970s [9].

Another adverse effect of chemotherapy is paralysis of extremities, fingers and palms in particular, which restricts a person's ability to independently perform Activities of Daily Living both during and after treatment. Peripheral nerve neuropathy induced by chemotherapy should be a kind of peripheral neuropathy. Many symptoms were able to reveal, such as muscle atrophy, less power of muscles, limitation of range of motion, imbalance of posture, or orthostatic hypotension. These symptoms could be reduced by rehabilitation intervention, which was prescribed by the attending physician, who worked together with rehabilitation team members, such as occupational therapists or physiotherapists [10].

21.4 Primary Impairment of Cancer Patients

There is no clear pathological evidence of symptoms because of a variety of investigations of bone metastases in advanced cancer patients in some subjective symptoms. Mostly patients with advanced cancer have bone metastases, especially lung cancer, breast cancer, and prostate cancer. This shows the complex situation of the cancer journey because many treatment options exist for patients to choose from or that the attending physician can recommend in advanced cancer cases. It depends on the stage of the primary cancer, whether or not the patients seeks to improve their daily life with cancer, not to stop any activities to prevent the risk of severe pain or pathologic fracture. Taking a bad selection of methods, then showing low Activities of Daily Living and/or poor Quality of Life should be occurring [11].

As acute symptoms experienced by patients and/or identified by medical staffs. Some options such as radiation therapy for cancer patients or paralysis control by medication, chemotherapy or immunotherapy for prevention of bone metastatis. When pathologic fractures breaking out locally, we make some surgery to prevent severe cancer pain or pathologic fractures. Because bone metastasis are very long sentence that should be broken down [12].

Pain is more complex because it is caused not only by the cancer itself but also by myofascial lower back pain as a non-malignancy. A cancer board should provide guidelines on how to handle bone metastases, because of the plethora of means available to the medical team members [13].

Simply an attending physician alone cannot cover the complex situation, as it involves making decisions for the patient with this situation. This needs to be some kind of staffs, such as oncologist, radiation oncologist, or surgeon, to reduce pain or paralysis. The other aim is to prevent pathological fracture for recovery of daily livings or better quality of life. There are many things to discuss among multidimensional staff and from many viewpoints, for example, "total pain" as pointed out by Dame Cicely Saunders in the 1970s. This is essential for the care of advanced cancer patients.

We need a multimodal medical team approach consisting of interdisciplinary staff; however, there are difficulties in communication. All members are specialists in their field, so they know useful technical terms, but those same terms could hinder team-building efforts as a result of misunderstanding among members or difficulties exchanging important information having to do with patient care. Thus, a common language would foster better understanding, and efforts made in the development of such a language would lead to much better patient outcomes with respect to improving their Activities of Daily Living and/or quality of life.

Cancer cachexia is common in patients with advanced cancer. Cachexia means the patient is closer to the end of life, and it has to be difficult to treat by any medical staffs because it showed a sign of far advanced cancer. The primary cancer has to be no effective treatment at the time of the days. [14]. Most of them has given up to cure cancer at all within the condition.

But it is quite similar in the clinical picture with arising disuse syndrome, i.e., muscle atrophy. When a patient with advanced cancer reduces physical activity for a period of time, some symptoms occur depending on the condition, such as decubitus those arise at least 2 hours, bone atrophy arising within 8 hours, and deep phlebothrombosis. These symptoms have taken place earlier than expectations of long bed-bounded of the patient. Then, bone atrophy or phlebothrombosis should be taken different approaches [15].

We watch very carefully the clinical picture of patients. When the patient seems to become thin, to lose weight, or to have a low activity level, then we implement a rehabilitation intervention regimen that is quite different with the goal of rehabilitation for the aim of the symptom. It is different to treat symptoms of the patient Table 21.3 shows a trade-off between cancer cachexia and disuse syndrome.

Table 21.3 A trade-off between cancer cachexia and disuse syndrome

Clinical picture	Cancer cachexia	Disuse syndrome
Basal metabolism	Increase	Decrease
Protein synthesis	Decrease	Increase with good nutrition
Muscle	Destroy	Could maintain but atrophic
Appetite	Increase	Decrease
Trophotherapy	Ineffective	Effective

Source: author original

21.5 Secondary Impairment of Cancer Patients

When disuse syndrome of a cancer patient breaks out, it leads to poor daily living because of a lower level of physical activity. The situation depends upon the cancer treatment itself, the adverse effects of anti-cancer therapy, or the depression experienced by the cancer patient.

Mostly anti-cancer treatment or some of therapies takes variety of the term. Surgical oncology takes some operational selection depending on bed-bound time. There is a challenge to shorten bed-boundness, but in more advanced stages, more time should be spent in bed. It is easy to understand for us such a situation after radical surgery or harsh chemotherapy.

When a cancer patient undergoes chemotherapy, the severity of the damage that can occur depends on the stage of the cancer. An outpatient on low-dose medication will face less severe adverse effects. However, high-dose chemotherapy, which should be an inpatient procedure for some time, carries the possibility of more severe adverse effects.

Patients who have undergone chemotherapy and who, over time engage in increasingly less physical activity should be prescribed rehabilitation intervention as soon as possible because stopping disuse syndrome depends upon the passage of time. Any chemotherapy should be prevent disuse syndrome because of its different physiological mechanisms of the body. Only physical activity reduces disuse symptoms, especially deconditioning [16].

Disuse syndrome has been impairments, some of them carry a severe threat to life expectancy, such as decubitus, which arises with sepsis, deep vein thrombosis with lung or cerebral infarction, hypostatic pneumonia with prolonged confinement to bed; all these symptoms or diseases are, in most cases, caused by hypoactivity or bed-boundness during or after chemotherapy. We can easily understand these clinical risks that result from deconditioning of patients or disuse syndrome.

A few articles in the literature address the relationship between radiation therapy and rehabilitation, especially the adverse effects of the former. It seems to be Japanese character between anti-cancer therapy and cancer rehabilitation. In one study, a male patient diagnosed with head and neck cancer (carcinoma of the oropharynx) undertook rehabilitation. He already received radiation therapy at 72 Gy. Then the skin on his neck became increasingly tough. The attending physician ordered rehabilitation intervention to improve the range of motion of his neck. The rehabilitation took place twice a week for a year, but the range of motion in his neck did not improve. He quit his job. He is a truck driver, so a short range of motion of the neck is likely a significant disadvantage for good job performance. The patient survived head and neck cancer but has been dealing with poor quality of daily life since his cancer treatment.

Several different rehabilitation measures are being discussed, but whatever measure are taken, patients with cancer will be no doubt continue to find out rebuilding their Activity of Daily Life as cancer survivors. Rehabilitation must be a key for these kinds of patients to recover in the post-treatment period. In fact, medical rehabilitation is limited.

21.6 Differences Between Supportive Care and Palliative Care Run by Rehabilitation Interventions

When a cancer patient gives up on finding a cure, the patient could opt for palliative care for end-of-life care. But during cancer treatment, rehabilitation may play a role in supportive care under some forms of therapy.

Cancer treatment can take many forms, and a variety of supportive care must be made available, such as nursing, counseling and rehabilitation. Patients should have access to nursing care in the ward, counseling to address any mental health issues they might be facing, and assistance with maintaining their Activities of Daily Living through rehabilitation.

Recall that palliative care is both a health issue that fall under primary care and a human rights issue, as revealed by stakeholders such as academic bodies, European Association of Palliative Care (EAPC) [17], or the World Health Organization [18].

When palliative care is a health issue, care should spread all over citizens in society. This applies not only to patients with cancer but all members of society. We should think about other diseases, such as organ failure, dementia, frailty and so on. Another perspective considers the human life cycle, young and old, male and female.

One issue is the difference between supportive care and palliative care. When we take supportive care, it adapts cancer treatment undergoing. But palliative care applies to all sorts of illness, especially life-threatening ones. Rehabilitation covers both factors of supportive care and palliative care. Many articles address the issue of rehabilitation of cancer patients, either in palliative care or supportive care and/or a combination of the two [19–22].

21.7 From Inpatient Care to Outpatient Care: Focusing on an Aging Society

Starting in the early 21st century, Japan has faced an aging society, and when there are more aged and fewer young people in the population, then there will be a shortage of institutions, including hospitals, hospice care providers, and support staff for oncological care or rehabilitation. However, life expectancy is increasing, and many generations are older than the mean age of life. We have greater need for rehabilitation for those generations and family and/or society, which means reducing social cost by rehabilitation interventions [23]. Figure 21.1 (below) shows live births and mortality in Japan, 1949–2018.

What are the secrets of Japan's aging society? It does not represent an increase in the number of senior citizens; the primary factor is a reduced birth rate. Older generations, meaning those over seventy, eighty, or even ninety years old, are growing. They have several diseases, such as different types of cancer, organ failure, diabetes, dementia, and frailty, which are chronic diseases with illness trajectories [24]. They require rehabilitation interventions in their institutions or home [25].

But a more serious issue is the lower birth rate. That means short of rehabilitation staffs. Rehabilitation consists of many different specialists, such as physicians, nurses, and therapists, not to mention patients and their family. If the younger population of our society grows smaller and smaller, there will be less and less staff to rehabilitate patients in need of rehabilitation. When the number of hospitals decreases, we should shift to a more institution-oriented approach. That increases in efficiency of rehabilitation in institution. Some respondents to our survey, however, said that most of the aging population (over 55%; a survey at the year 2007 by cabinet) or patients with chronic disease, including cancer, would like to spend the final stage of their lives at home and not receive treatment following diagnosis. Therefore, we will take a domestic-oriented approach to their rehabilitation.

We should find another solution to care for our aging population given the declining rehabilitation staff. Some countries have opted for policies that allow immigrant to perform rehabilitation, but Japan has little experience with such policies. We will seek to resolve the problem in a short amount of time as it is an urgent issue. The history of Japanese medicine after the Meiji Restoration in the late nineteenth century,

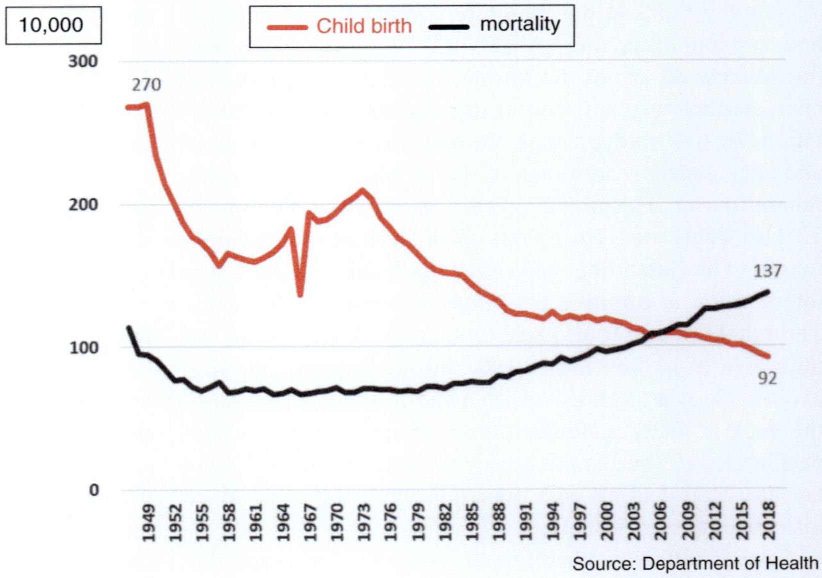

Fig. 21.1 Live births and mortality in Japan,1949–2018. (Source: Department of Health)

one strategy could be to develop some sort of advanced medication rather than through the rehabilitation of high-tech robots. Currently, no clear answer has presented itself.

21.8 Limitations of Cancer Rehabilitation in Japan

Generally speaking, Japan has been mostly cure-oriented when it comes to addressing cancer. Many efforts have been devoted to controlling cancer, simply because it is the primary cause of morbidity and mortality in Japan. The government has founded the National Cancer Centre sixty years ago, we have the history of cancer care. However, cancer rehabilitation in Japan has been underdeveloped compared with treatment or therapy. One of main factors are not to have close relationship between cancer and its treatment. Most rehabilitation personnel are oriented toward physical activity involving the upper or lower extremities. Physiotherapy must be implemented to build muscle mass or an ability to engage in physical activity, but not functioning or adverse effect caused by cancer itself or its treatment. Disuse syndrome leads to other important problems for cancer patients.

One researcher said that there exists a frontline of cancer rehabilitation [26]; unfortunately, I have never seen such a line personally. Few specialists working in rehabilitation have accepted patients with cancer in Japan. But I understand that some earnest soldiers cope with their way for rehabilitation of cancer patients in their everyday activities in hospitals or clinical settings and at home. I hope to further develop rehabilitation for patients with cancer and their family at any stage in Japan.

References

1. Katanoda K, et al. Updated trends in cancer in Japan: incidence in 1985-2015 and mortality in 1958-2018—a sign of decrease in cancer incidence. J Epidemiol. 2021;31(7):426–50.
2. Hamaguchi T, et al. Survey of the current status of cancer rehabilitation in Japan. Disabil Rehabil. 2008;30(7):559–64.
3. Okamura H. Importance of rehabilitation in cancer treatment and palliative medicine. Jpn J Clin Once. 2011;41(6):733–8.
4. Tsujimura H, et al. Successful treatment of histiolytic sarcoma with induction chemotherapy consisting of dose-escalated CHOP plus etoposide and upfront consolidation auto-transplantation. Int J Hematol. 2014;100(5):507–10.
5. Kotz R, et al. A modular femur-tibia reconstruction system. Orthopedics. 1986;9(12):1639–52.
6. Chan CM, et al. Why rotationplasty? A qualitative study of decision-making by families of patients with primary bone sarcoma. J Patient Exp. 2022;9:1–7.
7. Matsugaki R, et al. Immediate effects of exercise intervention on cancer-related fatigue. J Phys Ther Sci. 2018;30:262–5.
8. Anazawa S, Sakurai K. Stoma rehabilitation in Japan: in the past and at present. J Enterostomal Ther. 1989;16(2):72–5.
9. An K-Y, et al. Development process of an evidence-based exercise program for post-operative colorectal cancer patients. Support Care Cancer. 2020;28(2):755–65.
10. Lahart IM, et al. Physical activity for women with breast cancer after adjuvant therapy. Cochrane Database Syst Rev. 2018;1(1):CD011292.
11. Bunting RW, Shea B. Bone metastasis and rehabilitation. Cancer. 2001;92(4 Suppl):1020–8.
12. Shinoda Y, et al. Prediction of pathological fracture in patients with lower limb bone metastasis using computed tomography imaging. Clin Exp Metastasis. 2020;37(5):607–16.

13. Shibata H, et al. Diagnosis and treatment of bone metastasis: comprehensive guideline of the Japanese Society of Medical Oncology, Japanese Orthopedic Association, Japanese Urological Association, and Japanese Society for Radiation Oncology. ESMO Open. 2016;1(2):e000037.
14. Wakabayashi H, et al. The regulatory approval of anamorelin for treatment of cachexia in patients with non-small cell lung cancer, gastric cancer, pancreatic cancer, and colorectal cancer in Japan: facts and numbers. J Cachexia Sarcopenia Muscle. 2021;12:14–6.
15. Abe K, Okamura H. Development of a method for transferring paraplegic patients with advanced cancer from bed to wheelchair. J Palliat Med. 2016;19(6):656–60.
16. Tenconi S, et al. Rehabilitation for lung cancer patients undergoing surgery; results of the PUREAIR randomized trial. Eur J Phys Rehabil Med. 2021;57(6):1002–11.
17. Radbruch L, et al. The Lisbon challenge: acknowledging palliative care as a human right. J Palliat Med. 2013;16(3):301–4.
18. Clark J, et al. Reframing global palliative care advocacy for the sustainable development goal era: a qualitative study of the views of international palliative care experts. J Pain Symptom Manage. 2018;56(3):363–70.
19. Hui D, Bruera E. Integrating palliative care into the trajectory of cancer care. Nat Rev Clin Oncol. 2016;13(3):159–71.
20. Chan RJ, et al. Oncology practitioners' perspectives and practice patterns of post-treatment cancer survivorship care in the Asia-Pacific region: results from the STEP study. BMC Cancer. 2017;17:715.
21. Uster A, et al. Effects of nutrition and physical exercise intervention in palliative cancer patients: a randomized controlled trial. Clin Nutr. 2018;37(4):1202–9.
22. Kaasa S, et al. Integration of oncology and palliative care: a Lancet Oncology Commission. Lancet Oncol. 2018;19(11):e588–653.
23. Arai H, et al. Japan as the front-runner of super-aged societies: perspectives from medicine and medical care in Japan. Geriatr Gerontol Int. 2015;15:673–87.
24. Lunney JR, et al. Patterns of functional decline at the end of life. JAMA. 2003;289(18):2387–92.
25. Taylor DR, Murray SA. Improving quality of care for end-stage respiratory disease: changes in attitude, changes in service. Chron Respir Dis. 2018;15(1):19–25.
26. Tsuji T. The front line of cancer rehabilitation in Japan: current status and future issues. J Cancer Rehab. 2019;2:10–7.

22 Appearance-related Supportive Care

Rie Ozeki

Abstract

The majority of chemotherapy's side effects are nausea, alopecia, and myelosuppression. These phenomena are consequences of chemotherapy's mechanism of action: it targets cells with high proliferative potential, thus affecting not only malignant cells but also actively proliferating normal cells. While alopecia and nail changes are not typically prioritized as significant side effects in clinical practice, their potential impact on interpersonal relationships and employment warrants consideration, as these changes are often visible to others.

Keywords

Alopecia · Hand-foot syndrome · Nail toxicity · Pigmentation

22.1 Alopecia

For female breast cancer patients, alopecia is often considered the most distressing side effect, and many patients express reluctance toward chemotherapy because of it. Alopecia typically begins 2–3 weeks after the start of chemotherapy, with hair regrowth beginning approximately 1 month after treatment completion. It then takes about 6 months to a year for the hair to grow back to a short length. Regrown hair may differ from the original hair in terms of thickness, color, and texture, but it often returns to its previous state over time. However, some patients experience delayed or incomplete regrowth. Hair loss also affects the eyebrows and eyelashes.

To mitigate the effects of chemotherapy on hair matrix cells, scalp cooling was developed, and a cooling system was approved by the FDA in 2012. Two types of scalp cooling systems are currently available: DigniCap and PAXMAN, which are believed to have a preventive effect of approximately 50% for patients with early-stage breast cancer. As an example, the PAXMAN scalp cooling system is described here. A silicone cap is placed on the patient, and a cap cover is secured on top (Fig. 22.1). A cooling fluid at −4 °C is continuously supplied from the cooling system through the cap's lines, maintaining the scalp temperature at 20 °C. Cooling is applied for 30 min before, during, and for 90 min after chemotherapy administration. While some patients may experience chills, headaches, or jaw pain from the chin strap's tightness, these can be managed with an electric blanket or by adjusting the strap. Evidence on hair regrowth is insufficient, but there are reports that scalp cooling accelerates regrowth. The availability of this treatment is often limited by the financial burden on the patient and the staffing requirements for the medical facility, as it is not consistently covered by insurance across different healthcare systems. Patients are advised to verify insurance coverage within their specific national or private healthcare plans.

Given the risk of hair loss, patients are advised to prepare wigs and caps in advance. A wide variety of wigs is available for purchase from wig makers, beauty salons, or online retailers, with prices ranging from hundreds to thousands of dollars.

R. Ozeki (✉)
Faculty of Pharmacy, Juntendo University, Urayasu, Chiba, Japan
e-mail: r.ozeki.gs@juntendo.ac.jp

© The Author(s), under exclusive license to Springer Nature Singapore Pte Ltd. 2026
M. Endo et al. (eds.), *Cancer and Work in Asia Volume 2*, https://doi.org/10.1007/978-981-95-6537-5_22

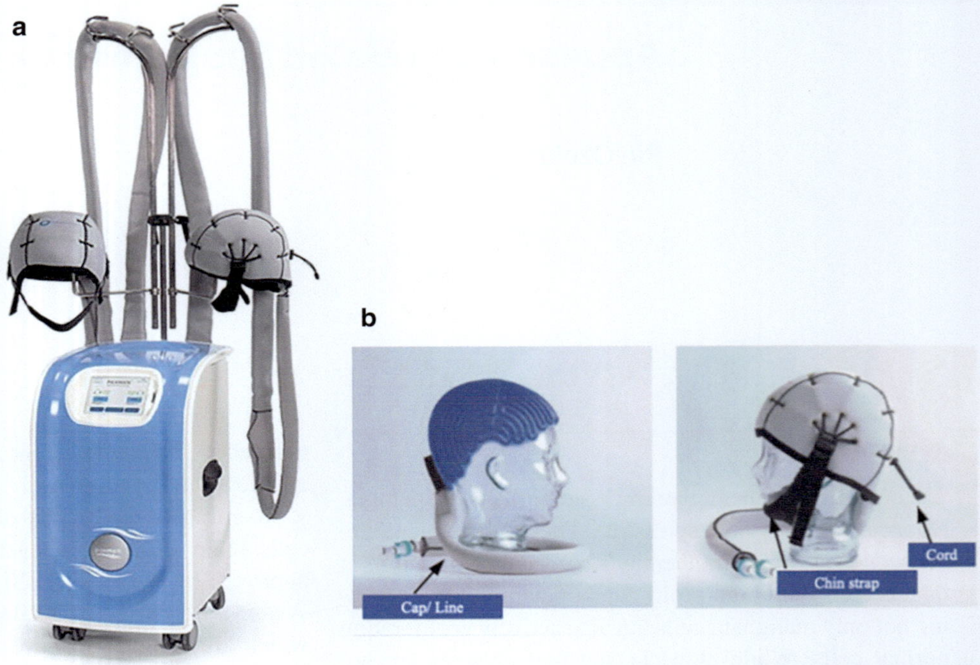

Fig. 22.1 The Paxman Scalp Cooling System (**a**) The compact refrigeration unit. This unit contains a specialized coolant that is circulated through the cooling cap to extract heat from the patient's scalp. (**b**) The Paxman cooling caps. The system features a lightweight, medical-grade silicone cold cap (inner) designed for a close fit, and a neoprene cover (outer) that insulates the cap and ensures consistent scalp contact using bungee-cord (chin strap) adjustments.

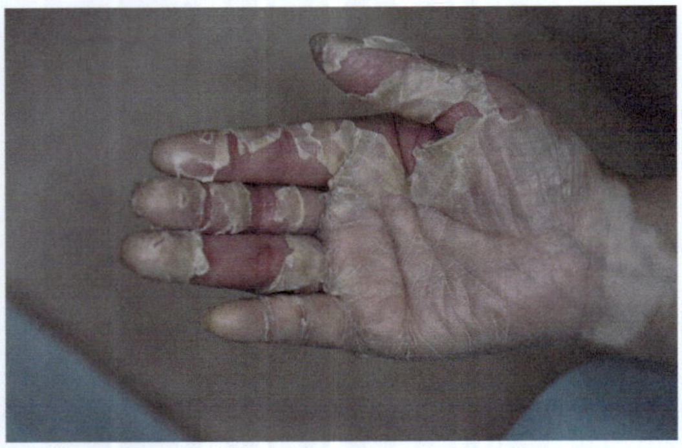

Fig. 22.2 An example of Grade III hand-foot syndrome in a breast cancer patient receiving docetaxel. (Courtesy of Satoshi Hirakawa, MD)

22.2 Hand-Foot Syndrome

Hand-foot syndrome (HFS) is a side effect of chemotherapy that causes symptoms such as stabbing pain, redness, numbness, swelling, dryness, itching, and skin discoloration on the palms of the hands and soles of the feet (Fig. 22.2).

It is known to occur frequently with fluoropyrimidine drugs like capecitabine, cytotoxic agents such as liposomal doxorubicin and docetaxel, and kinase inhibitors including sorafenib, sunitinib, and regorafenib. The onset of HFS varies by drug class. HFS caused by fluoropyrimidines often appears weeks to months after treatment initiation, while HFS from kinase inhibitors can occur within days of administration. In mild cases, symptoms may be managed with moisturizing creams and topical steroids, but for moderate or more severe cases, a dose reduction or discontinuation of chemotherapy may be necessary.

22.3 Nail Toxicity

Chemotherapy also affects nail matrix cells, the source of nail growth, which can lead to brittle, thin, and discolored fingernails and toenails (Fig. 22.3). To reduce pressure on the nails, it's recommended to use a nail file for gentle shaping rather than nail clippers. Maintaining short, neat nails, thoroughly drying hands after washing, and moisturizing the nail area with oil or cream are also important preventive measures. Nail toxicity caused by taxanes is a characteristic side effect, manifesting as melanonychia, onycholysis, and onychomadesis. The incidence and severity of these conditions increase with the frequency and cumulative duration of drug administration. Since most cases are reversible, they are typ-

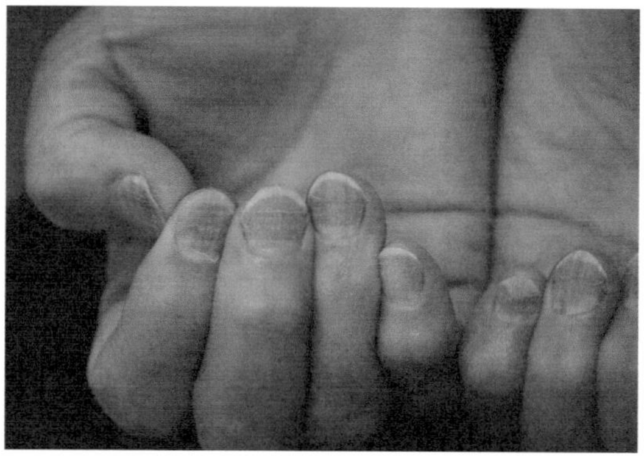

Fig. 22.3 An example of Grade I nail toxicity (Beau's lines) in a parotid cancer patient receiving docetaxel. (Courtesy of Satoshi Hirakawa, MD)

ically managed conservatively rather than with aggressive treatment. Symptomatic care includes the use of moisturizers, protective gloves, and hand-foot cooling.

Nail changes can cause significant psychological distress due to alterations in color and shape, and they may also lead to pain at pressure points. Topical antibacterial or antifungal medications are used when a local infection, such as paronychia, is suspected. To protect the nails, it is essential to gently remove any hangnails or cuticles and to wear gloves when hands are in water. Regular application of moisturizers to the nail and surrounding skin is also recommended, as dryness can lead to splitting and peeling.

22.4 Pigmentation

Chemotherapy-induced skin pigmentation is believed to be caused by the stimulation of melanocytes in the basal cell layer by chemotherapy drugs (Fig. 22.4). This side effect primarily appears on the palms of the hands and soles of the feet

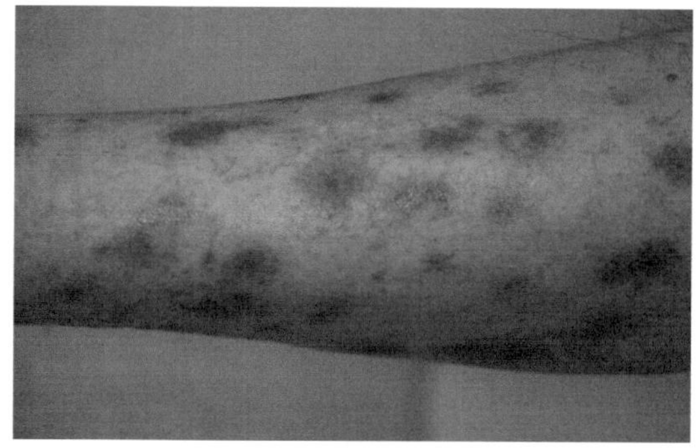

Fig. 22.4 An example of Grade I pigmentation in a lung cancer patient receiving osimertinib. (Courtesy of Satoshi Hirakawa, MD)

and is more likely to occur with 5-fluorouracil (5-FU). To camouflage nail discoloration, patients may use nail polish. Continued use of nail polish can help protect the nail bed and may reduce damage by providing a barrier that enhances the nail's texture and reduces physical contact.

22.5 Workplace Considerations

Patients receiving cancer treatment often experience adverse events while undergoing chemotherapy. Because there are many types of anticancer drugs, there are also many different side effects. Patients should feel comfortable discussing any concerns about their physical condition or appearance with their employer.

We ask that managers and colleagues listen to patients' concerns and offer support by accommodating their work arrangements. For example, if a patient is worried about sales activities due to changes in their appearance, consider offering them an alternative role, such as an office position, at their request. Allowing for flexible working hours or time off is also a crucial way to cooperate.

Fertility Management

23

Tadashi Maezawa, Yodo Sugishita, Tomoaki Ikeda, and Nao Suzuki

Abstract

In recent years, fertility preservation technology has improved remarkably, and not only sperm, oocyte, and embryo cryopreservation, but also ovarian tissue cryopreservation is becoming a common medical treatment. In order to efficiently provide this technology to patients, large organizations have been established to address fertility preservation, such as the ISFP (International Society for Fertility Preservation) and FertiPROTEKT in Europe and Oncofertility Consortium in the United States. Their activities include not only the medical aspect of fertility preservation, such as the creation of a system that facilitates the provision of fertility preservation to patients by consolidating at large facilities, but also the development of guidelines and the holding of symposiums. Fertility preservation is becoming popular in many Asian countries. The ASFP was established in 2015 by experts from 14 countries. In Japan, many activities, including nationwide educational campaigns, have resulted in the establishment of a nationwide registration system and government subsidies. This chapter will introduce a wide range of initiatives from various countries and organizations as well as efforts in Japan.

T. Maezawa
Department of Obstetrics and Gynecology, St. Marianna University School of Medicine, Kanagawa, Japan

Department of Obstetrics and Gynecology, Mie University School, Tsu, Japan
e-mail: tada-m@med.mie-u.ac.jp

Y. Sugishita · N. Suzuki (✉)
Department of Obstetrics and Gynecology, St. Marianna University School of Medicine, Kanagawa, Japan
e-mail: yodo@marianna-u.ac.jp; nao@marianna-u.ac.jp

T. Ikeda
Department of Obstetrics and Gynecology, Mie University School, Tsu, Japan
e-mail: t-ikeda@med.mie-u.ac.jp

Keyword

Fertility preservation · ASFP · Fertility preservation guideline · Oncofertility networks · Expenses for fertility preservation · Outcome after fertility preservation

23.1 Fertility Management

23.1.1 History of Fertility Preservation

In recent years, improved outcomes of cancer treatments have increased the survival rate in childhood, adolescent, and young adult (CAYA) cancer patients to above 80% [1, 2]. Late complications in cancer survivors vary widely, including neurological complications (posterior fossa syndrome, secondary malignancy, cognitive dysfunction, and cerebellar dysfunction, etc.) [3] and cerebrovascular disorders [4]. Infertility also can be a significant complication in many survivors, and the respective impacts of chemotherapy and irradiation therapy are described in another chapter. Because of these impacts, cryopreservation of sperms, oocytes, embryos, and ovarian tissues has been conducted for fertility preservation in CAYA cancer patients [5].

Fertility preservation began with the world's first live birth (Louise Brown) from in vitro fertilization and embryo transplantation, which was achieved by Robert Edwards and Patrick Steptoe in 1978 [6]. In vitro fertilization technologies subsequently spread across the world. These technologies include intracytoplasmic sperm injection (ICSI), which enables fertilization even when only a limited amount of sperm is available; the first pregnancy and delivery with an embryo fertilized by ICSI was reported in Belgium in 1942 [7].

The advancement of in vitro fertilization technologies has been accompanied by advances in sperm cryopreservation technologies. In 1949, glycerin was found to have a cryoprotective effect [8], and the first live birth from cryopreserved sperm was reported in 1953 [9]. Since then, cryopreservation of sperm has become a feasible procedure, and sperm cryo-

© The Author(s), under exclusive license to Springer Nature Singapore Pte Ltd. 2026

M. Endo et al. (eds.), *Cancer and Work in Asia Volume 2*, https://doi.org/10.1007/978-981-95-6537-5_23

preservation with liquid nitrogen vapor has become a standard method [10] that is widely used around the world.

Embryo cryopreservation by the slow freezing method was developed in 1972 [11]. Subsequently, in 1983, the world's first pregnancy and delivery from a human fertilized ovum (embryo) after cryopreservation and thawing was reported [12]. In 1985, a vitrification method was devised [13] that made rapid freezing possible without requiring special equipment, and vitrification started to be used worldwide. In the meantime, as a result of advancements in embryo cryopreservation technologies, surplus embryos that are not used for embryo transplantation after in vitro fertilization can be cryopreserved. Consequently, in Japan, single-embryo transplantation is now widely performed, contributing to a decrease in the number of multiple pregnancies [14]. Vitrification technologies have advanced, and more than 90% of embryos are reported to be viable after thawing [15–18].

The first pregnancy and delivery from in vitro fertilization with an unfertilized ovum after cryopreservation and thawing was reported in 1986 [19]. The survival rate of oocytes after thawing was lower than that of embryos because of the vulnerability of the transparent layer; however, it has been gradually increasing and is currently higher than 80% [20]. Because of the increased survival rate after thawing, cryopreservation of oocytes has become an option for fertility preservation in cancer patients [21]. Since Jack Donnez and his group in Belgium reported the first successful live childbirth after auto-transplantation of cryopreserved ovarian tissue in 2004 [22], this procedure has become widely clinically applied throughout the world.

23.2 Fertility Preservation in Europe and the United States

After the report by Jack Donnez and colleagues, researchers and physicians became more interested in fertility preservation for CAYA cancer patients. In 2006, the American Society of Clinical Oncology (ASCO) and the American Society for Reproductive Medicine (ASRM) jointly published the world's first guidelines on fertility preservation in young cancer patients [23]. In the same year, Teresa K. Woodruff and colleagues founded the Oncofertility Consortium in the United States, an association that works on fertility preservation in young cancer patients under the leadership of 4 universities (Northwestern University, University of California, the University of Pennsylvania, and the University of Oregon); the Consortium published the "Oncofertility Medical Practice" guidelines for treating patients [24]. In 2006 in Europe, von Wolff and others established FertiPROTEKT, an association that works on fertility preservation and currently includes about 155 institutions in Germany, Switzerland, and Austria [25]. In 2011, FertiPROTEKT published its guidelines, "Fertility Preservation in Women" [26] and initiated a cryopreservation bank for oocytes, embryos, and ovarian tissues, which has been operated under a rigid management scheme. Furthermore, in 2007, Jack Donnez and colleagues established the International Society for Fertility Preservation (ISFP) and, in 2012, published guidelines on fertility preservation in young cancer patients [27–30]. Since 2009, the ISFP has been holding a biennial World Congress of Fertility Preservation, where researchers in this field assemble from all over the world. The first congress was held in Brussels, Belgium, and the sixth was held in New York, USA (in November 2019). The 2021 congress, which was scheduled to be held in Belgium, was postponed because of the COVID-19 pandemic.

23.3 Fertility Preservation in Asia

In recent years, fertility preservation activities have also begun in Asia. In Japan, the Japan Society for Fertility Preservation (JSFP) was launched in 2012. In Korea, the Korean Society for Fertility Preservation (KSFP) was established in 2013 (by Seok Hyon Kim and colleagues), and in India, Fertility Preservation India was founded in 2014 (by Nalini Mahajan and colleagues). Samuel Kim in the United States, who is one of the legends in this field and a later advisor to the Asia Society for Fertility Preservation (ASFP), together with Nao Suzuki and Nalini Mahajan, proposed to establish an academic association specialized in oncofertility in Asia in order to promote awareness of this topic. Consequently, in 2015, the ASFP was established, with the participation of 14 countries (Australia, China, Hong Kong, India, Indonesia, Japan, the Republic of Korea, Pakistan, the Philippines, Singapore, Taiwan, Thailand, Turkey, and Vietnam) [31]. Subsequently, the Malaysian Fertility Society for Preservation (MFSP) was established in Malaysia in 2020 (by Mohd Faizal Achmad and colleagues). In the Philippines, the Philippine Society for Fertility Preservation was also founded in 2020 (by Virgilio M. Novero and colleagues). Malaysia joined the ASFP in 2020, and Bangladesh in 2021. Consequently, the ASFP currently includes 16 countries. Nao Suzuki from Japan served as the first president of the ASFP (from 2015 to 2020), and Nalini Kaul from India is currently serving as the second president. Since 2016, the ASFP has alternated between convening a scientific meeting and a symposium each year. In 2016, the first scientific meeting was held in Ho Chi Minh, Vietnam (hosted by Minh Chau and colleagues); in 2017, the first symposium was held in Shanghai, China (hosted by Ri-Cheng Chian and colleagues); in 2018, the 2nd scientific meeting was held in New Delhi, India (hosted by Nalini Mahajan and colleagues); and in 2019, the second symposium was held in Seoul, Korea (hosted by Seok Hyon Kim and colleagues). The 3rd scientific meeting was scheduled to be held in Bali, Indonesia, in 2020; however, it was postponed because of the COVID-19 pandemic and held online in 2021 (hosted by Budi Wiweko). In Japan, the JSFP has been convening an annual scientific meeting.

In 2017, the Japan Society of Clinical Oncology published its "Clinical Practice Guidelines for Fertility Preservation in Childhood, Adolescent, and Young Adult Cancer Patients" [32–34]. The guidelines were subsequently translated into Chinese and published in 2020 by Xu Cong Jian and his coworkers at Fudan University. In Korea, the KSFP published guidelines, "The Korean Society for Fertility Preservation clinical guidelines," in 2017.

23.4 Oncofertility Networks

Fertility preservation is a reproductive medicine treatment for cancer patients, and patients can undergo fertility preservation only when referred by an oncologist. Therefore, it is extremely important to raise oncologists' awareness of fertility preservation and systemize the issuance of referrals. Commonly, Oncofertility Networks play a role in increasing awareness. However, the location and scale of such networks vary because they are formed to match the actual situation in an individual area.

In Denmark, three university hospitals provide oncology medicine services, and each of these hospitals also has a department where in vitro fertilization is performed. For ovarian tissue cryopreservation, the ovaries are removed at the individual institutions and systematically shipped to Copenhagen University Hospital. Thus, in Denmark a system has been devised for coordinating fertility preservation [25].

As mentioned above, FertiPROTEKT is a network in German-speaking countries that comprises over 150 centers. It has a few central ovarian tissue cryopreservation banks and an established operational system in which ovaries are resected at individual facilities and systematically shipped to one of the central banks for cryopreservation. It is also equipped with counseling and psychotherapy centers, which can quickly provide patients with advice on fertility preservation.

The Oncofertility Consortium in the United States is a larger-scale network that connects researchers and clinical physicians in the United States and around the world. A meeting of the Oncofertility Consortium is held every year in Chicago to share research results and clinical experiences from all over the world. The meetings aim to raise the level of research and clinical practice in the field of oncofertility. The meeting offers an education program and conducts training to increase knowledge about oncofertility in reproductive medicine.

In some countries, fertility preservation is aggregated, as is the case in Denmark and FertiPROTEKT. In Japan, however, no aggregated system for fertility preservation exists. When an institution in Japan wishes to perform cryopreservation of oocytes, embryos, or ovarian tissue, it must file an application with and obtain authorization from the Japan Society of Obstetrics and Gynecology (as of November 2021, 160 institutions have been authorized). Thus, fertility preservation is independently conducted at individual facilities, and these facilities coordinate their activities with an oncology facility through inter-hospital collaborations.

To advance fertility preservation in Japan, the JSFP holds a scientific meeting once a year that enables information sharing and offers hands-on seminars aimed at improving practitioners' skills. The JSFP also conducts activities in individual sections for obstetricians, pharmacists, phychologists, nurses, and so on so that persons in each section can become more competent in their respective roles in fertility preservation. In addition, the JSFP announces local fertility preservation activities on their homepage. Furthermore, the JSFP has created a specialized qualification certification scheme for psychologists specializing in oncofertility, certified Oncofertility Navigators, and others to promote future leaders in oncofertility.

In Asia, few countries have Oncofertility Networks. In Korea, however, an inter-hospital network and referral system have been established [31]. The KSFP has published fertility preservation guidelines [31] and has been performing research on and improving domestic clinical practice programs.

Many aspects of the effectiveness and long-term safety of fertility preservation remain unclear because the treatment is new and because biological specimens for fertility preservation are stored for a long time. Although the safety and efficacy of fertility preservation are gradually becoming clearer thanks to reports from FertiPROTEKT and other networks, it remains important to study nation-specific outcomes that reflect ethnic and methodological differences. Among Asian countries, a patient registration system for fertility preservation is available in Australia [35]. And in Japan, the Japanese Oncofertility Registry (JOFR) was launched in 2016 by the leadership of the JSFP. In 2021, the JOFR became a national project and was subsequently linked with the cancer registry. Therefore, more accurate information on outcomes in Japan may be available in the future.

Table 23.1 The maximum amounts of financial assistance and number of times assistance was paid for fertility preservation in Japan (2021.4-)

Treatment	Maximum amount of assistance per treatment	Number of times of assistance paid
Embryo (fertilized egg) freezing	350,000 yen	Up to 2 times
Unfertilized egg freezing	200,000 yen	Up to 2 times
Ovarian tissue freezing	400,000 yen	Up to 2 times (once for tissue collection, once for re-transplantation)
Sperm freezing	25,000 yen	Up to 2 times
Sperm freezing (testicular sperm sampling)	350,000 yen	Up to 2 times

List of public subsidies from the government for fertility preservation that began in Japan in April 2021 (https://www.mhlw.go.jp/content/000913104.pdf)

23.5 Expenses for Fertility Preservation

Cancer patients carry a large financial burden because cancer treatment is expensive, and patients' ability to work is often affected during and after treatment. Although private health insurance and government support are often available for cancer treatment, each country has different attitudes toward fertility preservation. In Japan, public financial assistance began to be provided for fertility preservation in April 2021 (Table 23.1), and the burden on patients has since been reduced. In Denmark and Israel, there is no cost for fertility preservation [25, 36], and in Germany, Spain, and Belgium, the cost is covered by public insurance [37]. In Australia, financial assistance is available for oocyte freezing, and in South Korea, for embryo freezing [35].

23.6 Efforts to Improve Fertility Preservation in Cancer Patients in Japan

Having compared the situation between countries above, in this section we would like to discuss oncofertility in Japan. In Japan, a research group funded by the Ministry of Health, Labor, and Welfare is conducting various activities to help raise awareness of fertility preservation. Raising awareness requires research to investigate the current situation, identify the needs of medical institutions, and provide feedback to them. First, the research group estimated the annual budget based on the total number of patients across the country who need fertility preservation and the respective expenses and made recommendations to the national government; consequently, financial assistance, which previously differed between regions, is now paid by the national government with support from local governments. The group has conducted surveys of and given lectures to core hospitals for pediatric cancer (15 core facilities at hospitals across the country that treat children with cancer and are designated as providing seamless medical care for pediatric cancer patients) to enable a system of fertility preservation to be added to the medical care system led by the base hospitals. Because it is difficult to obtain informed consent or assent from pediatric cancer patients, the research group is now exploring how to gain the full understanding of patients themselves. The group is also verifying ways and creating explanatory materials to enable clear, age-appropriate explanations to be given to patients. Because the implementation system for fertility preservation differs between regions, the group is promoting the founding of networks of hospitals that provide fertility preservation for cancer patients throughout the country and establishing a coordination system between networks to ensure that all patients have access to equal treatment. Specimens for fertility preservation are stored for a prolonged period, so to standardize a secure management system across the country, the group is conducting surveys of long-term storage systems and making recommendations for standardizing them. It is conducting a nationwide perinatal prognosis survey of cancer survivors and establishing a support system for preconception care. Furthermore, it is promoting foster parenting and adoption for cancer survivor couples who cannot have their own children. To verify the prognosis of fertility preservation, the group is creating an application to establish a system that allows patients to enter information and healthcare professionals to track information. It is also reviewing the provision of easy-to-understand information to patients and promoting the involvement of genetic counseling of cancer patients interested in fertility preservation. Pharmacists are spreading awareness through lectures at academic meetings and at elementary/junior high schools and universities. The research group is also promoting and spreading awareness of women's health after cancer treatment. Furthermore, the group developed and performed a study to verify the usefulness of a psycho-educational program for fertility preservation in cancer patients, the O!PEACE program [38].

While various efforts are currently being made in Japan to create a system that enables patients to have equal access to fertility preservation across the country with the support of the national government, economic and medical disparities still exist in Asia, depending on the country. In vitro fertilization is an advanced medical treatment, and some countries have a level of medical care that is insufficient for enabling future pregnancies in CAYA cancer patients. The ASFP should play a major role in improving the level of fertility preservation in cancer patients in Asia, but at the same time, it is important to also establish a system of foster parenting and adoption. The adoption rate is much lower among cancer survivors than in the general population, not only in Japan but also in many other countries in Asia [39]. Because young female cancer patients have been reported to be more interested in adoption than women in general [40], development of this area is also an important challenge in Asia.

Oncofertility is an interdisciplinary field that saw a breakthrough with the live birth after transplantation of frozen-thawed ovarian tissue by Jack Donnez in 2004 and that has since made dramatic progress. Fertility preservation procedures have spread worldwide, and several countries have already established fertility preservation systems. However, such systems are still in development in many Asian countries, including Japan, and are needed to ensure that equal opportunities for fertility preservation are provided to all cancer patients.

References

1. Phillips SM, et al. Survivors of childhood cancer in the United States: prevalence and burden of morbidity. Cancer Epidemiol Biomarkers Prev. 2015;24(4):653–63.
2. Martinez F, E.-A. E. W. G. International Society for Fertility Preservation. Update on fertility preservation from the Barcelona International Society for Fertility Preservation-ESHRE-ASRM 2015 expert meeting: indications, results and future perspectives. Fertil Steril. 2017;108(3):407–15. e411
3. Sun LR, Cooper S. Neurological complications of the treatment of Pediatric neoplastic disorders. Pediatr Neurol. 2018;85:33–42.
4. Scholz-Kreisel P, et al. Prevalence of cardiovascular late sequelae in long-term survivors of childhood cancer: a systematic review and meta-analysis. Pediatr Blood Cancer. 2017;64(7) https://doi.org/10.1002/pbc.26428.
5. Harada M, Osuga Y. Fertility preservation for female cancer patients. Int J Clin Oncol. 2019;24(1):28–33.
6. Steptoe PC, Edwards RG. Birth after the reimplantation of a human embryo. Lancet. 1978;2(8085):366.
7. Palermo G, et al. Pregnancies after intracytoplasmic injection of single spermatozoon into an oocyte. Lancet. 1992;340:17–8.
8. Moore SG, Hasler JF. A 100-year review: reproductive technologies in dairy science. J Dairy Sci. 2017;100(12):10314–31.
9. Bunge RG, Sherman JK. Fertilizing capacity of frozen human spermatozoa. Nature. 1953;172(4382):767–8.
10. Hu J, et al. Liquid nitrogen vapor is comparable to liquid nitrogen for storage of cryopreserved human sperm: evidence from the characteristics of post-thaw human sperm. Fertil Steril. 2015;104(5):1253–1257 e1251-1252.
11. Whittingham DG, et al. Survival of mouse embryos frozen to −196 degrees and −269 degrees C. Science. 1972;178(4059):411–4.
12. Trounson A, Mohr L. Human pregnancy following cryopreservation, thawing and transfer of an eight-cell embryo. Nature. 1983;305(5936):707–9.
13. Rall WF, Fahy GM. Ice-free cryopreservation of mouse embryos at −196 degrees C by vitrification. Nature. 1985;313(6003):573–5.
14. Hayashi M, et al. The effect of single embryo transfer on perinatal outcomes in Japan. Int J Med Sci. 2015;12(1):57–62.
15. Abdelhafez FF, Desai N, Abou-Setta AM, Falcone T, Goldfarb J. Slow freezing, vitrification and ultra-rapid freezing of human embryos: a systematic review and meta-analysis. Reprod Biomed Online. 2010;20:209–22.
16. Lin TK, Su JT, Lee FK, Lin YR, Lo HC. Cryotop vitrification as compared to conventional slow freezing for human embryos at the cleavage stage: survival and outcomes. Taiwan J Obstet Gynecol. 2010;49:272–8.
17. Desai NN, Goldberg JM, Austin C, Falcone T. The new Rapid-I carrier is an effective system for human embryo vitrification at both the blastocyst and cleavage stage. Reprod Biol Endocrinol. 2013;11:41.
18. Kuwayama M. Highly efficient vitrification for cryopreservation of human oocytes and embryos: the Cryotop method. Theriogenology. 2007;67:73–80.
19. Chen C. Pregnancy after human oocyte cryopreservation. Lancet. 1986;1(8486):884–6.
20. Iussig B, et al. A brief history of oocyte cryopreservation: arguments and facts. Acta Obstet Gynecol Scand. 2019;98(5):550–8.
21. Tao T, Del Valle A. Human oocyte and ovarian tissue cryopreservation and its application. J Assist Reprod Genet. 2008;25(7):287–96.
22. Donnez J, Dolmans MM, Demylle D, Jadoul P, Pirard C, Squifflet J, et al. Livebirth after orthotopic transplantation of cryopreserved ovarian tissue. Lancet. 2004;364:1405–10.
23. ASCO recommendations on fertility preservation in cancer patients: guideline summary. J Oncol Pract. 2006;2(3):143–6.
24. Woodruff TK. The Oncofertility consortium–addressing fertility in young people with cancer. Nat Rev Clin Oncol. 2010;7(8):466–75.
25. von Wolff M, et al. FertiPROTEKT, Oncofertility consortium and the Danish fertility-preservation networks—what can we learn from their experiences? Clin Med Insights Reprod Health. 2019;13:1179558119845865.
26. von Wolff M, et al. Fertility preservation in women–a practical guide to preservation techniques and therapeutic strategies in breast cancer, Hodgkin's lymphoma and borderline ovarian tumours by the fertility preservation network FertiPROTEKT. Arch Gynecol Obstet. 2011;284(2):427–35.
27. Committee IP, et al. Recommendations for fertility preservation in patients with lymphoma, leukemia, and breast cancer. J Assist Reprod Genet. 2012;29(6):465–8.
28. Jadoul P, et al. Fertility considerations in young women with hematological malignancies. J Assist Reprod Genet. 2012;29(6):479–87.
29. Klemp JR, et al. Fertility preservation in young women with breast cancer. J Assist Reprod Genet. 2012;29(6):469–72.
30. Schmidt KT, et al. Recommendations for fertility preservation in patients with lymphomas. J Assist Reprod Genet. 2012;29(6):473–7.
31. Harzif AK, et al. Investigation of each Society for fertility preservation in Asia. Front Endocrinol (Lausanne). 2019;10:151.
32. Suzuki N. Clinical practice guidelines for fertility preservation in Pediatric, adolescent, and young adults with cancer. Int J Clin Oncol. 2019;24(1):20–7.
33. Suzuki N. Japan Society of Clinical Oncology Clinical Practice Guidelines 2017 for fertility preservation in childhood, adolescent, and young adult cancer patients: part 1. Int J Clin Oncol. 2021;27:265.
34. Suzuki N. Japan Society of Clinical Oncology Clinical Practice Guidelines 2017 for fertility preservation in childhood, adolescent, and young adult cancer patients: part 2. Int J Clin Oncol. 2021; https://doi.org/10.1007/s10147-021-02076-7.
35. Takae S, et al. Fertility preservation for child and adolescent cancer patients in Asian countries. Front Endocrinol (Lausanne). 2019;10:655.
36. Inhorn MC, et al. Medical egg freezing: the importance of a patient-centered approach to fertility preservation. J Assist Reprod Genet. 2018;35(1):49–59.
37. Kyono K, et al. A transportation network for human ovarian tissue is indispensable to success for fertility preservation. J Assist Reprod Genet. 2017;34(11):1469–74.
38. Suzuki N, et al. An intervention RCT-study aimed at improving mental health and increasing understanding of fertility preserva-

tion with Oncofertility! Psycho-Education and Couple Enrichment (O!PEACE) therapy. In: 2020 ASCO annual meeting; 2020.

39. Shiraishi E, et al. Study of the awareness of adoption as a family-building option among oncofertility stakeholders in Japan. JCO Glob Oncol. 2020;6:350.

40. Gorman JR, et al. Adoption consideration and concerns among young adult female cancer survivors. J Cancer Surviv. 2017;11(1):149–57.

24 Clinical Practice Guidelines

Akiko Okumura and Toshio Fukuoka

Abstract

In Japan, the Japan Council for Quality Health Care (https://jcqhc.or.jp/en/) has been operating the Evidence-Based Medicine (EBM) and Clinical Practice Guidelines (CPGs) Promoting Project, commonly known as "Minds" (hereafter referred to as "Minds"), since 2011 under commission from the Ministry of Health, Labour and Welfare.

The aim of this project is to improve the quality of healthcare by supporting decision-making by patients and healthcare providers through the dissemination of high-quality CPGs.

The project primarily focuses on evaluating and selecting CPGs, supporting their development, and promoting their implementation.

Through the "Minds Guideline Library" (https://minds.jcqhc.or.jp/), the project provides access to CPGs and related information.

Keywords

Clinical Practice Guidelines (CPGs) · Evidence-Based Medicine (EBM) · Decision-making · AGREE II · Cancer-Related Clinical Practice Guidelines (CPGs)

24.1 What Are Clinical Practice Guidelines?

Minds defines a clinical practice guideline as follows:

> A document that systematically reviews and evaluates the body of evidence, and presents recommendations considered optimal by balancing benefits and harms, in order to support decision-making by healthcare users and providers on important health issues. (Source: "Minds Clinical Practice Guidelines Development Handbook 2020," published March 22, 2021) https://minds.jcqhc.or.jp/docs/methods/cpg-development/minds-manual/pdf/chap1_manual_2020ver.pdf

Based on current conditions and trends both in Japan and internationally, the scope of CPGs has expanded beyond the treatment of diseases to encompass a wide range of topics, including disease prevention and health promotion, health checkups and screenings, rehabilitation, nursing and caregiving interventions, health education, and social support.

This definition frames the content of CPGs as addressing "important issues related to health."

CPGs differ from other medical literature and information sources in that they are specifically developed "to support decision-making by healthcare users and providers" and are required to "present recommendations" after "systematically reviewing and evaluating the body of evidence" and "balancing benefits and harms."

In *Clinical Practice Guidelines We Can Trust* (published in 2011), the National Academy of Medicine (NAM) proposed the following eight standards as essential requirements for CPGs:

① Establishing Transparency
② Management of Conflict of Interest (COI)
③ Guideline Development Group Composition
④ Clinical Practice Guideline–Systematic Review Intersection
⑤ Establishing Evidence Foundations for and Rating Strength of Recommendations
⑥ Articulation of Recommendations
⑦ External Review
⑧ Updating

Ensuring the transparency and appropriateness of the development process of CPGs is critically important, and strict measures are required for the management of conflicts of interest (COI).

In COI management, it is necessary to address not only financial interests but also academic and other types of interests.

A. Okumura (✉)
Japan Council for Quality Health Care, Tokyo, Japan
e-mail: a-okumura@jcqhc.or.jp

T. Fukuoka
Kurashiki Central Hospital, Okayama, Japan
e-mail: tf11308@kchnet.or.jp

© The Author(s), under exclusive license to Springer Nature Singapore Pte Ltd. 2026

M. Endo et al. (eds.), *Cancer and Work in Asia Volume 2*, https://doi.org/10.1007/978-981-95-6537-5_24

It is desirable to develop guidelines that incorporate the perspectives of a diverse range of stakeholders, including not only a limited group of experts but also patients and members of the public.

The methods used for developing CPGs should be clearly and transparently described in the guideline so that users can easily verify them.

24.2 Appraisal of Guidelines for Research and Evaluation II Instrument [2] (AGREE II)

CPGs selected for publication in the Minds Guideline Library are chosen based on the results of a two-step screening process and evaluation using the Appraisal of Guidelines for Research and Evaluation II (AGREE II) instrument and the AGREE Reporting Checklist, both of which are representative tools for the appraisal of CPGs.

The AGREE II is a widely used, internationally recognized evaluation tool applicable to all types of practice guidelines.

It assesses the method, development process, and reporting quality of guidelines, based on their content, and consists of 23 items across six domains, along with two items for overall evaluation.

Each item within the six domains is rated on a seven-point scale (1 = not at all applicable to 7 = strongly applicable), and it is recommended that each guideline be evaluated by at least two, and preferably four, independent reviewers to enhance the reliability of the assessment results (Table 24.1).

Table 24.1 Appraisal of guidelines for research and evaluation II instrument (AGREE II)

Domain 1. Scope and purpose	
1	The overall objective(s) of the guideline is (are) specifically described
2	The health question(s) covered by the guideline is (are) specifically described
3	The population (patients, public, etc.) to whom the guideline is meant to apply is specifically described
Domain 2. Stakeholder involvement	
4	The guideline development group includes individuals from all relevant professional groups
5	The views and preferences of the target population (patients, public, etc.) have been sought
6	The target users of the guideline are clearly defined
Domain 3. Rigour of development	
7	Systematic methods w ere used to search for evidence
8	The criteria for selecting the evidence are clearly described
9	The strengths and limitations of the body of evidence are clearly described
10	The methods for formulating the recommendations are clearly described
11	The health benefits, side effects, and risks have been considered in formulating the recommendations
12	There is an explicit link between the recommendations and the supporting evidence
13	The guideline has been externally reviewed by experts prior to its publication
14	A procedure for updating the guide line is provided
Domain 4. Clarity of presentation	
15	The recommendations are specific and unambiguous
16	The different options for management of the condition or health issue are clearly presented
17	Key recommendations are easily identifiable
Domain 5. Applicability	
18	The guideline describes facilitators and barriers to its application
19	The guideline provides advice and/or tools on how the recommendations can be put into practice
20	The potential resource implications of applying the recommendations have been considered
21	The guide line presents monitoring and/or auditing criteria
Domain 6. Editorial independence	
22	The views of the funding body have not influenced the content of the guideline
23	Competing interests of guideline development group members have been recorded and addressed
Overall guideline assessment	
1	Rate the overall quality of this guidelines the overall quality of this guideline
2	I would recommend this guideline for use. (Yes/Yes, with modifications/No)

24.3 Development and Updates of Cancer-Related Clinical Practice Guidelines in Japan

24.3.1 Trends in the Development of Cancer-Related Clinical Practice Guidelines in Japan

In Japan, the development and revision of cancer-related CPGs have been actively promoted, with each guideline prepared under the leadership of the relevant medical societies. In recent years, approximately 20% of all CPGs published in Japan have been related to cancer. Among these, guidelines concerning the digestive system represent the largest proportion, followed by those addressing women's health, such as breast cancer, and pediatrics.

24.3.2 Methodological Challenges in the Development of Cancer-Related CPGs in Japan

Based on the evaluation results using AGREE II, the CPGs assessment tool mentioned earlier, the methodological quality of cancer-related CPGs developed in Japan has been found to be significantly higher compared to that of CPGs across all medical fields.

However, this does not mean that there are no challenges. Below, the methodological issues associated with the development of cancer-related CPGs in Japan are outlined.

① *The views and preferences of the target population (patients, the public, etc.)*

In practice, only a small number of CPGs involve patients or the public in their development. Even when such participation occurs, few guidelines clearly describe how the views and preferences of the target population were gathered and how they were incorporated into the final recommendations.

To enhance the quality of cancer-related CPGs in the future, it is essential to gather the views and preferences of the target population and to develop the issues and recommendations to be addressed in the guidelines based on these perspectives and values.

② *Description of the criteria for selecting evidence and the strengths and limitations of the body of evidence*

In many cases, while the methods for searching evidence are described, the criteria used to select the evidence gathered are not clearly stated.

Furthermore, even when the evaluation of individual studies is provided, only a few guidelines clearly describe the assessment of the risk of bias for specific outcomes or for the overall body of evidence that synthesizes all studies, highlighting the need for further improvement.

③ *Description of external evaluation*

External evaluation should be conducted by individuals who were not involved in the development of the guideline. It is desirable to obtain feedback from diverse perspectives, including not only clinical experts in the relevant fields but also experts in guideline development methodology, patients, members of the public, and other stakeholders.

Only a few guidelines clearly report the results of external evaluations and explain how these results were incorporated into the finalization process. Conducting appropriate external evaluations and finalizing the guideline based on the findings will enhance its validity and strengthen public trust.

24.4 Introduction to Websites Providing Access to Clinical Practice Guidelines

As examples of websites where CPGs can be accessed, the following are introduced:

- *NICE (National Institute for Health and Care Excellence)*
  https://www.nice.org.uk/guidance
- *NCCN (National Comprehensive Cancer Network)*
  https://www.nccn.org/home/about#
- *GIN (Guidelines International Network)*
  https://g-i-n.net/international-guidelines-library
- *ECRI*
  https://guidelines.ecri.org/
- *SIGN (Scottish Intercollegiate Guidelines Network)*
  https://www.sign.ac.uk/our-guidelines/

These websites provide access to a wide range of CPGs, including those related to cancer.

References

1. AGREE Next Steps Consortium. The AGREE II instrument [Electronic version]. 2017. Retrieved April 27, 2025 from http://www.agreetrust.org.
2. Institute of Medicine. Clinical practice guidelines we can trust. Washington, DC: National Academies Press; 2011.

Cancer Survivors

25

Laureline Gatellier, Bandana Kumari Khand, V. L. Hmangaihzuali, Komal Syed, Ayaka Koizumi, Toru Kishida, David Ong, and Abhishek Shankar

Abstract

Background
Cancer is a public health issue in all Asian countries, as it is in other parts of the world. In the Asian region, major differences are observed across a broad range of factors, strongly affecting healthcare systems as well as cancer patients' unmet needs.

Method
Six patient representatives from the region were interviewed to explore unmet needs. Each patient representative described key challenges and opportunities, including those already achieved, currently in progress, or planned for the future.

Review of the Cancer Burden in Asia—the End-Use Perspective
Despite advances in managing cancer as a public health issue in the region, gaps remain between the availability of prevention, diagnosis, treatment, survivorship structures, economic and financial toxicities, and the actual unmet needs of patients. These include long-term side effects as well as social, cultural, behavioral, and spiritual factors. Addressing such gaps is likely to decrease the burden not only on patients but also on the healthcare system as a whole.

Challenges and Opportunities Proposed by the 6 End-User Patient Representatives
Concrete examples of challenges faced by cancer patients in low-and middle-income countries as well as high-income countries revealed both similarities and differences across contexts. All patients representatives reported major mental, physical, spiritual, and quality-of-life impact on their cancer journey.Examples include health camps and patient counselling initiatives to promote prevention and early detection, implemented in collaboration with the government. Additionally, opportunities were highlighted to further take actions related to fertility preservation for adolescents and young adults and to strenghten return-to-work systems benefiting cancer patients, workplace, and healthcare systems.

Conclusion and Future Directions
Awareness leads to empowerment. Including patient representatives in this chapter is key to giving a voice to patient representatives from the Asian region. This work represents a starting point toward more systematic inclusion, highlighting the need for greater visibility of patient representatives to better address region-specific unmet needs.

Keywords

Cancer patients · Patient perspective · Asia · Low Middle Income Country (LMIC) · High income country · Cancer and work · Survivorship · Needs

L. Gatellier (✉)
Division of International Health Policy Research, Institute for Cancer Control, National Cancer Center Japan, Tokyo, Japan

Japan Brain Tumor Alliance, Yokohama, Japan
e-mail: lgatelli@ncc.go.jp

B. K. Khand
NGO-Parichaya, Chitwan, Nepal

V. L. Hmangaihzuali
All India Institute of Medical Sciences, Delhi, India

K. Syed
Brain Tumour Foundation of Pakistan, Karachi, Pakistan
e-mail: Info@braintumour.pk

A. Koizumi
Japan Brain Tumor Alliance, Yokohama, Japan

T. Kishida
Cancer Note, Tokyo, Japan
e-mail: kishida_toru@gannote.com

D. Ong
The Lazarus Generation, Singapore, Singapore

A. Shankar
Department of Radiation Oncology, All India Institute of Medical Sciences, Delhi, India

© The Author(s), under exclusive license to Springer Nature Singapore Pte Ltd. 2026

M. Endo et al. (eds.), *Cancer and Work in Asia Volume 2*, https://doi.org/10.1007/978-981-95-6537-5_25

25.1 Background

Cancer burden, as a public health issue, corresponds to around half of the cancer burden worldwide (more than 18 million new cancer cases and almost 10 million cancer deaths estimated in 2020) [1]. Asia represents a wide range of countries, from low-income countries to high-income countries, and gaps in incidence and mortality are still very apparent [2]. In this very diverse continent, a key message from the end-users, who are patients and families, will focus on a review of unmet needs in the region. Unmet needs include the current education for healthcare professionals to patients and their families, as well as raising awareness in the community, which will contribute to better prevention and more focused treatment (by delivering adapted anti-cancer drugs while decreasing treatment-related side effects from early to late stages of the disease). The current management of physical, mental, social, and quality of life of patients and their families represents another essential unmet need from the end-user's perspective [3, 4]. In addition, economic, social, and socio-psychological systems, as well as cultural, religious, and ideological beliefs surrounding cancer, are considered as other unmet needs to be taken into consideration to comprehend the scope and limits of national and regional healthcare systems and public health [5].

With the development in technology and new drug development in cancer management, people are surviving longer with cancer. Cancer survivorship has become an important issue with the increasing survival in different cancer types. The singularity of this chapter is the uniqueness of the viewpoint from the end-users who are cancer patients, survivors, caregivers, and bereaved (various cancer types and stages in different cultural as well as geographical backgrounds), mainly addressing five major gaps in unmet needs, namely (1) economic and financial challenges, (2) work-related challenges, (3) social and cultural challenges, (4) mental, physical, and spiritual challenges and quality of life, and (5) availability of relevant information.

The next subchapter will focus on an overview of the scientific Asian cancer landscape from the perspective of the cancer patient as end-user. The following subchapter summarizes an Asian map of unmet patient needs based on 6 end-user interviews from the Asian region.

25.2 Method

Six patient representatives were selected based on their officially recognized implication in the cancer field, such as the establishment of a patient group or active advocacy toward screening beyond their personal disease area. Direct qualitative interviews were performed to highlight their unmet needs related to their cancer type, aspects of prevention, diagnosis, mental and physical struggles, survivorship, as well as spiritual aspects where relevant. Challenges and opportunities, whether achieved, in progress, or upcoming, were proposed by each patient representative.

25.3 Review of the Current Burden Of Cancer in Asia—the End-User Perspective

In recent years, the cancer burden has increased in Asia, a continent with a growing population, changing lifestyle, urbanization, and increasing lifespan. This cancer burden cannot be separated from continental, regional, and national variable healthcare infrastructures, healthcare policies, and investments [6]. In such a landscape, Asians have been focusing on and tackling Asian cancer-related public health issues [7], and achievements are being observed in the region (e.g., the Asian National Cancer Centers Alliance and the Asian Fund for Cancer Research are starting to show concrete achievements [8]. Asia is a wide continent in which countries are at different stages of implementing relevant actions.

Gaps related to diagnosis, treatment, and post-treatment cancer survivorship care have been observed in comparisons between LMICs and HICs and also comparatively with Western countries [9, 10]. In a broader perspective on Southeast Asia, a low GDP seems to be correlated to limited research productivity, as has been shown elsewhere for brain tumor research in the region [11]. Diagnostic and treatment gaps are widely observed in the region. Due to significant wage gaps between patients and doctors, many patients or families don't feel comfortable asking doctors for clarifying questions or for second opinions and simply go ahead with whatever the doctor suggests (K. Syed).

From an economical and financial perspective, financial toxicity is widely known in Asia as well as in other parts of the globe to be a potential consequence of costly cancer treatment and to decrease the quality of life of cancer patients and their families [12, 13]. Especially in LMICs, due to many basic needs not even being met, such as being able to cover the financial burden of treatments/lack of health care insurance/risk of losing jobs and no replacement income available, most patients and families are not able to focus on mental health and well-being or take time to understand treatment plans in detail (K. Syed). In addition, access to universal health coverage is limited in quite a few Asian countries [14]. On top of that, due to exchange rates, accessing medical drugs is not financially possible for many, and patients depend on drug coverage through donors/funds (K. Syed). Issues are not limited to geographically or economically underserved countries in Asia, as in Japan, even with an established Universal Health Coverage [15], a national survey showed that 4.9% of all cancer patients

(3.4% of those under insurance coverage) changed or abandoned some form of treatment. Of those, 20% said they had to cut into their long-term savings, and 8.0% had to cut back on food, medical care, and other daily expenses [16].

Work-related issues are tremendously affecting cancer patients, as the return to work is a challenge for most of them, with an estimation of 57% in Asia [17]. A faster diagnosis and regular screening could improve the survival rate of cancer patients and the increase of return-to-work. In addition, the return-to-work of cancer patients would gain to obtain more support from health care providers as well as the public, as previously exemplified in Asian countries (Iran, Korea, Japan) [18–20]. In Nepal, an initiation of awareness programs; screening camps by local government, government and private hospitals; and cancer survivor's networks and organizations for information, awareness, prevention, and early detection has been established. However, the number of cancer hospitals and health institutions are mainly in urban areas, and people who come for diagnosis, treatment, and regular follow-up need a long duration, which impacts their regular works, such as having to sell their livestock and stop their agriculture works and businesses (B. Khand). In India, cancer treatment requires regular visits to the hospital for longer periods. As most of the cancer centers are located in urban areas, whereas most patients are located in rural areas, this largely affects the work. Many of the cancer patients are forced to discontinue jobs in view of their engagement with cancer treatment (VL Hmangaihzuali). Return to work for brain cancer has also shown limitations due to cognitive and neurological dysfunctions, in turn impacting the quality of life of patients and their families [21]. In Japan, more than half of those working had to take a leave due to cancer treatment, while around 20% had to retire or close their business [16].

A major barrier in overcoming mental barriers and other quality of life (QOL) aspects (including long-term side effects and impact on the family) has previously been explained through culture and ethnicity gaps in the communication between healthcare professionals and cancer patients about mental health distress in Asia, as a general tendency and in relation with cancer [22–24]. In Japan, based on a national survey, less than half of respondents received sufficient advice for physical pain related to cancer, while it was even lower for mental distress (only one-third), highlighting the gap between expectation and level of healthcare support [16].

Social, cultural, structural, and behavioral factors have been shown to influence all aspects of cancer, which affects all patients and families from the initial phase of the disease up to supportive care, starting with disbelief, shock, and panic at diagnosis, usually followed by anger, hostility, and a decrease in self-control [25]. Taboos related to cancer are still widely spread, particularly in South Asia, affecting awareness, prevention, screening, detection, and treatment [26–28]. One example is medical help-seeking decisions by patients are particularly low in low- and lower-middle-income countries (LMIC), which goes in line with poor cancer outcomes [29]. In Nepal, due to patriarchal mindsets and behavior, women's economic dependency on men and family, and gender differences, women have limited access to healthcare, self-care, and healthy food, which delays cancer diagnosis (B. Khand) [30]. In addition, belief in traditional healers is still engraved in some rural areas, which negatively impacts early detection, treatment, and also awareness campaigns (B. Khand) [31]. In Singapore, cultural effects such as fatalistic cancer beliefs and risk optimism have been shown to affect cancer prevention [32], and due to a higher education on cancer by Singaporeans, the stigma toward cancer is on the down, as one in 3–4 persons in Singapore do get cancer (D. Ong).

Last but not least, the spiritual aspect is essential to reach a holistic view of cancer care, together with all the aspects above, as spiritual faith does play a major role in helping people to overcome the tremendous burden of cancer, as shown for breast cancer in Asia [33] and as an unmet need for myeloma [34] (D. Ong). Spiritual care, as part of clinical care, should be considered more as a need than an option, as it decreases symptoms of severity and improves QOL, among other things, while it is mostly not addressed in medical settings [35]. Spiritual faith can definitely contribute to a more holistic cancer care [36] (D. Ong).

25.4 Challenges and Opportunities Proposed by 6 End-User Patient Representatives

The selected 6 end-users represent both low-middle-income countries (Nepal, Pakistan, and India) as well as high-income countries (Japan and Singapore). The individuals are as follows: one Nepalese and one Indian female survivor with breast cancer, one Pakistani brain tumor bereaved woman from Pakistan, one brain cancer female Adolescent-Young Adult (AYA) survivor from Japan, one germ cell tumor AYA male survivor with metastasis in the testis, and one myeloma male survivor from Singapore.

Each cancer, at each stage, impacts patients and their families in a specific way, leading to shock and loneliness, known in the literature and illustrated in Table 25.1 below and elsewhere [37]. Asia as a broad continent is worth being compared through the eyes of cancer patients as end-users, which will reflect current gaps and hurdles within and beyond healthcare systems in the region. The results in Table 25.1 below further highlights challenges and opportunities com-

Table 25.1 Summary of real-life cancer patient challenges and proposed opportunities

Cancers	Challenges (commonalities and gaps experienced by responders)	Opportunities
Diagnosis and treatment	Diagnosis, as the first encounter of patients to cancer, tremendously impacted them, regardless of cancer type or stage. Most responders underwent surgery. Cancer treatment affected their health by creating pain and weaknesses, decreasing the energy of most patients *Breast cancer survivor (Nepal)*: She was diagnosed with breast cancer in 2015 and underwent chemotherapy from September 2015 to February 2016 at BP Koirala Memorial Cancer Hospital, Chitwan, receiving nearby treatment from her regular work and home *Breast cancer survivor (India)*: Being a nursing officer in Medical Oncology department at the apex medical center of India, i.e., All India Institute of Medical Sciences in Delhi, she had an easy access to treatment and understanding from her work environment *Brain tumor bereaved wife (Pakistan)*: Treatment options were limited and encouraged them to look for, travel and undergo treatment in Singapore, with the use of their personal savings and the medical insurance coverage. Most clinical trials are developed keeping HIC in mind. As a result, no clinical trial for brain cancers are available in Pakistan today *Brain tumor survivor (Japan)*: The brain tumor was diagnosed at age 2. She is now 27 years old, still in treatment, suffering of hypopituitarism and higher brain dysfunctions, visiting the hospital every 2 months *Germ-cell tumor survivor (Japan)*: The first symptoms at age 25 (swollen neck and feeling unwell) first led to misdiagnosis. When later diagnosed of germ cell tumor, six months later, the cancer had already spread to the lymph nodes. At the time of recurrence in the testis, at age 27, he again underwent surgery and is currently under observation, with a follow-up every 6 months Diagnosed and treated as AYA generation, his fertility preservation was performed before the start of his anti-cancer treatment, as anti-cancer treatment may impair sexual functions *Myeloma survivor (Singapore)*: After his diagnosis of myeloma, he had to undergo a stem cell transplant (GVHD/graft), with bleeding, multiple ulcers, and excruciating pain in the mouth. He also very much struggled with major side effects of anti-cancer medications and had to use morphine to help him overcome the major additional pain in his ribs	Cancer awareness (prevention and early detection) campaigns have been established in different parts of Asia. In Nepal, health camps, screening, and patient counselling are created, focusing on women and children to promote cancer prevention and early detection In addition, cancer survivor's networks for cancer prevention programs are being promoted jointly with the government. As a concrete example, B. Khand established a non-profit organization focusing on awareness, prevention, early detection, and counselling [38] Another opportunity to be taken in consideration is a network of hospitals/cancer centers, which would allow cancer patients to reach appropriate facilities in their own country or neighboring countries To provide more opportunities for cancer patients in clinical research from LMICs, more clinical trials should expand their scope beyond HICs so new drugs could also be taken into consideration the needs of LMIC patients For the AYA generation, fertility should be seriously taken into consideration prior to or around the start of the treatment, as anti-cancer treatments are known to impair the reproductive ability of cancer patients [39]. In Japan, systems subsidizing fertility preservation have been recently established, an initiative to be considered in other parts of Asia

(continued)

Table 25.1 (continued)

Cancers	Challenges (commonalities and gaps experienced by responders)	Opportunities
Financial impact	All patients experienced issues paying for their treatment (even more acute in LMICs, where governmental subsidies are much less available, limiting treatment availabilities) *Breast cancer survivor (Nepal)*: She had worked at an organization, as of now, healthcare system treatment expenses are covered by her organization. The Nepal government provides 1 lakh Nepali rupees (.1 million) to cancer patient, whereas support is insufficient for treatment *Breast cancer survivor (India)*: Working in a governmental institution, her medical expenses have been covered so far, but such coverage is not guaranteed while the treatment is dragging on *Brain tumor bereaved wife (Pakistan)*: For those who do not have personal savings or medical insurance coverage, access to treatment is very limited *Brain tumor survivor (Japan)*: As she was diagnosed as a small child (2 years old), she used to benefit from a system specific to children, the "Childhood specific chronic diseases." However, after 16 years old, she gave up the treatment, as the treatment cost became too high. She is currently using the "universal health care system". She had to search by herself for which system was available to manage to apply and benefit from them *Germ-cell tumor survivor (Japan)*: Prior to treatment, he was an office worker. The healthcare system allowed him to benefit of the "Universal health care system," and "High-cost medical care reimbursement system," two systems available for patients to support undergoing treatments. Despite these two systems, it was financially very hard for him to manage the cost of treatment, as income was very limited While his treatment was dragging on, he could benefit from his company system (sickness support for company employees, guaranteeing up to one and a half years of two-thirds of their salary) *Myeloma survivor (Singapore)*: while being hospitalized, he could benefit from governmental support and insurance policies, but after 90 days (when he became an outpatient, he could only afford a limited amount (around 600 USD) per year to offset his bills	From a financial perspective, each country experiences a different insurance coverage system, not always known by the population. Awareness programs allowing cancer patients (including patients from HICs) to be aware of basic financial support would be essential, as such major steps make the cancer patient's journey relentlessly challenging

(continued)

Table 25.1 (continued)

Cancers	Challenges (commonalities and gaps experienced by responders)	Opportunities
Cancer and Work	Cancer impacted almost all responders from the time of diagnosis through their survival journey. Some, to afford the treatment, were compelled to continue working all the way through treatment and side effects. Others did not have the opportunity to return back to work due to the heavy toll that cancer represented *Breast cancer survivor (Nepal)*: She was at a management-level position with heavy responsibilities at the time of diagnosis and treatment. After the project phase–out, just 2 months after the completion of her treatment, she started working as a freelancer for the government and related stakeholders. She also established an NGO and is involved in cancer prevention works *Breast cancer survivor (India)*: Prior to the treatment, she was a nurse. She resumed in between treatments to pay for her treatments. Her employer agreed to adapt her workload to better fit the change in capacities due to the treatment *Brain tumor survivor (Japan)*: Higher brain dysfunctions heavily impact her job-seeking strategy. If considered in the general category of job seekers, she could not find a job matching her skills and limitations due to illness. After obtaining a certificate as a "disabled person's framework," she eventually found a job as support working in a welfare office for disabled people. To overcome memory loss and time taken to remember things due to higher brain dysfunction, she frequently takes notes. She also purchased a wristwatch with notification functions. Furthermore, to decrease her symptoms of brain fatigue, she frequently refreshes herself by drinking tea *Germ-cell tumor survivor (Japan)*: After returning to work at his company as a salesman, he had to shift to inside duties to address his physical fitness *Myeloma survivor (Singapore)*: He was a pastor before being diagnosed with myeloma. During his lengthy and highly physically impacting treatment, he stopped working for six years. He then restarted as part-time, a pace more adapted to his health conditions, also allowing him to take care of his son (4 years old at time of diagnosis) with the financial and mental support of his understanding wife	Even though cancer patients tend to live longer than in the past, depending on the location and the stage of their cancer, returning to work is still a challenge for most of them. One major opportunity is that cancer allows survivors to advocate for a better environment for themselves and cancer fellows. A more standardized "return-to-work" guideline or guidebook may be beneficial in the future to lead the path in the cancer journey
Mental, physical, spiritual, and QOL	All 6 patients experienced pain and a major decrease in their physical capacities in short and longer terms during and after chemotherapies In addition, the lack of interaction with other cancer patients with the same disease impacted the quality of life of most responders, irrespective of the country's standard of living *Brain tumor responders (Pakistan and Japan)*: two types of mental issues could be extracted for brain tumors: (1) mental disabilities such as memory, brain dysfunctions, dizziness, and delayed responses and (2) mental health and emotions. The proportion of both depended on the personal experience and challenges of each patient *Myeloma survivor (Singapore)*: The physical struggles strongly affected his mental health, leading to a whirlwind of negative emotions. To maintain his quality of life after cancer, he changed his lifestyle intentionally, learning to surrender to losses such as meeting with friends to avoid being immunocompromised. As such, he gets to spend more precious time with his family, reaching a different stage of maturity. He also kept his spiritual faith strong as part of recovery and healing while going through this never-ending physically and mentally tough journey	Despite the significant number of physical, mental, and QOL challenges experienced by the responders, they all tended to cope with this stress in personal ways, with no optimal way. Opportunities remain to be explored as a major concern for patients, with a need to decrease stress, while cancer patients tend to live longer [40, 41]. From a spiritual perspective, cancer can be turned around and conquered to reach good achievements. Cancer teaches patients to cherish their loved ones while facing their own mortality (D. Ong)

(continued)

Table 25.1 (continued)

Cancers	Challenges (commonalities and gaps experienced by responders)	Opportunities
Availability of information	Availability of information was one of the major gaps experienced by the cancer patients. Except for one, in Singapore, all mentioned not only a lack of information they could reach but also the issue of misleading information, which also generated inappropriate support and advice from families and friends On specific matters, access to accurate information by the younger generation or on sensitive matters such as sex, money, and family adds to the lack of sound and scientific information related to cancers, as per the natural tendency of human beings *Breast cancer survivor (Nepal)*: She got the required information using related websites herself and from her family members and friends who are in medical fields *Breast cancer survivor (India)*: Overwhelming support from friends and families may be too much of a burden when not adequately provided, which puts in light the inadequate cancer awareness in India *Brain tumor bereaved wife (Pakistan)*: Due to the rarity of brain cancers, there is a lack of interaction with patients with the same disease. Access to accurate and relevant information on this cancer also highly hampers the cancer journey *Brain tumor survivor (Japan)*: Being an AYA generation, in addition to the limited information on her disease, she struggled and is still struggling a lot, not only about the lack of availability of information on her disease but also about life-stage events, such as education, employment, marriage, and childbearing. Struggles related to these life stages are mostly not understood by her "healthy" friends and acquaintances *Germ-cell tumor survivor (Japan)*: As germ-cell tumor is a rare cancer, accurate information is not easily available. Families, sometimes with good intentions, provided misleading information to him due to the limited availability of sound information on their types of cancer. Since the cancer AYA generation is very limited, a community is needed, as well as outpatient clinics specializing in the AYA generation *Myeloma survivor (Singapore)*: While being treated by a renowned physician at a renowned cancer center, he did not feel any necessity for additional information	Actions should be taken to allow the establishment of and/or an increased focus on education, awareness, peer support (including groups specializing in unmet needs such as AYA generation), and fundraising groups Examples (Nepal) B. Khand established an NGO promoting cancer prevention programs, information, awareness, psychosocial counseling, peer support, media mobilization, health education, and cancer screening camps (Pakistan) Brain Tumour Pakistan was established in September 2020 by Komal Syed, after her husband passed away in 2015, with the mission of reaching every individual in Pakistan impacted by a brain tumor with support, education, information, and research through (1) awareness, (2) non-medical support, and (3) funding and supporting research While raising advocacy, K. Syed stays widely aware that due to low literacy in the region, raising awareness for cancer-related topics is difficult (Japan) Cancer Note was established in 2014 by Toru Kishida using interviews to disseminate the voices of cancer patients to cancer patients, including sensitive cancer types for which patients used to be embarrassed about in the past

mon to cancer patients irrespective of or closely related to the cancer type, geographical location, or other relevant features specific to the Asian region.

25.5 Conclusions and Future Directions

Cancer directly impacts patients from all possible aspects in a lifetime. Patients, survivors, and caregivers can and should play a major role by sharing their own experience with cancer with health care providers, researchers, experts, policy makers, the pharmaceutical and device industry, and the public as an essential contribution to short-, medium-, and long-term cancer control nationally and regionally in the Asian region. The awareness of the actual experience of cancer patients by clinicians, researchers, cancer patients, policy-makers, and industry, as well as the general public, is essential to address the real needs of patients.

In line with limited awareness, the access to relevant information and institutions is limited for cancer patients and their families, even more so in low- and lower-middle-income countries in Asia [42], highlighting the need to increase views of cancer patients and their caregivers with regard to access, adherence, and disruption to cancer care.

In LMICs, such as Pakistan and India, the poor awareness level among the population shows the need for health education and sensitization regarding cancer and its different aspects (including early detection and better health-seeking behavior). As a result, cancer patients are diagnosed at an advanced stage, leading to unfavorable outcomes and difficult survivorship (VL Hmangaihzuali).

The way forward, from the views of end-users' patient representatives, should include empowering actions initiated by patients. Figure 25.1 below illustrates patients' experiences at different stages of their journey, a journey that has empowered them first to be strong enough and then to become stronger for others. These actions include promoting, advocating for, and, where possible, establishing awareness campaigns on aspects not taken sufficiently into consideration by other related stakeholders. Survivorship for patients includes access to appropriate awareness, prevention, diagnostics, treatment, and clinical trials in all parts of

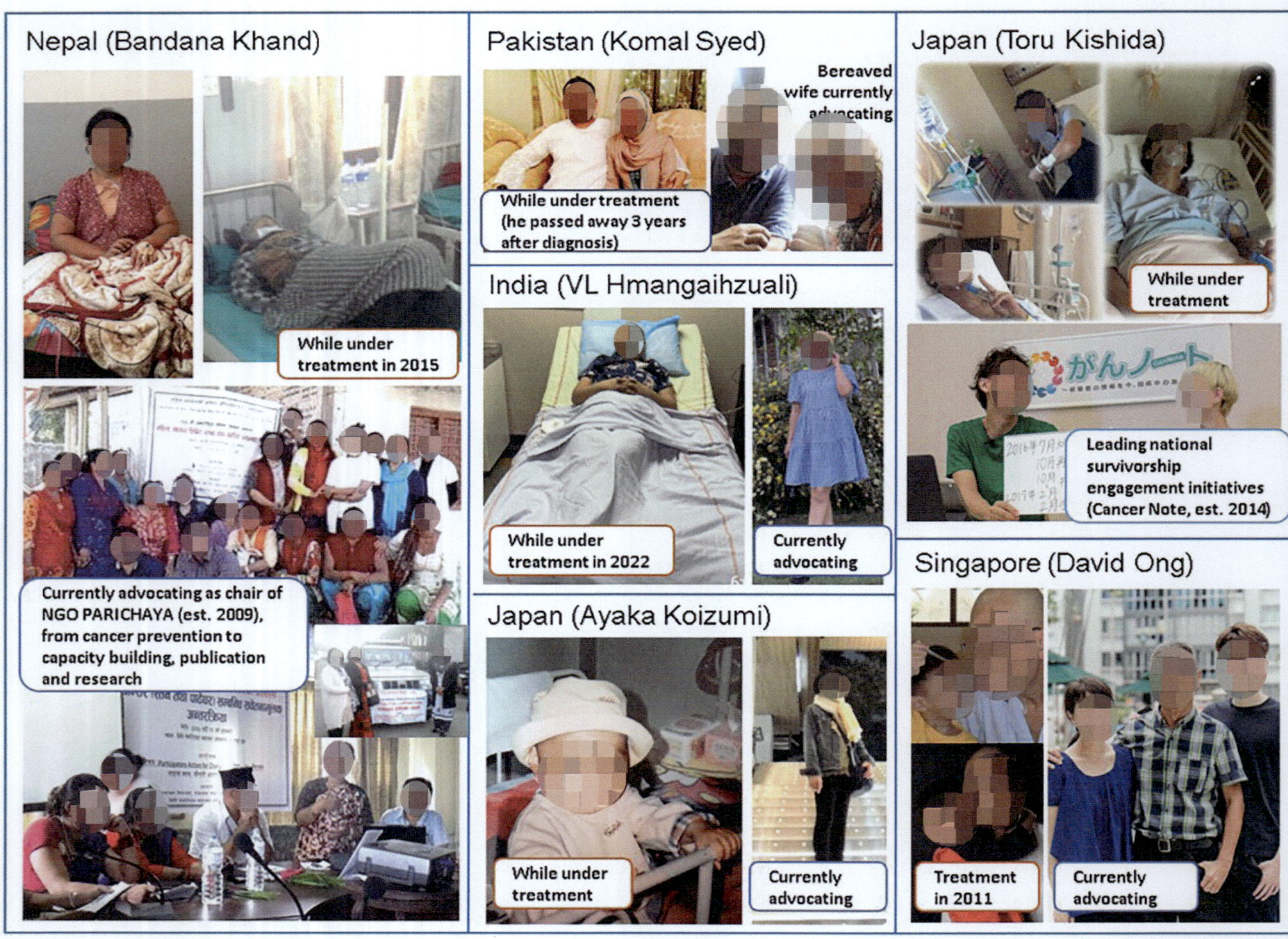

Fig. 25.1 Cancer patients' journey in Asia: from "being strong to survive" to "being strong for others"

Asia. It also includes other matters such as spiritual matters and personal matters such as money, family, and sex, as well as aspects impacting the younger generations that are mostly ignored by governmental bodies, healthcare professionals, the media, and all relevant stakeholders. Increased multi-stakeholder collaboration and empowerment of patients in all aspects of survivorship is the way forward.

References

1. Cancer Today. https://gco.iarc.fr/today/home2020. Available from: https://gco.iarc.fr/today/home.
2. Global Burden of Disease Cancer C, Kocarnik JM, Compton K, Dean FE, Fu W, Gaw BL, et al. Cancer incidence, mortality, years of life lost, years lived with disability, and disability-adjusted life years for 29 cancer groups from 2010 to 2019: a Systematic Analysis for the Global Burden of Disease Study 2019. JAMA Oncol. 2022;8(3):420–44.
3. Rana S, Gupta R, Chaudhary P, Khurana D, Mishra S, Bhatnagar S. Cancer pain management: basic information for the young pain physicians. Indian J Palliat Care. 2011;17(2):127–30.
4. Kilic ST, Oz F. Family caregivers' involvement in caring with cancer and their quality of life. Asian Pac J Cancer Prev. 2019;20(6):1735–41.
5. Copur MS. State of cancer research around the globe. Oncology (Williston Park). 2019;33(5):181–5.
6. Sankaranarayanan R, Ramadas K, Qiao YL. Managing the changing burden of cancer in Asia. BMC Med. 2014;12:3.
7. Goh BC, Lim JF. Cancer drugs in Asian populations: availability, accessibility, and affordability. Cancer J. 2020;26(4):323–9.
8. Gatellier L, Matsuda T, Sabapathy K, Dai M, Dewi LKM, Huong TT, et al. An Asian body to tackle cancers in Asia—the Asian National Cancer Centers Alliance. Asian Pac J Cancer Prev. 2020;21(5):1207–12.
9. Kingham TP, Alatise OI. Establishing translational and clinical cancer research collaborations between high- and low-income countries. Ann Surg Oncol. 2015;22(3):741–6.
10. Chan RJ, Yates P, Li Q, Komatsu H, Lopez V, Thandar M, et al. Oncology practitioners' perspectives and practice patterns of post-treatment cancer survivorship care in the Asia-Pacific region: results from the STEP study. BMC Cancer. 2017;17(1):715.
11. Mondia MWL, Espiritu AI, Jamora RDG. Primary brain tumor research productivity in Southeast Asia and its association with socioeconomic determinants and burden of disease. Front Oncol. 2020;10:607777.
12. Boby JM, Rajappa S, Mathew A. Financial toxicity in cancer care in India: a systematic review. Lancet Oncol. 2021;22(12):e541–e9.
13. Bhoo-Pathy N, Ng CW, Lim GC, Tamin NSI, Sullivan R, Bhoo-Pathy NT, et al. Financial toxicity after cancer in a setting with universal health coverage: a call for urgent action. J Oncol Pract. 2019;15(6):e537–e46.
14. Matsuda T. Lecture No. 3 Current status and future outlook for collection of cancer-related data in Asia. Jpn J Clin Oncol. 2021;51(12 Suppl 2):i14–6.
15. Welfare MoHLa. Japan Universal Health Insurance System. Available from: https://www.mhlw.go.jp/stf/seisakunitsuite/bunya/kenkou_iryou/iryouhoken/iryouhoken01/index.html.
16. Ministry of Health Labour and Welfare. Patient Experience Survey Report 2018. 2020.
17. Tavan H, Azadi A, Veisani Y. Return to work in cancer patients: a systematic review and meta-analysis. Indian J Palliat Care. 2019;25(1):147–52.
18. Mardani-Hamooleh M, Heidari H. Cancer patients' effort to return to normal life: a hermeneutic study. Scand J Caring Sci. 2017;31(2):351–8.
19. Shim HY, Lee CW, Yu ES, Park BY, Yang EJ. Cancer survivors and returning to work perspectives from occupational health physicians in Korea. J Korean Med Sci. 2019;34(11):e98.
20. Ota A, Fujisawa A, Kawada K, Yatsuya H. Recent status and methodological quality of return-to-work rates of cancer patients reported in Japan: a systematic review. Int J Environ Res Public Health. 2019;16(8):1461.
21. Basalathullah MAR, Malik M, Valiyaveettil D, Elizabeth NB, Ahmed SF. Return to work in survivors of primary brain tumours treated with intensity modulated radiotherapy. Cancer Treat Res Commun. 2021;26:100302.
22. Kikuzawa S, Pescosolido B, Kasahara-Kiritani M, Matoba T, Yamaki C, Sugiyama K. Mental health care and the cultural toolboxes of the present-day Japanese population: examining suggested patterns of care and their correlates. Soc Sci Med. 2019;228:252–61.
23. Granek L, Nakash O, Ariad S, Shapira S, Ben-David MA. The role of culture/ethnicity in communicating with cancer patients about mental health distress and suicidality. Cult Med Psychiatry. 2020;44(2):214–29.
24. Granek L, Nakash O, Ariad S, Shapira S, Ben-David M. Strategies and barriers in addressing mental health and Suicidality in patients with cancer. Oncol Nurs Forum. 2019;46(5):561–71.
25. Ozkan S, Ozkan M, Armay Z. Cultural meaning of cancer suffering. J Pediatr Hematol Oncol. 2011;33(Suppl 2):S102–4.
26. Anderson de Cuevas RM, Saini P, Roberts D, Beaver K, Chandrashekar M, Jain A, et al. A systematic review of barriers and enablers to South Asian women's attendance for asymptomatic screening of breast and cervical cancers in emigrant countries. BMJ Open. 2018;8(7):e020892.
27. Zamanzadeh V, Rahmani A, Valizadeh L, Ferguson C, Hassankhani H, Nikanfar AR, et al. The taboo of cancer: the experiences of cancer disclosure by Iranian patients, their family members and physicians. Psychooncology. 2013;22(2):396–402.
28. Kaul P, Kumar R, Singh MP, Garg PK. Social taboos: a formidable challenge in cancer care. BMJ Case Rep. 2021;14(1):e236095.
29. McCutchan G, Weiss B, Quinn-Scoggins H, Dao A, Downs T, Deng Y, et al. Psychosocial influences on help-seeking behaviour for cancer in low-income and lower middle-income countries: a mixed-methods systematic review. BMJ Glob Health. 2021;6(2):e004213.
30. Nepal A, Dangol SK, van der Kwaak A. Improving maternal health services through social accountability interventions in Nepal: an analytical review of existing literature. Public Health Rev. 2020;41(1):31.
31. Pham TV, Koirala R, Kohrt BA. Satisfaction in the soul: common factors theory applied to traditional healers in rural Nepal. Ethos. 2020;48(1):93–128.
32. Kim HK, Lwin MO. Cultural effects on cancer prevention Behaviors: fatalistic cancer beliefs and risk optimism among Asians in Singapore. Health Commun. 2017;32(10):1201–9.
33. Wei D, Liu XY, Chen YY, Zhou X, Hu HP. Effectiveness of physical, psychological, social, and spiritual intervention in breast cancer survivors: an integrative review. Asia Pac J Oncol Nurs. 2016;3(3):226–32.

34. Tsatsou I, Konstantinidis T, Kalemikerakis I, Adamakidou T, Vlachou E, Govina O. Unmet supportive care needs of patients with Hematological malignancies: a systematic review. Asia Pac J Oncol Nurs. 2021;8(1):5–17.
35. Ripamonti CI, Giuntoli F, Gonella S, Miccinesi G. Spiritual care in cancer patients: a need or an option? Curr Opin Oncol. 2018;30(4):212–8.
36. Shimazono S. Development of spiritual Care in Cancer Treatment in Japan. Gan To Kagaku Ryoho. 2017;44(1):1–6.
37. Deckx L, van den Akker M, van Driel M, Bulens P, van Abbema D, Tjan-Heijnen V, et al. Loneliness in patients with cancer: the first year after cancer diagnosis. Psychooncology. 2015;24(11):1521–8.
38. Khand B. PARICHAYA – participatory action for change 2009. Available from: parichaya.org.np.
39. Del-Pozo-Lerida S, Salvador C, Martinez-Soler F, Tortosa A, Perucho M, Gimenez-Bonafe P. Preservation of fertility in patients with cancer (Review). Oncol Rep. 2019;41(5):2607–14.
40. Rick O, Dauelsberg T, Kalusche-Bontemps EM. Oncological rehabilitation. Oncol Res Treat. 2017;40(12):772–7.
41. Surman M, Janik ME. Stress and its molecular consequences in cancer progression. Postepy Hig Med Dosw (Online). 2017;71:485–99.
42. Datta SS, Ghose S, Ghosh M, Jain A, Mandal S, Chakraborty S, et al. Journeys: understanding access, affordability and disruptions to cancer care in India. Ecancermedicalscience. 2022;16:1342.

MIX
Papier aus verantwortungsvollen Quellen
Paper from responsible sources
FSC® C105338

If you have any concerns about our products,
you can contact us on
ProductSafety@springernature.com

In case Publisher is established outside the EU,
the EU authorized representative is:
Springer Nature Customer Service Center GmbH
Europaplatz 3, 69115 Heidelberg, Germany

Printed by Libri Plureos GmbH
in Hamburg, Germany